The World Health Report 2005

Make every mother and child count

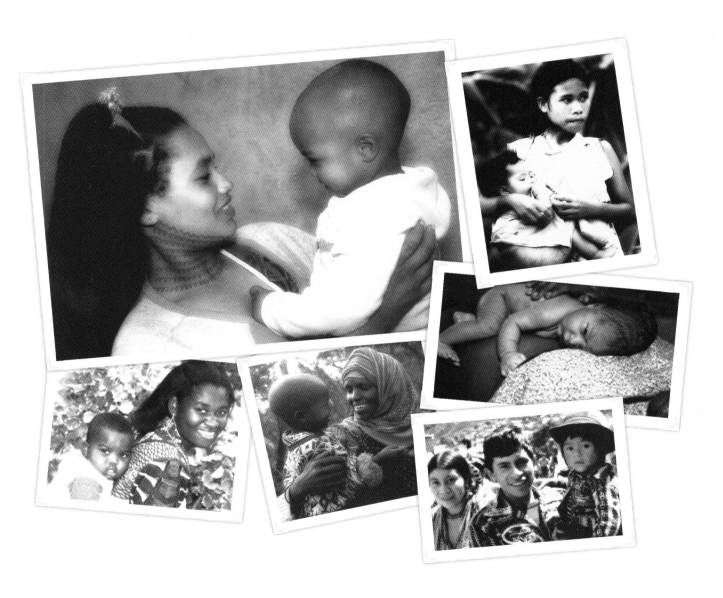

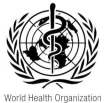

World Health Organization

WHO Library Cataloguing-in-Publication Data

World Health Organization.
    The World health report : 2005 : make every mother and child count.

    1.World health - trends 2.Maternal welfare 3.Child welfare. 4.Maternal health services - organization and administration.
    5.Child health services - organization and administration 6.World Health Organization I.Title II.Title: Make every mother and child count.

    ISBN 92 4 156290 0   (NLM Classification: WA 540.1)
    ISSN 1020-3311

Information concerning this publication can be obtained from:
World Health Report
World Health Organization
1211 Geneva 27, Switzerland
E-mail: whr@who.int

Copies of this publication can be ordered from: bookorders@who.int

This report was produced under the overall direction of Joy Phumaphi (Assistant Director-General, Family and Child Health), Tim Evans (Assistant Director-General, Evidence and Information for Policy) and Wim Van Lerberghe (Editor-in-Chief). The principal authors were Wim Van Lerberghe, Annick Manuel, Zoë Matthews and Cathy Wolfheim. Thomson Prentice was the Managing Editor.

Valuable inputs (contributions, background papers, analytical work, reviewing, suggestions and criticism) were received from Elisabeth Aahman, Carla Abou-Zahr, Fiifi Amoako Johnson, Fred Arnold, Alberta Bacci, Rajiv Bahl, Rebecca Bailey, Robert Beaglehole, Rafael Bengoa, Janie Benson, Yves Bergevin, Stan Bernstein, Julian Bilous, Ties Boerma, Jo Borghi, Paul Bossyns, Assia Brandrup-Lukanov, Eric Buch, Flavia Bustreo, Meena Cabral de Mello, Virginia Camacho, Guy Carrin, Andrew Cassels, Kathryn Church, Alessandro Colombo, Jane Cottingham, Bernadette Daelmans, Mario Dal Poz, Catherine d'Arcangues, Hugh Darrah, Luc de Bernis, Isabelle de Zoysa, Maria Del Carmen, Carmen Dolea, Gilles Dussault, Steve Ebener, Dominique Egger, Gerry Eijkemans, Bjorn Ekman, Zine Elmorjani, Tim Ensor, Marthe Sylvie Essengue, David Evans, Vincent Fauveau, Paulo Ferrinho, Helga Fogstad, Marta Gacic Dobo, Ulf Gerdham, Adrienne Germain, Peter Ghys, Elizabeth Goodburn, Veloshnee Govender, Metin Gulmezoglu, Jean-Pierre Habicht, Sarah Hall, Laurence Haller, Steve Harvey, Peggy Henderson, Patricia Hernández, Peter Hill, Dale Huntington, Julia Hussein, Guy Hutton, Mie Inoue, Monir Islam, Christopher James, Craig Janes, Ben Johns, Rita Kabra, Betty Kirkwood, Lianne Kuppens, Joy Lawn, Jerker Liljestrand, Ornella Lincetto, Craig Lissner, Alessandro Loretti, Jane Lucas, Doris Ma Fat, Carolyn Maclennan, Ramez Mahaini, Sudhansh Malhostra, Adriane Martin Hilber, José Martines, Elizabeth Mason, Matthews Mathai, Dileep Mavalankar, Gillian Mayers, Juliet McEachren, Abdelhai Mechbal, Mario Merialdi, Tom Merrick, Thierry Mertens, Susan Murray, Adepeju Olukoya, Guillermo Paraje, Justin Parkhurst, Amit Patel, Vikram Patel, Steve Pearson, Gretel Pelto, Jean Perrot, Annie Portela, Dheepa Rajan, K.V. Ramani, Esther Ratsma, Linda Richter, David Sanders, Parvathy Sankar, Robert Scherpbier, Peelam Sekhri, Gita Sen, Iqbal Shah, Della Sherratt, Kenji Shibuya, Kristjana Sigurbjornsdottir, Angelica Sousa, Niko Speybroeck, Karin Stenberg, Will Stones, Tessa Tan-Torres Edejer, Petra Ten Hoope-Bender, Ann Tinker, Wim Van Damme, Jos Vandelaer, Paul Van Look, Marcel Vekemans, Cesar Victora, Eugenio Villar Montesinos, Yasmin Von Schirnding, Eva Wallstam, Steve Wiersma, Karl Wilhelmson, Lara Wolfson, Juliana Yartey and Jelka Zupan.

Contributers to statistical tables were: Elisabeth Aahman, Dorjsuren Bayarsaikhan, Ana Betran, Zulfiqar Bhutta, Maureen Birmingham, Robert Black, Ties Boerma, Cynthia Boschi-Pinto, Jennifer Bryce, Agnes Couffinhal, Simon Cousens, Trevor Croft, David D. Vans, Charu C. Garg, Kim Gustavsen, Nasim Haque, Patricia Hernández, Ken Hill, Chandika Indikadahena, Mie Inoue, Gareth Jones, Betty Kirkwood, Joseph Kutzin, Joy Lawn, Eduardo Levcovitz, Edilberto Loaiza, Doris Ma Fat, José Martines, Elizabeth Mason, Colin Mathers, Saul Morris, Kim Mulholland, Takondwa Mwase, Bernard Nahlen, Pamela Nakamba-Kabaso, Agnès Prudhomme, Rachel Racelis, Olivier Ronveaux, Alex Rowe, Hossein Salehi, Ian Scott, U Than Sein, Kenji Shibuya, Rick Steketee, Rubén Suarez, Tessa Tan-Torres Edejer, Nathalie van de Maele, Tessa Wardlaw, Neff Walker, Hongyi Xu, Jelka Zupan, and many staff in WHO country offices, governmental departments and agencies, and international institutions.

Valuable comments and guidance were provided by Denis Aitken and Michel Jancloes. Additional help and advice were kindly provided by Regional Directors and members of their staff.

The report was edited by Leo Vita-Finzi, assisted by Barbara Campanini. Editorial, administrative and production support was provided by Shelagh Probst and Gary Walker, who also coordinated the photographs. The web site version and other electronic media were provided by Gael Kernen. Proofreading was by Marie Fitzsimmons. The index was prepared by Kathleen Lyle.

Front cover photographs (clockwise from top left): L. Gubb/WHO; Pepito Frias/WHO; Armando Waak/WHO/PAHO; Carlos Gaggero/WHO/PAHO; Liba Taylor/WHO; Pierre Virot/WHO. Back cover photographs (left to right): Pierre Virot/WHO; J. Gorstein/WHO; G. Diez/WHO; Pierre Virot/WHO. This report contains several photographs from "River of Life 2004" – a WHO photo competition on the theme of sexual and reproductive health.

Design: Reda Sadki
Layout: Steve Ewart and Reda Sadki
Figures: Christophe Grangier
Photo retouching: Reda Sadki and Denis Meissner
Printing coordination: Keith Wynn
Printed in France

contents

Boxes

Tables

message from the
director-general

Parenthood brings with it the strong desire to see our children grow up happily and in good health. This is one of the few constants in life in all parts of the world. Yet, even in the 21st century, we still allow well over 10 million children and half a million mothers to die each year, although most of these deaths can be avoided. Seventy million mothers and their newborn babies, as well as countless children, are excluded from the health care to which they are entitled. Even more numerous are those who remain without protection against the poverty that ill-health can cause.

Leaders readily agree that we cannot allow this to continue, but in many countries the situation is either improving too slowly or not improving at all, and in some it is getting worse. Mothers, the newborn and children represent the well-being of a society and its potential for the future. Their health needs cannot be left unmet without harming the whole of society.

Families and communities themselves can do a great deal to change this situation. They can improve, for example, the position of women in society, parenting, disease prevention, care for the sick, and uptake of services. But this area of health is also a public responsibility.

Public health programmes need to work together so that all families have access to a continuum of care that extends from pregnancy (and even before), through childbirth and on into childhood, instead of the often fragmented services available at present. It makes no sense to provide care for a child while ignoring the mother's health, or to assist a mother giving birth but not the newborn child.

To ensure that all families have access to care, governments must accelerate the building up of coherent, integrated and effective health systems. This means tackling the health workforce crisis, which in turn calls for a much higher level of funding and better organization of it for these aspects of health. The objective must be health systems that can respond to these needs, eliminate financial barriers to care, and protect people from the poverty that is both a cause and an effect of ill-health.

The world needs to support countries striving to achieve universal access and financial protection for all mothers and children. Only by doing so can we make sure that every mother, newborn baby and child in need of care can obtain it, and no one is driven into poverty by the cost of that care. In this way we can move not only towards the Millennium Development Goals but beyond them.

LEE Jong-wook
Director-General
World Health Organization
Geneva, April 2005

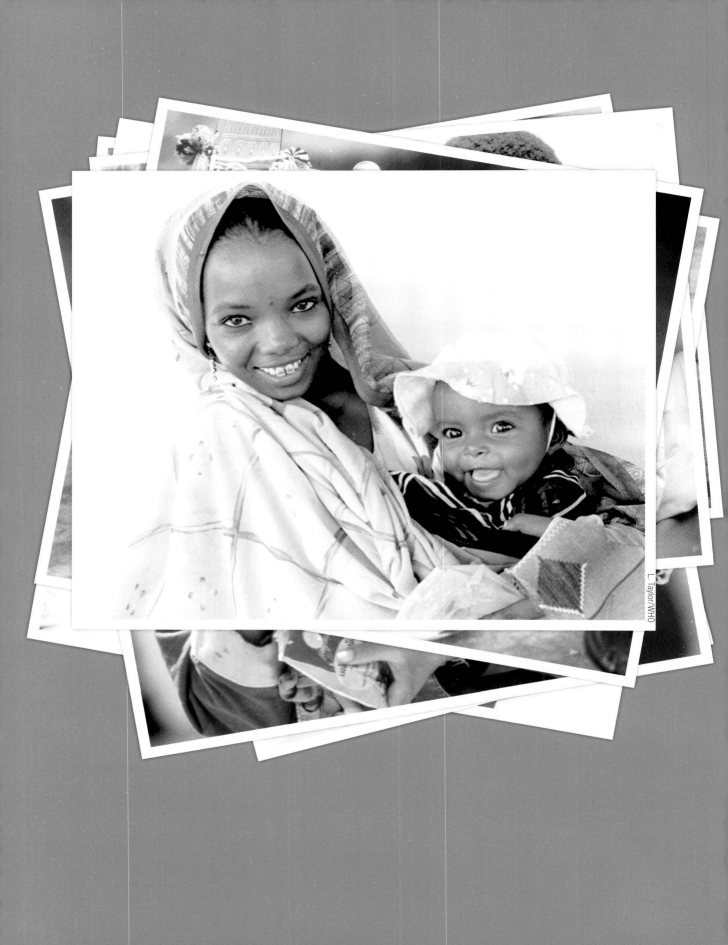

overview

This year's *World Health Report* comes at a time when only a decade is left to achieve the Millennium Development Goals (MDGs), which set internationally agreed development aspirations for the world's population to be met by 2015. These goals have underlined the importance of improving health, and particularly the health of mothers and children, as an integral part of poverty reduction.

The health of mothers and children is a priority that emerged long before the 1990s – it builds on a century of programmes, activities and experience. What is new in the last decade, however, is the global focus of the MDGs and their insistence on tracking progress in every part of the world. Moreover, the nature of the priority status of maternal and child health (MCH) has changed over time. Whereas mothers and children were previously thought of as targets for well-intentioned programmes, they now increasingly claim the right to access quality care as an entitlement guaranteed by the state. In doing so, they have transformed maternal and child health from a technical concern into a moral and political imperative.

This report identifies exclusion as a key feature of inequity as well as a key constraint to progress. In many countries, universal access to the care all women and children are entitled to is still far from realization. Taking stock of the erratic progress to date, the report sets out the strategies required for the accelerated improvements that are known to be possible. It is necessary to refocus the technical strategies developed within maternal and child health programmes, and also to put more emphasis on the importance of the often overlooked health problems of newborns. In this regard, the report advocates the repositioning of MCH as M*N*CH (maternal, *newborn* and child health).

The proper technical strategies to improve MNCH can be put in place effectively only if they are implemented, across programmes and service providers, throughout pregnancy and childbirth through to childhood. It makes no sense to provide care for a child and ignore the mother, or to worry about a mother giving birth and fail to pay attention to the health of the baby. To provide families universal access to such a continuum of care requires programmes to work together, but is ultimately dependent on extending and strengthening health systems. At the same time, placing MNCH at the core of the drive for universal access provides a platform for building sustainable health systems where existing structures are weak or fragile. Even where the MDGs will not be fully achieved by 2015, moving towards universal access has the potential to transform the lives of millions for decades to come.

PATCHY PROGRESS AND WIDENING GAPS – WHAT WENT WRONG?

Each year 3.3 million babies – or maybe even more – are stillborn, more than 4 million die within 28 days of coming into the world, and a further 6.6 million young children die before their fifth birthday. Maternal deaths also continue unabated – the annual total now stands at 529 000 often sudden, unpredicted deaths which occur during pregnancy itself (some 68 000 as a consequence of unsafe abortion), during childbirth, or after the baby has been born – leaving behind devastated families, often pushed into poverty because of the cost of health care that came too late or was ineffective.

How can it be that this situation continues when the causes of these deaths are largely avoidable? And why is it still necessary for this report to emphasize the importance of focusing on the health of mothers, newborns and children, after decades of priority status, and more than 10 years after the United Nations International Conference on Population and Development put access to reproductive health care for all firmly on the agenda?

Although an increasing number of countries have succeeded in improving the health and well-being of mothers, babies and children in recent years, the countries that started off with the highest burdens of mortality and ill-health made least progress during the 1990s. In some countries the situation has actually worsened, and worrying reversals in newborn, child and maternal mortality have taken place. Progress has slowed down and is increasingly uneven, leaving large disparities between countries as well as between the poor and the rich within countries. Unless efforts are stepped up radically, there is little hope of eliminating avoidable maternal and child mortality in all countries.

Countries where health indicators for mothers, newborns and children have stagnated or reversed have often been unable to invest sufficiently in health systems. The health districts have had difficulties in organizing access to effective care for women and children. Humanitarian crises, pervasive poverty, and the HIV/AIDS epidemic have all compounded the effect of economic downturns and the health workforce crisis. With widespread exclusion from care and growing inequalities, progress calls for massively strengthened health systems.

Technical choices are still important, though, as in the past programmes have not always pursued the best approaches to make good care accessible to all. Too often, programmes have been allowed to fragment, thus hampering the continuity of care, or have failed to give due attention to professionalizing services. Technical experience and the successes and failures of the recent past have shown how best to move forward.

MAKING THE RIGHT TECHNICAL AND STRATEGIC CHOICES

There is no doubt that the technical knowledge exists to respond to many, if not most, of the critical health problems and hazards that affect the health and survival of mothers, newborns and children. The strategies through which households and health systems together can make sure these technical solutions are put into action for all, in the right place and at the right time, are also becoming increasingly clear.

Antenatal care is a major success story: demand has increased and continues to increase in most parts of the world. However, more can be made of the considerable potential of antenatal care by emphasizing effective interventions and by using it as a platform for other health programmes such as HIV/AIDS and the prevention and treatment of sexually transmitted infections, tuberculosis and malaria initiatives, and family planning. Health workers, too, can make more use of antenatal care to help mothers prepare for birthing and parenting, or to assist them in dealing with an environment that does not always favour a healthy and happy pregnancy. Pregnant women, adolescents in particular, may be exposed to violence, discrimination in the workplace or at school, or marginalization. Such problems need to be dealt with also, but not only, by improving the social, political and legal environments. A case in point is how societies face up to the problem of the many millions of unintended, mistimed and unwanted pregnancies. There remains a large unmet need for contraception, as well as for more and better information and education. There is also a real need to facilitate access to responsive post-abortion care of high quality and to safe abortion services to the fullest extent allowed by law.

Attending to all of the 136 million births every year is one of the major challenges that now faces the world's health systems. This challenge will increase in the near future as large cohorts of young people move into their reproductive years, mainly in those parts of the world where giving birth is most dangerous. Women risk death to give life, but with skilled and responsive care, at and after birth, nearly all fatal outcomes and disabling sequelae can be averted – the tragedy of obstetric fistulas, for example – and much of the suffering can be eased. Childbirth is a central event in the lives of families and in the construction of communities; it should remain so, but it must be made safe as well. For optimum safety, every woman, without exception, needs professional skilled care when giving birth, in an appropriate environment that is close to where she lives and respects her birthing culture. Such care can best be provided by a registered midwife or a health worker with midwifery skills, in decentralized, first-level facilities. This can avert, contain or solve many of the life-threatening problems that may arise during childbirth, and reduce maternal mortality to surprisingly low levels. Skilled midwifery professionals do need the back-up only a hospital can provide, however, for women with problems that go beyond the competency or equipment available at the first level of care. All women need first-level maternal care and back-up care is only necessary for a minority, but to be effective both levels need to work in tandem and both must be put in place simultaneously.

The need for care does not stop as soon as the birth is over. The hours, days and weeks that follow birth can be dangerous for women as well as for their babies. The welcome emphasis, in recent years, on improving skilled attendance at birth should not divert attention from this critical period, during which half of maternal deaths occur as well as a considerable amount of illness. There is an urgent need to develop effective ways of organizing continuity of care during the first weeks after birth, when health service responsibilities are often ill-defined or ambiguous.

The postpartum gap in providing care for women is also a postnatal gap. Although the picture of the unmet need in caring for newborns is still very incomplete, it shows that the health problems of newborns have been unduly neglected and underestimated. Newborn babies seem to have fallen between the cracks of safe motherhood programmes on one side and child survival initiatives on the other. Newborn mortality is a sizeable proportion of the mortality of children under five years of age. It has become clear that the MDG for child mortality will not be reached without substantial advances for the newborn. Although modest declines in neonatal mortality have occurred worldwide (for example, vaccination is well on the way to eliminating tetanus as a cause of neonatal death), in sub-Saharan Africa some countries have seen reversals that are both unusual and disturbing.

Progress in newborn health does not require expensive technology. It does however require health systems that provide continuity of care starting from the beginning of pregnancy (and even before) and continuing through professional skilled care at birth into the postnatal period. Most crucially, there is a need to ensure that the delicate and often overlooked handover between maternal and child services actually takes place. Newborns who are breastfed, loved and kept warm will mostly be fine, but problems can and do occur. It is essential to empower households – mothers and fathers in particular – so that they can take good care of their babies, recognize dangers early, and get professional help immediately when difficulties arise.

The greatest risks to life are in its beginning, but they do not disappear as the newborn grows into an infant and a young child. Programmes to tackle vaccine-preventable diseases, malnutrition, diarrhoea, or respiratory infections still have a large unfinished agenda. Immunization, for example, has made satisfactory progress in some regions, but in others coverage is stagnating at levels between 50% and 70% and has to find a new momentum. These programmes have, however, made such inroads on the burden of ill-health that in many countries its profile has changed. There is now a need for more integrated approaches: first, to deal efficiently with the changing spectrum of problems that need attention; second, to broaden the focus of care from the child's survival to its growth and development. This is what is needed from a public health point of view; it is also what families expect.

The Integrated Management of Childhood Illness (IMCI) combines a set of effective interventions for preventing death and for improving healthy growth and develop-ment. More than just adding more subsets to a single delivery channel, IMCI has transformed the way the health system looks at child care – going beyond the mere treatment of illness. IMCI has three components: improving the skills of health workers to treat diseases and to counsel families, strengthening the health system's support, and helping households and communities to bring up their children healthily and deal with ill-health when it occurs. IMCI has thus moved beyond the traditional notion of health centre staff providing a set of technical interventions to their target population. It is bringing health care closer to the home, while at the same time improving refer-ral links and hospital care; the challenge now is to make IMCI available to all families with children, and create the conditions for them to avail themselves of such care whenever needed.

MOVING TOWARDS UNIVERSAL COVERAGE: ACCESS FOR ALL, WITH FINANCIAL PROTECTION

There is a strong consensus that, even if all the right technical choices are made, maternal, newborn and child health programmes will only be effective if together, and with households and communities, they establish a continuum of care, from pregnancy through childbirth into childhood. This continuity requires greatly strengthened health systems with maternal, newborn and child health care at the core of their develop-ment strategies. It is forcing programmes and stakeholders with different histories, interests and constituencies to join forces. The common project that can pull together the different agendas is universal access to care. This is not just a question of fine-tuning advocacy language: it frames the health of mothers, babies and children within a broader, straightforward political project, responding to society's claim for the pro-tection of the health of its citizens and for access to care – a claim that is increasingly seen as legitimate. The magnitude of the challenge of scaling up services towards universal access, however, should not be underestimated.

Reaching all children with a package of essential child health interventions necessary to comply with and even go beyond the MDGs is technically feasible within the next decade. In the 75 countries that account for most of child mortality this will require US$ 52.4 billion, in addition to current expenditure, of which US$ 25 billion represents additional costs for human resources. This US$ 52.4 billion corresponds to an increase as of now of 6% of current median public expenditure on health in these countries, rising to 18% by 2015. In the 21 countries facing the greatest constraints and where a long lead time is likely, current public expenditure on health would have to grow by 27% as of 2006, rising to around 76% in 2015.

For maternal and newborn care, universal access is further away. It is possible to envisage various scenarios for scaling up services, taking into account the specific circumstances in each of the same 75 countries. At present, some 43% of mothers and newborns receive some care, but by no means the full range of what they need even just to avoid maternal deaths. Adding up the optimistic – but also realistic – scenarios for each of the 75 countries gives access to a full package of first-level and back-up care to 101 million mothers (some 73% of the expected births) in 2015, and to their babies. If these scenarios were implemented, the MDG for maternal health would not be reached in every country, but the reduction of maternal and perinatal mortality globally would be well on the way. The costs of implementing these 75 country scenarios would be in the region of US$ 39 billion additional to current expenditure. This corresponds to a growth of 3%, in 2006, rising to 14% over the years, of current median public expenditure on health in these countries. In the 20 countries with currently the lowest coverage and facing the greatest constraints, current public expenditure on health would have to grow by 7% in 2006, rising to 43% in 2015.

Putting in place the health workforce needed for scaling up maternal, newborn and child health services towards universal access is the first and most pressing task. Making up for the staggering shortages and imbalances in the distribution of health workers in many countries will remain a major challenge for years to come. The extra work required for scaling up child care activities requires the equivalent of 100 000 full-time multipurpose professionals, supplemented, according to the scenarios that have been costed, by 4.6 million community health workers. Projected staffing requirements for extending coverage of maternal and newborn care assumes the production in the coming 10 years of at least 334 000 additional midwives – or their equivalents – as well as the upgrading of 140 000 health professionals who are currently providing first-level maternal care and of 27 000 doctors who currently do not have the competencies to provide back-up care.

Without planning and capacity-building, at national level and within health districts, it will not be possible to correct the shortages and to improve the skills mix and the working environment. Planning is not enough, however, to put right disruptive histories that have eroded workforce development. After years of neglect there are problems that require immediate attention: first and foremost is the nagging question of the remuneration of the workforce.

In many countries, salary levels are rightfully considered unfair and insufficient to provide for daily living costs, let alone to live up to the expectations of health professionals. This situation is one of the root causes of demotivation, lack of productivity and the various forms of brain-drain and migration: rural to urban, public to private and from poorer to richer countries. It also seriously hampers the correct functioning of services as health workers set up in dual practice to improve their living conditions or merely to make ends meet – leading to competition for time, a loss of resources for the public sector, and conflicts of interest in dealing with their clients. There are even more serious consequences when health workers resort to predatory behaviour: financial exploitation may have catastrophic effects on patients who use the services, and create barriers to access for others; it contributes to a crisis of trust in the services to which mothers and children are entitled.

There is an urgent need to invent and deploy a whole range of measures to break the vicious circle, and bring productivity and dedication back to the level the population expects and to which most health workers aspire. Among these, one of the most challenging is rehabilitating the workforce's remuneration. Even a modest attempt to do so, such as doubling or even tripling the total workforce's salary mass and benefits in the 75 countries for which scenarios were developed, might still be insufficient to attract, retain and redeploy quality staff. But it would correspond to an increase of 2% rising, over 10 years, to 17% of current public expenditure on health, merely for payment of the MNCH workforce. Such a measure would have political and macro-economic implications and is something that cannot be done without a major effort, not only by governments but by international solidarity as well. On the eve of a decade that will be focused on human resources for health, this will require a fundamental debate, in countries as well as internationally, on the volume of the funds that can be allocated and on the channelling of these funds. This is all the more important because rehabilitating the remuneration of the workforce is only one part of the answer: establishing an atmosphere of stability and hope is also needed to give health professionals the confidence they need to work effectively and with dedication.

At the same time, ensuring universal access is not merely a question of increasing the supply of services and paying health care providers. For services to be taken up, financial barriers to access have to be eliminated and users given predictable financial protection against the costs of seeking care, and particularly against the catastrophic payments that can push households into poverty. Such catastrophic payments occur wherever user charges are significant, households have limited ability to pay, and pooling and prepayment is not generalized. To attain the financial protection that has to go with universal access, countries throughout the world have to move away from user charges, be they official or under-the-counter, and generalize prepayment and pooling schemes. Whether they choose to organize financial protection on the basis of tax-generated funds, through social health insurance or through a mix of schemes, two things are important: first, that ultimately no population groups are excluded; second, that maternal and child health services are at the core of the health entitlements of the population, and that they be financed in a coherent way through the selected system. While it can take many years to move from a situation of a limited supply of services, high out-of-pocket payments and exclusion of the poorest to a situation of universal access and financial protection, the extension of health care supply networks has to proceed in parallel with the construction of such insurance mechanisms.

Financing is the killer assumption underlying the planning of maternal, newborn and child health care. First, increased funding is required to pay for building up the supply of services towards universal access. Second, financial protection systems have to be built at the same time as access improves. Third, the channelling of increased funds, both domestic and international, has to guarantee the flexibility and predictability that make it possible to cope with the principal health system constraints – particularly the problems facing the workforce.

Channelling increased funding flows through national health insurance schemes – be they organized as tax-based, social health insurance, or mixed systems – offers the best avenue to meet these three challenges simultaneously. It requires major capacity-building efforts, but it offers the possibility of protecting the funding of the workforce in public sector and health sector reform policies and in the forums where macroeconomic and poverty-reduction policies are decided. It offers the possibility of tackling the problem of the remuneration and the working conditions of health workers in a way that gives them long-term, credible prospects, which traditional budgeting or the stopgap solutions of project funding do not offer.

While the financing effort seems to be within reasonable reach in some countries, in many it will go beyond what can be borne by governments alone. Both countries and the international community will need to show a sustained political commitment to mobilize and redirect the considerable resources that are required, to build the institutional capacity to manage them, and to ensure that maternal, newborn and child health remains at the core of these efforts. This decade can be one of accelerating the move towards universal coverage, with access for all and financial protection. That will ensure that no mother, no newborn, and no child in need remains unattended – because every mother and every child counts.

CHAPTER SUMMARIES

Chapter 1. Mothers and children matter – so does their health

This chapter recalls how the health of mothers and children became a public health priority during the 20th century. For centuries, care for mothers and young children was regarded as a domestic affair, the realm of mothers and midwives. In the 20th century this purely domestic concern was transformed into a public health priority. In the opening years of the 21st century, the MDGs place it at the core of the struggle against poverty and inequality, as a matter of human rights. This shift in emphasis has far-reaching consequences for the way the world responds to the very uneven progress in different countries.

The chapter summarizes the current situation regarding the health of mothers, newborns and children. Most progress has been made by countries that were already in a relatively good position in the early 1990s, while countries that started with the highest mortality rates are also those where improvements have been most disappointing.

Globally, mortality rates in children under five years of age fell throughout the latter part of the 20th century: from 146 per 1000 live births in 1970 to 79 in 2003. Towards the turn of the millennium, however, the overall downward trend started to falter in some parts of the world. Improvements continued or accelerated in the WHO Regions of the Americas, South-East Asia and Europe, while the African, Eastern Mediterranean and Western Pacific Regions experienced a slowing down of progress. In 93 countries, totalling 40% of the world population, under-five mortality is decreasing fast. A further 51 countries, with 48% of the world population, are making slower progress: they will only reach the MDGs if improvements are accelerated significantly. Even more worrying are the 43 countries that contain the remaining 12% of the world population, where under-five mortality was high or very high to start with and is now stagnating or reversing.

Reliable data on newborns are only recently becoming available and are more difficult to interpret. The most recent estimates show that newborn mortality is considerably higher than usually thought and accounts for 40% of under-five deaths; less than 2% of newborn deaths currently occur in high income countries. The difference between rich and poor countries seems to be widening.

Over 300 million women in the world currently suffer from long-term or short-term illness brought about by pregnancy or childbirth. The 529 000 annual maternal deaths, including 68 000 deaths attributable to unsafe abortion, are even more unevenly spread than newborn or child deaths: only 1% occur in rich countries. There is a sense of progress, backed by the tracking of indicators that show increases in the uptake of care during pregnancy and childbirth in all regions except sub-Saharan Africa during the 1990s, but the overall picture shows no spectacular improvement, and the lack of reliable information on the fate of mothers in many countries – and on that of their newborns – remains appalling.

Chapter 2. Obstacles to progress: context or policy?

This chapter seeks to explain why progress in maternal and child health has apparently stumbled so badly in many countries. Slow progress, stagnation and reversal are clearly related to poverty, to humanitarian crises, and, particularly in sub-Saharan Africa, to the direct and indirect effects of HIV/AIDS. These operate, at least in part, by fuelling or maintaining exclusion from care. In many countries numerous women and children are excluded from even the most basic health care benefits: those that are important for mere survival.

The specific causes, manifestations and patterns of exclusion vary from country to country. Some countries show a pattern of marginal exclusion: a majority of the population enjoys access to service networks, but substantial groups remain excluded. Other countries, often the poorest ones, show a pattern of massive deprivation: only a small minority, usually the urban rich, enjoys reasonable access, while an overwhelming majority is excluded. These countries have low density, weak and fragile health systems.

The policy challenges vary according to the different patterns of exclusion. Many countries have organized their health care systems as health districts, with a backbone of health centres and a referral district hospital. These strategies have often been so under-resourced that they failed to live up to expectations. The chapter argues that the health district model still stands as a rational way for governments to organize decentralized health care delivery, but that long-term commitment and investment are required to obtain sustained results.

Chapter 3. Great expectations: making pregnancy safer

This chapter reviews the three most important ways in which the outcomes of pregnancies can be improved: providing good antenatal care, finding appropriate ways of preventing and dealing with the consequences of unwanted pregnancies, and improving the way society looks after pregnant women.

Antenatal care is a success story: coverage throughout the world increased by 20% during the 1990s and continues to increase in most parts of the world. Concern for a good outcome of pregnancy has made women the largest group actively seeking care. Antenatal care offers the opportunity to provide much more than just pregnancy-related care. The potential to promote healthy lifestyles is insufficiently exploited, as is the use of antenatal care as a platform for programmes that tackle malnutrition, HIV/AIDS, sexually transmitted infections, malaria and tuberculosis and promote family planning. Antenatal consultations are the ideal occasion to establish birth plans that can make sure the birth itself takes place in safe circumstances, and to help mothers prepare for parenting.

The chapter sets out critical directions for the future, including the need to improve the quality of care and to further increase coverage.

Even in societies that value pregnancy highly, the position of pregnant women is not always enviable. In many places there is a need to improve the social, political and legal environments so as to tackle the low status of women, gender-based violence, discrimination in the workplace or at school, or marginalization. Eliminating sources of social exclusion is as important as providing antenatal care.

Unintended, mistimed or unwanted pregnancies are estimated to number 87 million per year. There remains a huge unmet need for investment in contraception, information and education to prevent unwanted pregnancy, though no family planning policy will prevent it all. More than half of the women concerned, 46 million per year, resort to induced abortion: that 18 million do so in unsafe circumstances constitutes a major public health problem. It is possible, however, to avoid all of the 68 000 deaths as well as the disabilities and suffering that go with unsafe abortions. This is not only a question of how a country defines what is legal and what is not, but also of guaranteeing women access, to the fullest extent permitted by law, to good quality and responsive abortion and post-abortion care.

Chapter 4. Attending to 136 million births, every year

This chapter analyses the major complications of childbirth and the main causes of maternal mortality. Direct causes of maternal mortality include haemorrhage, infection, eclampsia, obstructed labour and unsafe abortion. Childbirth is a moment of great risks, but in many situations over half of maternal deaths occur during the postpartum period. Effective interventions exist to avoid most of the deaths and long-term disabilities attributable to childbirth. The history of successes in reducing maternal and newborn mortalities shows that skilled professional care during and after childbirth can make the difference between life and death for both women and their newborn babies. The converse is true as well: a breakdown of access to skilled care may rapidly lead to an increase of unfavourable outcomes.

All mothers and newborns, not just those considered to be at particular risk of developing complications, need skilled maternal and neonatal care: close to where and how they live, close to their birthing culture, but at the same time safe, with a skilled professional able to act immediately when complications occur. Such birthing care can best be provided by a registered midwife or a professional health worker with equivalent skills, in midwife-led facilities. These professionals can avert, contain or solve many of the largely unpredictable life-threatening problems that may arise during childbirth and thus reduce maternal mortality to surprisingly low levels. But they do need the back-up only a hospital can provide to help mothers who present problems that go beyond their competency or equipment. All women need first-level maternal care, and only in a minority of cases is back-up care necessary, but to be effective both need to work in tandem, and have to be extended simultaneously. In many countries uptake of postpartum care is even lower than of care at childbirth. This is an area of crucial importance with much scope for improvement.

Chapter 5. Newborns: no longer going unnoticed

Until recently, there has been little real effort to tackle the specific health problems of newborns. A lack of continuity between maternal and child health programmes has allowed care of the newborn to fall through the cracks.

Each year nearly 3.3 million babies are stillborn, and over 4 million more die within 28 days of coming into the world. Deaths of babies during this neonatal period are as numerous as those in the following 11 months or those among children aged 1–4 years. Skilled professional care during pregnancy, at birth and during the postnatal period is as critical for the newborn baby as it is for its mother. The challenge is to find a better way of establishing continuity between care during pregnancy, at birth, and when the mother is at home with her baby. While the weakest link in the care chain is skilled attendance at birth, care during the early weeks of life is also problematic because professional and programmatic responsibilities are often not clearly delineated.

The chapter presents a set of benchmarks for the needs in human resources and service networks to provide first level and back-up maternal and newborn care to all. In many countries there are major shortages in facilities and, crucially, human resources. Using a set of scenarios to scale up towards universal access to both first-level and back-up maternal and newborn care in 75 countries, it seems realistic for coverage to increase from its present 43% (with a limited package of care) to around 73% (with a full package of care) in 2015. Implementing these scenarios would cost US$ 1 billion in 2006, increasing, as coverage expands, to US$ 6 billion in 2015: a total of US$ 39 billion over ten years, in addition to present expenditure on maternal and newborn health. This corresponds to an extra outlay of around US$ 0.22 per inhabitant per year initially, increasing to US$ 1.18 in 2015. A preliminary estimate of the potential impact of this scaling up suggests a reduction of maternal mortality, in these 75 countries, from a 2000 aggregate level of 485 to 242 per 100 000 births, and of neonatal mortality from 35 to 29 per 1000 live births by 2015.

Chapter 6. Redesigning child care: survival, growth and development

Increased knowledge means that technically appropriate, effective interventions for reducing child mortality and improving child health are available. It is now necessary to implement them on a much larger scale.

This chapter explains how in the 1970s and 1980s vertical programmes have undeniably allowed fast and significant results. The Expanded Programme on Immunization and initiatives to implement oral rehydration therapy, for example, with a combination of state-of-the-art management and simple technologies based on solid research, were adopted and promoted to great effect.

For all their impressive results, however, the inherent limitations of vertical approaches became apparent. At the same time, it became clear that a more comprehensive approach to the needs of the child was desirable, both to improve outcomes and to respond to a genuine demand from families. The response was to package a set of simple, affordable and effective interventions for the combined management of the major childhood illnesses and malnutrition, under the label of Integrated Management of Childhood Illness (IMCI). IMCI combined interventions designed to prevent deaths, taking into account the changing profile of mortality causes, but it also comprised of interventions and approaches to improve children's healthy growth and development. More than just adding extra programmes to a single delivery channel, IMCI has gone a step further and has sought to transform the way the health system looks at child care, spanning a continuum of care from the family and community to the first-level health facility and on to referral facilities, with an emphasis on counselling and problem-solving.

Many children still do not benefit from comprehensive and integrated care. As child health programmes continue to move towards integration it is necessary to progress towards universal coverage. Scaling up a set of essential interventions to full coverage would bring down the incidence and case fatality of the conditions causing children under five years of age to die, to a level that would permit countries to move towards and beyond the MDGs. This will not be possible without a massive increase of expenditure on child health. Implementing scenarios to reach full coverage in 75 countries would cost US$ 2.2 billion in 2006, increasing, as coverage expands, to US$ 7.8 billion in 2015: a total of US$ 52.4 billion over 10 years, in addition to present expenditure on child health. This corresponds to an extra outlay of around US$ 0.47 per inhabitant per year initially, expanding to US$ 1.48 in 2015.

Chapter 7. Reconciling maternal, newborn and child health with health system development

This last chapter looks at the place of maternal, newborn and child health within the broader context of health system development. Today, the maternal, newborn and child health agendas are no longer discussed in purely technical terms, but as part of a broader agenda of universal access. This frames it within a straightforward political project: responding to society's demand for the protection of the health of citizens and access to care, a demand that is increasingly seen as legitimate.

Universal access requires a sufficiently dense health care network to supply services. The critical challenge is to put in place the health workforce required for scaling up. The most visible features of the health workforce crisis in many countries are the staggering shortages and imbalances in the distribution of health workers. Filling these gaps will remain a major challenge for years to come. Part of the problem is that sustainable ways have to be devised of offering competitive remuneration and incentive packages that can attract, motivate and retain competent and productive health workers. In many of the countries where progress towards the MDGs is disappointing, very substantial increases in the remuneration packages of health personnel are urgently needed, a challenge of a magnitude that many poor countries cannot face alone.

Universal access, however, is more than deploying an effective workforce to supply services. For health services to be taken up, financial barriers to access have to be reduced or eliminated and users given predictable protection against the costs of seeking care. The chapter shows that by and large the introduction of user fees is not a viable answer to the underfunding of the health sector, and institutionalizes exclusion of the poor. It does not accelerate progress towards universal access and financial protection; this can be guaranteed only through generalized prepayment and pooling schemes. Whichever system is adopted to organize these schemes, two things are important. First, ultimately no population groups should be excluded; second, maternal, newborn and child health services should be at the core of the set of services to which citizens are entitled and which are financed in a coherent way through the selected system.

With time, most countries move towards universal coverage, widening prepayment and pooling schemes, in parallel with the extension of their health care supply networks. This also has consequences for the funding flows directed towards maternal, newborn and child health. In most countries, financial sustainability for maternal, newborn and child health can best be achieved in the short and middle term by looking at all sources of funding: external and domestic, public and private. Channelling funds towards generalized insurance schemes that both fund the expansion of health care networks and provide financial protection, offers most guarantees for sustainable financing of maternal, newborn and child health and of the health systems on which it depends.

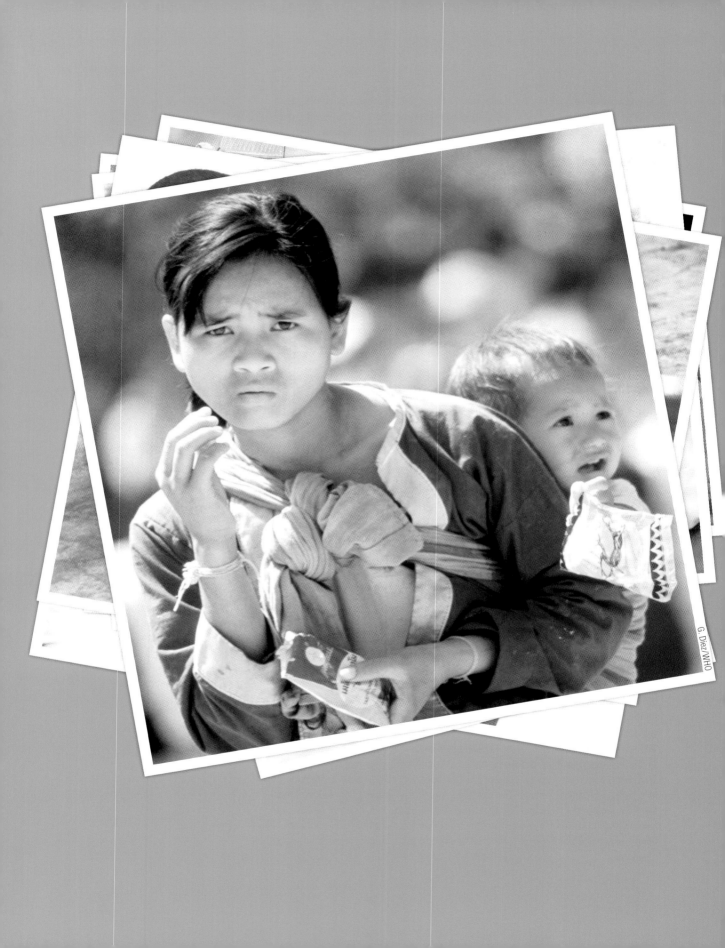

G. Diez/WHO

chapter one

mothers and children matter – so does their health

The healthy future of society depends on the health of the children of today and their mothers, who are guardians of that future. However, despite much good work over the years, 10.6 million children and 529 000 mothers are still dying each year, mostly from avoidable causes. This chapter assesses the current status of maternal and child health programmes against their historical background. It then goes on to examine in more detail the patchwork of progress, stagnation and reversals in the health of mothers and children worldwide and draws attention to the previously underestimated burden of newborn mortality.

Most pregnant women hope to give birth safely to a baby that is alive and well and to see it grow up in good health. Their chances of doing so are better in 2005 than ever before – not least because they are becoming aware of their rights. With today's knowledge and technology, the vast majority of the problems that threaten the world's mothers and children can be prevented or treated. Most of the millions of untimely deaths that occur are avoidable, as is much of the suffering that comes with ill-health. A mother's death is a tragedy unlike others, because of the deeply held feeling that no one should die in the course of the normal process of reproduction and because of the devastating effects on her family *(1)*. In all cultures, families and communities acknowledge the need to care for mothers and children and try to do so to the best of their ability.

An increasing number of countries have succeeded in improving the health and well-being of mothers, babies and children in recent years, with noticeable results. However, the countries with the highest burden of mortality and ill-health to start with made little progress during the 1990s. In some, the situation has actually worsened in recent years. Progress has therefore been patchy and unless it is accelerated significantly, there is little hope of reducing maternal mortality by three quarters and child mortality by two thirds by the target date of 2015 – the targets set by the Millennium Declaration *(2, 3)*.

In too many countries the health of mothers and children is not making the progress it should. The reasons for this are complex and vary from one country to another. They include the familiar, persistent enemies of health – poverty, inequality, war and civil unrest, and the destructive influence of HIV/AIDS – but also the failure to translate life-saving knowledge into effective action and to invest adequately in public health and a safe environment. This leaves many mothers and children, particularly the poorest among them, excluded from access to the affordable, effective and responsive care to which they are entitled.

For centuries, care for childbirth and young children was regarded as a domestic affair, the realm of mothers and midwives. In the 20th century, the health of mothers and children was transformed from a purely domestic concern into a public health priority with corresponding responsibilities for the state. In the opening years of the 21st century, the Millennium Development Goals place it at the core of the struggle against poverty and inequality, as a matter of human rights. This shift in emphasis has far-reaching consequences for the way the world responds to the very uneven progress in different countries.

THE EARLY YEARS OF MATERNAL AND CHILD HEALTH

The creation of public health programmes to improve the health of women and children has its origins in Europe at the end of the nineteenth century. With hindsight, the reasons for this concern look cynical: healthy mothers and children were seen by governments at that time to be a resource for economic and political ambitions. Many of Europe's politicians shared a perception that the ill-health of the nation's children threatened their cultural and military aspirations *(4)*. This feeling was particularly strong in France and Britain, which had experienced difficulties in recruiting soldiers fit enough for war. Governments saw a possible solution in the pioneering French experiments of the 1890s, such as Léon Dufour's *Goutte de lait* (drop of milk) clinics and Pierre Budin's *Consultations de nourrissons* (infant welfare clinics) *(5)*. These programmes offered a scientific and convincing way to produce healthy children who would become productive workers and robust soldiers. The programmes also increasingly found support in the emerging social reform and charitable movements of the time. As a result, all industrialized countries and their colonies, as well as Thailand and many Latin American countries, had instituted at least an embryonic form of maternal and infant health services by the onset of the 20th century *(6)*. The First World War accelerated the movement. Josephine Baker, then Chief of the Division of Child Hygiene of New York, summed it up as follows:

One of the first maternal and child health clinics, in the late 19th century, was
'L'Œuvre de la goutte de lait': Dr Variot's consultation at the Belleville Dispensary, Paris.

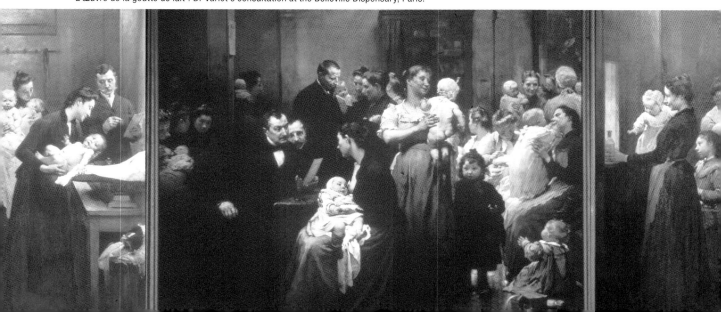

"It may seem like a cold-blooded thing to say, but someone ought to point out that the World War was a back-handed break for children ... As more and more thousands of men were slaughtered every day, the belligerent nations, on whatever side, began to see that new human lives, which could grow up to replace brutally extinguished adult lives, were extremely valuable national assets. [The children] took the spotlight as the hope of the nation. That is the handsomest way to put it. The ugliest way – and, I suspect, the truer – is to say flatly that it was the military usefulness of human life that wrought the change. When a nation is fighting a war or preparing for another ... it must look to its future supplies of cannon fodder" (7).

Caring for the health of mothers and children soon gained a legitimacy of its own, beyond military and economic calculations. The increasing involvement of a variety of authorities – medical and lay, charitable and governmental – resonated with the rising expectations and political activism of civil society *(1)*. Workers' movements, women's groups, charities and professional organizations took up the cause of the health of women and children in many different ways. For example, the International Labour Organization proposed legal standards for the protection of maternity at work in 1919; the *New York Times* published articles on maternal mortality in the early 1930s; and in 1938 the Mothers' Charter was proclaimed by 60 local associations in the United Kingdom. Backed by large numbers of official reports, maternal and child health became a priority for ministries of health. Maternal and child health programmes became a public health paradigm alongside that of the battle against infectious diseases *(8)*.

These programmes really started to gain ground after the Second World War. Global events precipitated public interest in the roles and responsibilities of governments, and the Universal Declaration of Human Rights in 1948 by the newly formed United Nations secured their obligation to provide "special care and assistance" for mothers and children *(9)*. This added an international and moral dimension to the issue of the health of mothers and children, representing a huge step forward from the political and economic concerns of 50 years earlier.

One of the core functions assigned to the World Health Organization (WHO) in its Constitution of 1948 was "to promote maternal and child health and welfare" *(10)*. By the 1950s, national health plans and policy documents from development agencies invariably stressed that mothers and children were vulnerable groups and therefore priority "targets" for public health action. The notion of mothers and children as vulnerable groups was also central to the primary health care movement launched at Alma-Ata (now Almaty, Kazakhstan) in 1978. This first major attempt at massive scaling up of health care coverage in rural areas boosted maternal and child health programmes by its focus on initiatives to increase immunization coverage and to tackle malnutrition, diarrhoea and respiratory diseases. In practice, child health programmes were usually the central – often the only – programmatic content of early attempts to implement primary health care *(11)*.

WHERE WE ARE NOW: A MORAL AND POLITICAL IMPERATIVE

The early implementation of primary health care often had a narrow focus, but among its merits was the fact that it laid the groundwork for linking health to development and to a wider civil society debate on inequalities. The plight of mothers and children soon came to be seen as much more than a problem of biological vulnerability. The 1987 Call to Action for Safe Motherhood explicitly framed it as "deeply rooted in the adverse social, cultural and economic environments of society, and especially the environment that societies create for women" *(12)*. Box 1.1 recalls some important milestones in establishing the rights of women and children.

In this more politicized view, women's relative lack of decision-making power and their unequal access to employment, finances, education, basic health care and other resources are considered to be the root causes of their ill-health and that of their children. Poor nutrition in girls, early onset of sexual activity and adolescent pregnancy all have consequences for well-being during and after pregnancy for both mothers and children. Millions of women and their families live in a social environment that works against seeking and enjoying good health. Women often have limited exposure to the education, information and new ideas that could spare them from repeated childbearing and save their lives during childbirth. They may have no say in decisions on whether to use contraception or where to give birth. They may be reluctant to use health services where they feel threatened and humiliated by the staff, or pressured to accept treatments that conflict with their own values and customs *(13)*. Poverty, cultural traditions and legal barriers restrict their access to financial resources, making it even more difficult to seek health care for themselves or for their children. The unfairness of this situation has made it obvious that the health of mothers and children is an issue of rights, entitlements and day-to-day struggle to secure these entitlements.

The shift to a concern for the rights of women and children was accelerated by the International Conference on Population and Development, held in Cairo, Egypt, in

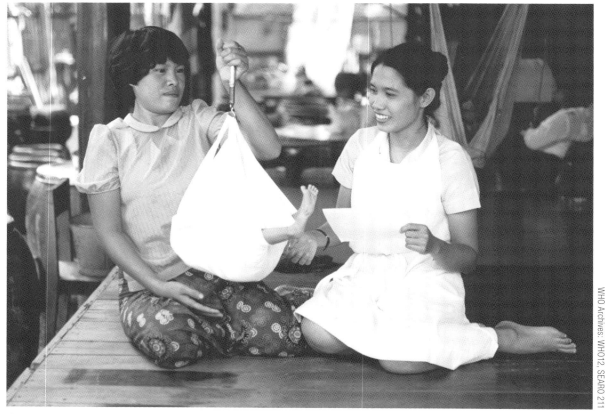

WHO Archives: WHO12, SEARO 211

Child health programmes were central to early attempts to implement primary health care.
Here a community nurse in Thailand watches as a mother weighs her baby.

Box 1.1 Milestones in the establishment of the rights of women and children

In the 20th century several international treaties came into being, holding signatory countries accountable for the human rights of their citizens. Over the past two decades United Nations bodies, as well as international, regional and national courts, have increasingly focused on the human rights of mothers and children.

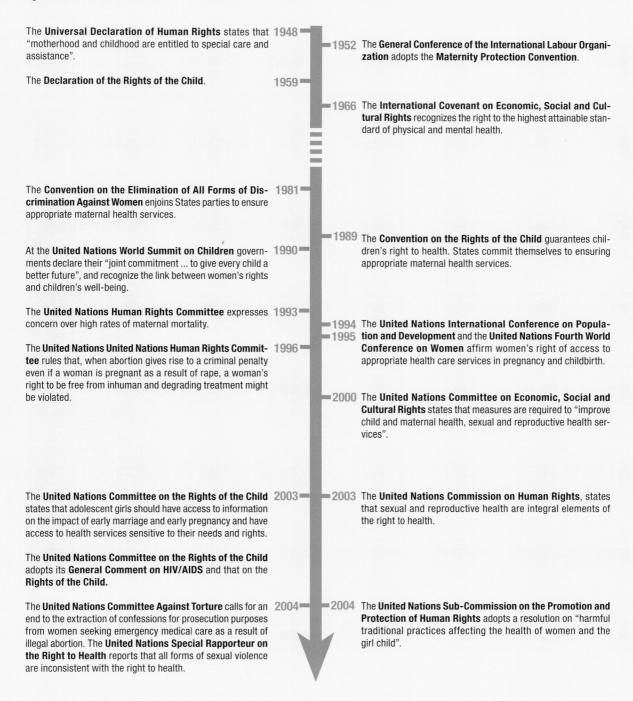

The **Universal Declaration of Human Rights** states that "motherhood and childhood are entitled to special care and assistance". **1948**

1952 The **General Conference of the International Labour Organization** adopts the **Maternity Protection Convention**.

The **Declaration of the Rights of the Child.** **1959**

1966 The **International Covenant on Economic, Social and Cultural Rights** recognizes the right to the highest attainable standard of physical and mental health.

The **Convention on the Elimination of All Forms of Discrimination Against Women** enjoins States parties to ensure appropriate maternal health services. **1981**

1989 The **Convention on the Rights of the Child** guarantees children's right to health. States commit themselves to ensuring appropriate maternal health services.

At the **United Nations World Summit on Children** governments declare their "joint commitment ... to give every child a better future", and recognize the link between women's rights and children's well-being. **1990**

The **United Nations Human Rights Committee** expresses concern over high rates of maternal mortality. **1993**

1994 The **United Nations International Conference on Population and Development** and the **United Nations Fourth World Conference on Women** affirm women's right of access to appropriate health care services in pregnancy and childbirth. **1995**

The **United Nations United Nations Human Rights Committee** rules that, when abortion gives rise to a criminal penalty even if a woman is pregnant as a result of rape, a woman's right to be free from inhuman and degrading treatment might be violated. **1996**

2000 The **United Nations Committee on Economic, Social and Cultural Rights** states that measures are required to "improve child and maternal health, sexual and reproductive health services".

The **United Nations Committee on the Rights of the Child** states that adolescent girls should have access to information on the impact of early marriage and early pregnancy and have access to health services sensitive to their needs and rights. **2003**

2003 The **United Nations Commission on Human Rights**, states that sexual and reproductive health are integral elements of the right to health.

The **United Nations Committee on the Rights of the Child** adopts its **General Comment on HIV/AIDS** and that on the **Rights of the Child.**

The **United Nations Committee Against Torture** calls for an end to the extraction of confessions for prosecution purposes from women seeking emergency medical care as a result of illegal abortion. The **United Nations Special Rapporteur on the Right to Health** reports that all forms of sexual violence are inconsistent with the right to health. **2004**

2004 The **United Nations Sub-Commission on the Promotion and Protection of Human Rights** adopts a resolution on "harmful traditional practices affecting the health of women and the girl child".

1994. The conference produced a 20-year plan of action that focused on universal access to reproductive health services (of which maternal and child health care became a subset), which was grounded in individual choices and rights. This change in perspective is important, because it alters the rationale for investing in the health of mothers and children.

Today, more is known than ever before about what determines the health of women and children and about which interventions bring about improvements most cost-effectively. This knowledge makes investment more successful, and withholding care even less acceptable. The health of mothers and children satisfies the classical criteria for setting public health priorities (see Box 1.2). Compelling as these arguments may be, however, they miss two vital points.

Box 1.2 Why invest public money in health care for mothers and children?

Modern states guarantee health entitlements for mothers, newborns and children that are grounded in human rights conventions. Ensuring them access to care has become a moral and political imperative, which also has a strong rational basis.

From a public health point of view an important criterion for priority setting and public funding is that cost-effective intervention packages exist. Such packages are well documented in the case of maternal and child health *(14, 15)*. But cost-effectiveness is only one of the criteria for public investment. Others commonly used include: the generation of positive externalities; the production of public goods and the rule of rescue; and the potential to increase equity and avoid catastrophic expenditure *(16)*. Any of these criteria can be a sufficient condition for public investment on its own. When more than one is present, as in maternal and child health interventions, the case for public funding is even stronger.

Health care for mothers and children produces obvious positive externalities through vaccination or the treatment of the infectious diseases of childhood, and through the improved child health that follows improvement of maternal health. There has been little systematic research on the human, social and economic capital generated by improving the health of mothers and children, but the negative externalities of ill-health are clear.

The health of mothers is a major determinant of that of their children, and thus indirectly affects the formation of human capital. Motherless children die more frequently, are more at risk of becoming malnourished and less likely to enrol at school *(17, 18)*. The babies of ill or undernourished pregnant women are more likely to have a low birth weight *(19–21)* and impaired development *(19, 22–24)*. Low-

birth-weight children in turn are at greater risk of dying and of suffering from infections and growth retardation *(25)*, have lower scores on cognitive tests *(26–28)* and may be at higher risk of developing chronic diseases in adulthood *(29, 30)*.

Healthy children are at the core of the formation of human capital. Child illnesses and malnutrition reduce cognitive development and intellectual performance *(31–33)*, school enrolment and attendance *(34, 35)*, which impairs final educational achievement. Intrauterine growth retardation and malnutrition during early childhood have long-term effects on body size and strength *(36, 37)* with implications for productivity in adulthood.

In addition, with the death or illness of a woman, society loses a member whose labour and activities are essential to the life and cohesion of families and communities. Healthy mothers have more time and are more available for the social interaction and the creation of the bonds that are the prerequisite of social capital. They also play an important social role in caring for those who are ill.

The economic costs of poor maternal and child health are high *(38)*; substantial savings in future expenditure are likely through family planning programmes *(39, 40)* and interventions that improve maternal and child health in the long term. Consequent gains in human and social capital translate into long-term economic benefits *(41)*. There is evidence of economic returns on investment in immunization *(42)*, nutrition programmes *(41, 43)*, interventions to reduce low birth weight *(36)*, and integrated health and social development programmes *(44, 45)*.

Maternal and child health programmes are also prime candidates for public funding because they produce public goods. Although many

maternal and child health interventions can be classified as private goods, a comprehensive programme also includes components such as information on contraception, on sexual health and rights, on breastfeeding and child care, that are obvious public goods. Moreover, the rule of rescue, which gives priority to interventions that save lives, applies to many maternal and child health interventions.

Finally, public funding for maternal and child health care is justified on grounds of equity. Motherhood and childhood are periods of particularly high vulnerability that require "special care and assistance" *(19)*; they are also periods of high vulnerability because women and children are more likely to be poor. Although systematic documentation showing that they are overrepresented among the poor is scarce *(46)*, women are more likely to be unemployed, to have lower wages, less access to education and resources and more restricted decision-making power, all of which limit their access to care. Public investment in maternal and child health care is justified in order to correct these inequities.

In addition, where women and children represent a large proportion of the poor, subsidizing health services for them can be an effective strategy for income redistribution and poverty alleviation *(14)*. Ill-health among mothers and children, and particularly the occurrence of major obstetric problems, is largely unpredictable and can lead to catastrophic expenditures *(47)* that may push households into poverty. The risk of catastrophic expenditures is often a deterrent for the timely uptake of care – a major argument, technically and politically, for public investment.

First, children are the future of society, and their mothers are guardians of that future. Mothers are much more than caregivers and homemakers, undervalued as these roles often are. They transmit the cultural history of families and communities along with social norms and traditions. Mothers influence early behaviour and establish lifestyle patterns that not only determine their children's future development and capacity for health, but shape societies. Because of this, society values the health of its mothers and children for its own sake and not merely as a contribution to the wealth of the nation *(48)*.

Second, few consequences of the inequities in society are as damaging as those that affect the health and survival of women and children. For governments that take their function of reducing inequality and redistributing wealth seriously, improving the living conditions and providing access to health care for mothers and children are good starting points. Improving their health is at the core of the world's push to reduce poverty and inequality.

MOTHERS, CHILDREN AND THE MILLENNIUM DEVELOPMENT GOALS

In his report to the Millennium Summit, the Secretary-General of the United Nations, Kofi Annan, called on "the international community at the highest level – the Heads of State and Government convened at the Millennium Summit – to adopt the target of halving the proportion of people living in extreme poverty, and so lifting more than 1 billion people out of it, by 2015" *(49)*. He further urged that no effort be spared to

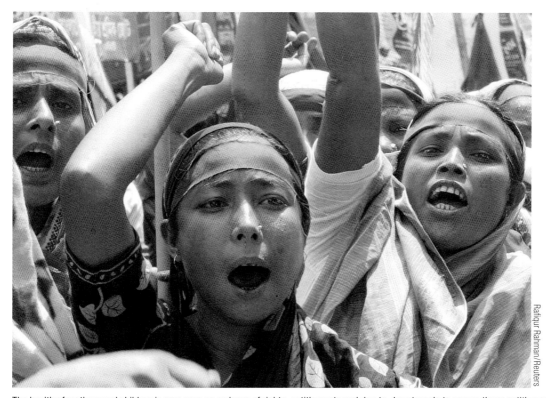

Rafiqur Rahman/Reuters

The health of mothers and children is now seen as an issue of rights, entitlements and day-to-day struggle to secure these entitlements.

reach this target by that date in every region, and in every country. The Millennium Declaration *(50)*, coming after a decade of "unprecedented stagnation and deterioration" *(51)*, set out eight specific Millennium Development Goals (MDGs), each with its numerical targets and indicators for monitoring progress. The MDGs galvanized countries and the international community in a global partnership that, for the first time, articulated a commitment by both rich and poor countries to tackle a whole range of dimensions of poverty and inequality in a concerted and integrated way.

The health agenda is very much in evidence in the MDGs: it is explicit in three of the eight goals, eight of the 18 targets, and 18 of the 48 indicators. This emphasis on health reflects a global consensus that ill-health is an important dimension of poverty in its own right. Ill-health contributes to poverty. Improving health is a condition for poverty alleviation and for development. Sustainable improvement of health depends on successful poverty alleviation and reduction of inequalities.

It is no accident that the formulation of the MDG targets and indicators reveals the special priority given to the health and well-being of women, mothers and children. Mother and child health is clearly on the international agenda even in the absence of universal access to reproductive health services as a specific Millennium Development Goal. Globally, we are making progress towards the MDGs in maternal and child health. Success is overshadowed, however, by the persistence of an unacceptably high mortality and the increasing inequity in maternal and child health and access to health care worldwide.

UNEVEN GAINS IN CHILD HEALTH

Being healthy means much more than merely surviving. Nevertheless, the mortality rates of children under five years of age provide a good indicator of the progress made – or the tragic lack of it. Under-five mortality rates fell worldwide throughout the latter part of the 20th century: from 146 per 1000 in 1970 to 79 per 1000 in 2003. Since 1990, this rate has dropped by about 15%, equating to more than two million lives

Figure 1.1 Slowing progress in child mortality: how Africa is faring worst

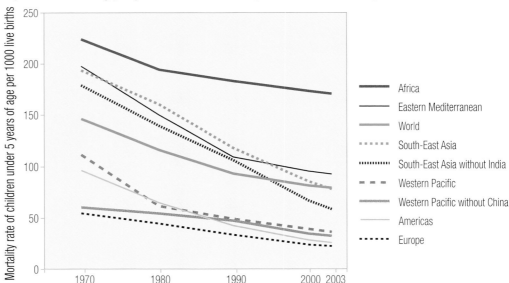

saved in 2003 alone. Towards the turn of the millennium, however, the overall downward trend was showing signs of slowing. Between 1970 and 1990, the under-five
mortality rate dropped by 20% every decade; between 1990 and 2000 it dropped by
only 12% (see Figure 1.1).

The global averages also hide important regional differences. The slowing down of
progress started in the 1980s in the WHO African and Western Pacific Regions, and
during the 1990s in the Eastern Mediterranean Region. The African Region started out
at the highest levels, saw the smallest reductions (around 5% by decade between
1980 and 2000) and the most marked slowing down. In contrast, progress continued
or accelerated in the WHO Region of the Americas, and the South-East Asia and
European Regions.

The result is that the differences between regions are growing. The under-five mortality rate is now seven times higher in the African Region than in the European Region;
the rate was "only" 4.3 times higher in 1980 and 5.4 times higher in 1990. Child
deaths are increasingly concentrated in the African Region (43% of the global total in
2003, up from 30% in 1990). As 28% of child deaths still occur in South-East Asia,
two of the six WHO regions – Africa and South-East Asia – account for more than
70% of all child deaths. Looking at it another way, more than 50% of all child deaths
are concentrated in just six countries: China, the Democratic Republic of the Congo,
Ethiopia, India, Nigeria and Pakistan.

The fortunes of the world's children have also been mixed in terms of their nutritional
status. Overall, children today are better nourished: between 1990 and 2000 the
global prevalence of stunting and underweight declined by 20% and 18%, respectively. Nevertheless, children across southern and central Asia continue to suffer very
high levels of malnutrition, and throughout sub-Saharan Africa the numbers of children
who are stunted and underweight increased in this period *(52)*.

THE NEWBORN DEATHS THAT WENT UNNOTICED

If further progress is to be made in reducing child mortality, increased efforts are
needed to bring about a substantial reduction in deaths among newborns. The first
global estimates of neonatal mortality, dating from 1983 *(53)*, were derived using
historical data and are generally considered to give only a rough indication of the
magnitude of the problem. More rigorous estimates became available for 1995 and
for 2000. These are based on national demographic surveys as well as on statistical
models. The new estimates show that the burden of newborn mortality is considerably
higher than many people realize.

Each year, about four million newborns die before they are four weeks old: 98% of
these deaths occur in developing countries. Newborn deaths now contribute to about
40% of all deaths in children under five years of age globally, and more than half of
infant mortality *(54, 55)*. Rates are highest in sub-Saharan Africa and Asia. Two thirds
of newborn deaths occur in the WHO Regions of Africa (28%) and South-East Asia
(36%) *(56)*. The gap between rich and poor countries is widening: neonatal mortality is now 6.5 times lower in the high-income countries than in other countries. The
lifetime risk for a woman to lose a newborn baby is now 1 in 5 in Africa, compared
with 1 in 125 in more developed countries *(57)*.

The above figures do not include the 3.3 million stillbirths per year. Data on stillbirths
are even more scarce than those on newborn deaths. This is not surprising, as only
14% of births in the world are registered. Both live births and deaths of newborns go
underreported; fetal deaths are even more likely to go unreported, particularly early
fetal deaths.

While the burden of neonatal deaths and stillbirths is very substantial, it is in many ways only part of the problem, as the same conditions that contribute to it also cause severe and often lifelong disability. For example, over a million children who survive birth asphyxia each year develop problems such as cerebral palsy, learning difficulties and other disabilities *(58)*. For every newborn baby who dies, at least another 20 suffer birth injury, infection, complications of preterm birth and other neonatal conditions. Their families are usually unprepared for such tragedies and are profoundly affected.

The health and survival of newborn children is closely linked to that of their mothers. First, because healthier mothers have healthier babies; second, because where a mother gets no or inadequate care during pregnancy, childbirth and the postpartum period, this is usually also the case for her newborn baby. Figure 1.2 shows that both mothers and newborns have a better chance of survival if they have skilled help at birth.

FEW SIGNS OF IMPROVEMENT IN MATERNAL HEALTH

Pregnancy and childbirth and their consequences are still the leading causes of death, disease and disability among women of reproductive age in developing countries – more than any other single health problem. Over 300 million women in the developing world currently suffer from short-term or long-term illness brought about by pregnancy and childbirth; 529 000 die each year (including 68 000 as a result of an unsafe abortion), leaving behind children who are more likely to die because they are motherless *(59)*.

There have been few signs of global improvement in this situation. However, during the 1960s and 1970s, some countries did reduce their maternal mortality by half over

Figure 1.2 **Neonatal and maternal mortality are related to the absence of a skilled birth attendant**

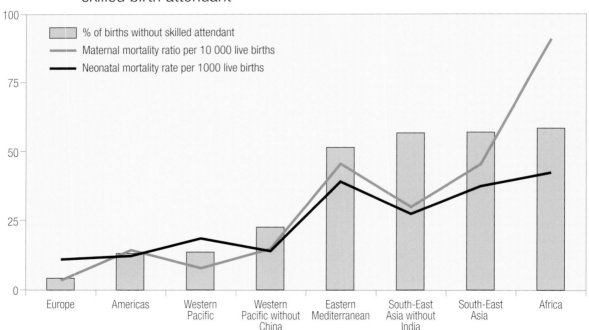

a period of 10 years or less. A few countries such as Bolivia and Egypt have managed this in more recent years. Other countries appear to have suffered reversals (see Box 1.3). Recent success stories in maternal health are less often heard than those for child health. This is partly because it takes longer to show results, partly because changes in maternal mortality are much more difficult to measure with the sources of information available at present.

Today, predictably, most maternal deaths occur in the poorest countries. These deaths are most numerous in Africa and Asia. Less than 1% of deaths occur in high-income countries. Maternal mortality is highest by far in sub-Saharan Africa, where the lifetime risk of maternal death is 1 in 16, compared with 1 in 2800 in rich countries.

Information on maternal mortality remains a serious problem. In the late 1970s, less than one developing country in three was able to provide data – and these were usually only partial hospital statistics. The situation has now improved but births and deaths in developing countries are often only registered for small portions of the population except in some Asian and Latin American countries. Cause of death is routinely reported for only 100 countries of the world, covering one third of the world's population. It is even difficult to obtain reliable survey data that are nationally representative. For 62 developing countries, including most of those with very high levels of mortality, the only existing estimates are based on statistical modelling. These are even more hazardous to interpret than those from surveys or partial death registration. The countries that rely on these modelled estimates represent 27% of the world's births. Effectively, this leaves no record of the fate of 36 million – about 1 out of 4 – of the women who give birth every year.

Gradual improvements in data availability, however, mean that a growing database now exists of maternal mortality by country. Since 1990, a joint working group of WHO, the United Nations Children's Fund (UNICEF) and the United Nations Population Fund (UNFPA) has been regularly assessing and synthesizing the available information *(60)*. It has not been possible, though, to assess changes over time with any confidence: the uncertainty associated with maternal mortality estimates makes it difficult to say whether that mortality has gone up or down, so no global downturn in maternal mortality ratios can yet be asserted.

Nevertheless, there is a sense of progress, backed by the tracking of indicators that point to significant increases in the uptake of care during pregnancy and childbirth

Box 1.3 A reversal of maternal mortality in Malawi

Malawi is one country that experienced a significant reversal in maternal mortality: from 752 maternal deaths per 100 000 live births in 1992 to 1120 in 2000, according to the Malawi Demographic and Health Surveys. According to confidential enquiries into maternal deaths in health facilities in 1989 and 2001, three factors apparently contributed to this increase. First, there was a sharp proportional increase in deaths from AIDS. This is not surprising since Malawi's national HIV prevalence has now reached 8.4%. Second, fewer mothers gave birth in health facilities: the proportion dropped from 55% to 43% between 2000 and 2001. Third, the quality of care within health facilities deteriorated. Between 1989 and 2001 the proportion of deaths associated with deficient health care increased from 31% to 43%. In 2001 only one mother out of four who died in the hospital had received standard care. Wrong diagnosis (11% of deaths), delays in starting treatment (19%), wrong treatment (16%), or lack of blood for transfusion (18%): deficient hospital care was the leading principal avoidable factor in 38% of deaths.

The diminishing coverage and the worsening of the quality of care are related to the deteriorating situation of the health workforce (itself not independent from the HIV/AIDS epidemic). In remote areas one midwife often has to run the entire rural health centre and is expected to be available for work day and night, seven days a week. One maternity unit out of 10 is closed for lack of staff. Hospitals also experience severe shortages of midwives, and unskilled cleaners often conduct deliveries. The shortage of staff in maternity units is catastrophic and rapidly getting worse; the chances of Malawi women giving birth in a safe environment diminish accordingly.

in all regions except sub-Saharan Africa during the 1990s. The proportion of births assisted by a skilled attendant rose by 24% during the 1990s, caesarean sections tripled and antenatal care use rose by 21%. Since professional care is known to be crucial in averting maternal deaths as well as in improving maternal health, maternal mortality ratios are likely to be declining everywhere except for those countries which started the 1990s at high levels. For these, which are mainly in sub-Saharan Africa, there has been no sign of progress.

A PATCHWORK OF PROGRESS, STAGNATION AND REVERSAL

The slowing down of improvement of global indicators that so worries policy-makers *(67)* hides a patchwork of countries that are on track, show slow progress, are stagnating or are going into reverse. As most progress is being made in countries that already have relatively low levels of maternal and child deaths, while the worst-off stagnate, the gaps between countries are inevitably widening.

A total of 93 countries, including most of those in the high income bracket, are "on track" to reduce their 1990 under-five mortality rates by two thirds by 2015 or sooner. The on-track countries are those that already had the lowest rates in 1990 (taken together they had a rate of 59 in 1990).

Box 1.4 Counting births and deaths

If nobody keeps track of their births and deaths, women and children simply do not count *(61)*. Mortality rates are frequently only rough estimates, of varying reliability. This is because the ways of estimating mortality are far from perfect and, in many cases, insufficient priority is given to obtaining such vital information.

It is often assumed that the quoted numbers of maternal and child deaths rely on **hospital statistics**. But apart from the problems of maintaining reporting systems, only a fraction of events takes place in facilities. Hospital information is currently the most flawed source of data on births and deaths.

The best approach to estimating maternal and child mortality is to count births and deaths through **vital registration systems**. In many developing countries, however, such systems are still incomplete. The births and deaths that are registered under-represent the rural population and the socioeconomically disadvantaged. In 47 countries of the world, less than 50% of the population registers their deaths. A reliable neonatal mortality rate, for example, can therefore be calculated for only 72 countries – less than 14% of births in the world. Internationally recommended definitions of what constitutes a neonatal death are not always used *(62, 63)*. The calculated rates, especially in central Asia, are therefore not always comparable across countries *(64)*. Vital registration systems are currently even less satisfactory for estimat-

ing maternal mortality. Ascertaining cause of death and relating it to pregnancy is difficult, particularly where most deaths occur at home. Misclassified or undercounting is frequent in countries with fully functioning vital registration systems – between 17% and 63% *(65)* – let alone in those where such systems cover only part of the population.

Many developing countries where births and deaths are not routinely counted conduct **sample surveys** asking women for their "birth histories" and how many of their children have died, when and at what age. These surveys yield estimates of child mortality. Often quite robust, they can be biased or inaccurate when the surveys are badly sampled and not representative of the population at large. Information on a deceased child whose mother has died herself will simply not be gathered. Mothers often do not know exact dates of birth or may be unwilling or unable to recall at what age a child has died. Completeness and accuracy very much depend on the skills and the cultural sensitivity of the interviewer. Unfortunately, finding out about the quality of survey data in the public domain is often not possible.

Maternal mortality is even more difficult to estimate from sample surveys. Information must be gleaned from relatives. Generally, women are asked whether their sisters died during pregnancy or shortly afterwards *(66)*. This presupposes that each woman who dies

in childbirth had a sister, that her sister is alive to tell the tale, that she knows of her sister's death, and knows her sister's age and pregnancy status at death. As maternal deaths are statistically rare, it is difficult to obtain reports on enough deaths to estimate the maternal mortality ratio with sufficient precision and reliability without undertaking more expensive studies such as a reproductive age mortality survey *(60)*. The result is that levels and trends are often very difficult to interpret.

In countries where registration is incomplete and where no survey has been conducted, the only remaining option for assessing mortality is to construct a **modelled estimate**. This is effectively an educated guess based on information from similar or neighbouring countries. A total of 28 countries rely only on such estimates for neonatal mortality, 62 for maternal mortality. These modelled estimates should be treated with great caution, but may be the only information available.

For the first time, this *World Health Report* presents, separately, tables with country estimates of mortality derived from surveys or vital registration, where these are available, and tables for all countries with country estimates that have been modelled and adjusted. These estimates can be found in Annex Tables 2a, 2b and 8.

A total of 51 other countries are showing slower progress: the number of deaths among children under five years of age is going down and the mortality rates are dropping, but not fast enough to reach one third of their 1990 level by 2015 unless they significantly accelerate progress during the coming 10 years. These countries started from a somewhat higher level than those that are on track: an average under-five mortality rate of 92 per 1000.

More problematic are the 29 countries where mortality rates are "stagnating" – where the number of deaths continues to grow, because modest reductions of mortality rates are too small to keep up with the increasing numbers of births. These are the countries that had the highest levels (207 on average) in 1990. Finally, there are 14 "reversal" countries, where under-five mortality rates went down to an average of 111 in 1990 but have increased since. During the 1990s there were more such countries than during the two previous decades combined. These reversals were also more pronounced than before. Countries that show reversal or stagnation are overwhelmingly in the African Region.

This grouping of countries,[1] categorized according to progress in under-five mortality during the 1990s, roughly corresponds to what happened in terms of neonatal and maternal health in these same countries. Although trend data are not available, neonatal and maternal mortality is highest in the countries with reversal and stagnation in under-five mortality (see Table 1.1 and Figures 1.3–1.6).

THE NUMBERS REMAIN HIGH

As the situation improves at a slower pace than expected – and hoped for – the gains in avoided deaths are partially offset by the demographic momentum. The numbers of untimely deaths of mothers and children could well be on the increase, because while rates are dropping, the numbers of mothers, births and children continue to grow. Worldwide, the number of live births will peak at 137 million per year towards 2015 *(68)*: 3.5 million more than at present. Most of the increase will be in sub-Saharan Africa and in parts of Asia – Pakistan and northern India – where the number of births will continue to grow well into the 2020s, even if fertility continues to drop. These are areas where the protection of adolescents and young women against early or unwanted pregnancy is most inadequate, mortality from unsafe abortion most pronounced, giving birth most hazardous and childhood most difficult to survive.

Why is it still necessary for this report to emphasize the importance of focusing on the health of mothers and children, after decades of priority status, and more than 10 years after the United Nations International Conference on Population and Development? Progress has slowed down and is increasingly uneven, with a widening gap between rich and poor countries as well as, often, between the poor and the rich within countries. The reasons for this patchy progress are examined in the next chapter.

---

[1] No data available for five countries.

Figure 1.3 Changes in under-5 mortality rates, 1990–2003:
countries showing progress, stagnation or reversal

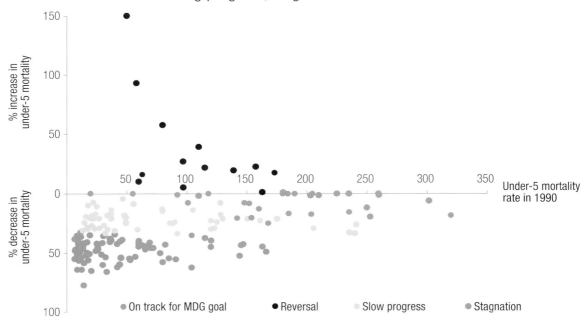

Figure 1.4 Patterns of reduction of under-5 mortality rates, 1990–2003

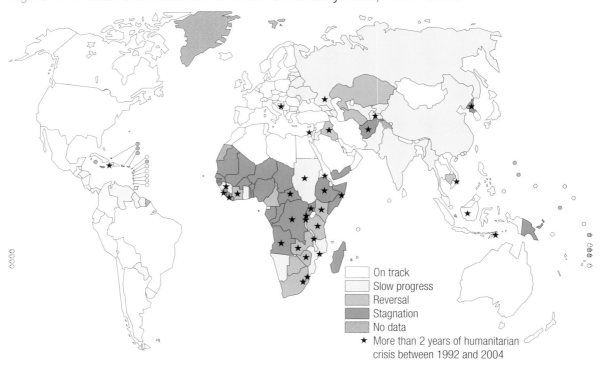

Figure 1.5 Maternal mortality ratio per 100 000 live births in 2000

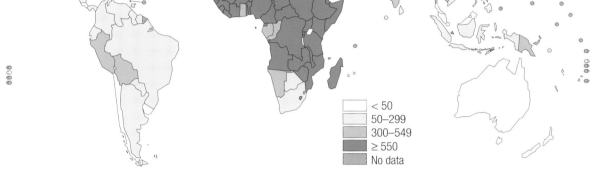

	< 50
	50–299
	300–549
	≥ 550
	No data

Figure 1.6 Neonatal mortality rate per 1000 live births in 2000[a]

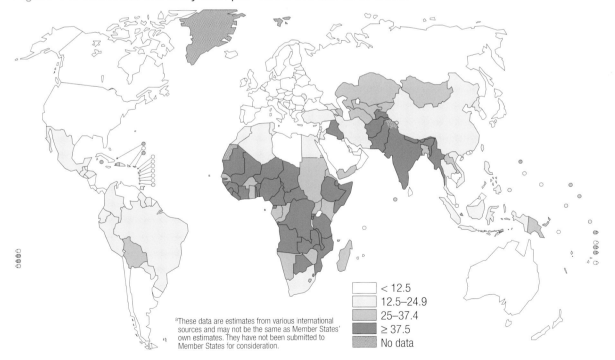

[a]These data are estimates from various international sources and may not be the same as Member States' own estimates. They have not been submitted to Member States for consideration.

	< 12.5
	12.5–24.9
	25–37.4
	≥ 37.5
	No data

Table 1.1   Neonatal and maternal mortality in countries where the decline in child mortality has stagnated or reversed

Decline of child mortality (1990–2003)	No. of countries	Population (2003)[a]	Average live births per year (2000–2005)[a]	Under-5 mortality rate (1990)[b]	Under-5 mortality rate (2003)[b]	No. of under-5 deaths (2003)[a]	Neonatal mortality rate (2000)[b]	No. of newborn deaths (2000)[a]	Maternal mortality ratio (2000)[c]	No. of maternal deaths (2000)[a]
On track	30 (OECD)	1 155 219 (18%)	14 980 (11%)	22	13	190.5 (2%)	7	110.5 (3%)	29	4.3 (1%)
	63 (non-OECD)	1 386 579 (22%)	30 782 (23%)	78	39	1200.5 (12%)	19	591.6 (15%)	216	65 (12%)
Slow progress	51	3 011 922 (48%)	58 858 (44%)	92	72	4 185.5 (40%)	35	2 069.5 (52%)	364	212.9 (40%)
In reversal	14	241 209 (4%)	7 643 (6%)	111	139	1 046.9 (10%)	41	305.4 (8%)	789	59.9 (11%)
Stagnating	29	487 507 (8%)	20 678 (16%)	207	188	3 773.9 (36%)	47	921.3 (23%)	959	185.8 (35%)

[a] Numbers in thousands.
[b] Per 1000 live births.
[c] Per 100 000 live births.

References

1. Loudon I. Childbirth. In: Bynum WF, Porter R, eds. *Companion encyclopedia of the history of medicine*. London and New York, NY, Routledge, 1993:1050–1071.
2. Haines A, Cassels A. Can the Millennium Development Goals be attained? *BMJ*, 2004, 329:394–397.
3. Nullis-Kapp C. The knowledge is there to achieve development goals, but is the will? *Bulletin of the World Health Organization*, 2004, 82:804–805.
4. Dwork D. *War is good for babies and other young children*. London, Tavistock, 1987.
5. Budin P. La mortalité infantile de 0 à 1 an [Infant mortality from 0 to 1 year]. *L'Obstétrique*, 1903:1–44.
6. Ungerer RLS. *Comecar de novo: Uma revisao historica sobre a crianca e o alojamento conjunto mae-filho [Starting afresh: a historical overview of children and keeping mothers and newborns together in hospital]*. Rio de Janeiro, Papel Virtual Editora, 2000.
7. Baker SJ. *Fighting for life*. New York, NY, Macmillan, 1939.
8. Van Lerberghe W, De Brouwere V. Of blind alleys and things that have worked: history's lessons on reducing maternal mortality. In: De Brouwere V, Van Lerberge W., eds. *Safe motherhood strategies: a review of the evidence*. Antwerp, ITG Press, 2001 (Studies in Health Organisation and Policy, 17:7–33).
9. *United Nations Universal Declaration of Human Rights*. New York, NY, United Nations, 1948.
10. Constitution of the World Health Organization, Article 2. Geneva, World Health Organization, 1948 (http://policy.who.int/cgi-bin/om_isapi.dll?infobase=Basicdoc&softpage=Browse_Frame_Pg42, accessed 22 November 2004).
11. Walsh JA, Warren K. Selective primary health care: an interim strategy for disease control in developing countries. *New England Journal of Medicine*, 1979, 301:967–974.
12. Mahler H. The Safe Motherhood Initiative: a call to action. *Lancet*, 1987,1:668–670.
13. Jaffré Y, Olivier de Sardan JP. *Une médecine inhospitalière: les difficiles relations entre soignants et soignés dans cinq capitales d'Afrique de l'Ouest [Inhospitable medicine: difficult relations between carers and cared for in five West African capital cities]*. Paris, Karlhala, 2003.

14. Jowett M. Safe Motherhood interventions in low-income countries: an economic justification and evidence of cost effectiveness. *Health Policy*, 2000, 53:201–228.

15. *The world health report 2002 – Reducing risks, promoting healthy life*. Geneva, World Health Organization, 2002.

16. Musgrove P. Public spending on health care: how are different criteria related? *Health Policy*, 1999, 47:207–223.

17. Strong MA. *The effects of adult mortality on infant and child mortality*. Unpublished paper presented at the Committee on Population Workshop on the Consequences of Pregnancy, Maternal Morbidity and Mortality for Women, their Families, and Society, Washington, DC, 19–20 October 1998.

18. Ainsworth M, Semali I. The impact of adult deaths on the nutritional status of children. In: *Coping with AIDS: the economic impact of adult mortality on the African household*. Washington, DC, World Bank, 1998.

19. Reed HE, Koblinsky MA, Mosley WH. *The consequences of maternal morbidity and maternal mortality: report of a workshop*. Washington, DC, National Academy Press, 1998.

20. Kramer MS. Determinants of low birth weight: methodological assessment and meta-analysis. *Bulletin of the World Health Organization*, 1987, 65:663–737.

21. Prada JA, Tsang RC. Biological mechanisms of environmentally induced causes of IUGR. *European Journal of Clinical Nutrition*, 1998, 52(Suppl. 1):S21–S27.

22. Murphy JF, O'Riordan J, Newcombe RG, Coles EC, Pearson JF. Relation of haemoglobin levels in first and second trimesters to outcome of pregnancy. *Lancet*, 1986, 1(8488):992–995.

23. Zhou LM, Yang WW, Hua JZ, Deng CQ, Tao X, Stoltzfus RJ. Relation of hemoglobin measured at different times in pregnancy to preterm birth and low birth weight in Shanghai, China. *American Journal of Epidemiology*, 1998, 148:998–1006.

24. Merialdi M, Caulfield LE, Zavaleta N, Figueroa A, DiPietro JA. Adding zinc to prenatal iron and folate tablets improves fetal neurobehavioral development. *American Journal of Obstetrics and Gynecology*, 1999, 180:483–490.

25. Ferro-Luzzi A, Ashworth A, Martorell R, Scrimshaw N. Report of the IDECG Working Group on Effects of IUGR on Infants, Children and Adolescents: immunocompetence, mortality, morbidity, body size, body composition, and physical performance. *European Journal of Clinical Nutrition*, 1998, 52(Suppl. 1):S97–S99.

26. Grantham-McGregor SM. Small for gestational age, term babies, in the first six years of life. *European Journal of Clinical Nutrition*, 1998, 52(Suppl. 1):S59–S64.

27. Grantham-McGregor SM, Lira PI, Ashworth A, Morris SS, Assuncao AM. The development of low-birth-weight term infants and the effects of the environment in northeast Brazil. *Journal of Pediatrics*, 1998, 132:661–666.

28. Goldenberg R, Hack M, Grantham-McGregor SM, Schürch B. *Report of the IDECG/IUNS Working Group on IUGR: effects on neurological, sensory, cognitive, and behavioural function*. Lausanne, IDECG Secretariat, c/o Nestlé Foundation, 1999.

29. Barker DJP. *Mothers, babies and health in later life*, 2nd ed. Sydney, Churchill Livingstone, 1998.

30. Grivetti L, Leon D, Rasmussen K, Shetty PS, Steckel R, Villar J. Report of the IDECG Working Group on Variation in Fetal Growth and Adult Disease. *European Journal of Clinical Nutrition*, 1998, 52(Suppl. 1):S102–S103.

31. Bhargava A. *Nutrition, health and economic development: some policy priorities*. Geneva, World Health Organization, 2001 (Commission on Macroeconomics and Health, CMH Working Paper Series, Paper No. WG1:14).

32. Scrimshaw NS. Malnutrition, brain development, learning, and behavior. *Nutrition Research*, 1998, 18:351–379.

33. Grantham-McGregor SM, Ani CC. *Undernutrition and mental development*. Lausanne, Nestlé, 2001 (Nutrition Workshop Series, Clinical Performance Programme, 5:1–14).

34. Alderman H, Behrman JR, Lavy V, Menon R. *Child nutrition, child health, and school enrollment: a longitudinal analysis*. Washington, DC, World Bank (Policy Research Department, Poverty and Human Resources Division), 1997.

35. Glewwe P, Jacoby HG, King EM. Early childhood nutrition and academic achievement: A longitudinal analysis. *Journal of Public Economics*, 2001, 81:345–368.

36. Alderman H, Behrman JR. *Estimated economic benefits of reducing low birth weight in low-income countries*. Washington, DC, World Bank, 2004 (Health, Nutrition and Population Discussion Paper).

37. Martorell R, Ramakrishnan U, Schroeder DG, Melgar P, Neufeld L. Intrauterine growth retardation, body size, body composition and physical performance in adolescence. *European Journal of Clinical Nutrition*, 1998, 52(Suppl. 1):S43–S52.

38. Islam MK, Gerdtham U-G. *A systematic review of the estimation of costs-of-illness associated with maternal newborn ill-health*. Geneva, World Health Organization, 2004. Maternal-Newborn Health and Poverty (MNHP) Project.

39. Legislator's Committee on Population and Development. Family planning saves lives and P303 million for the Philippine Government. *People Count*, 1993, 3:1–4.

40. Martinez Manautou J. *Analisis del costo beneficio del programa de planificacion familiar del Instituto Mexicano del Seguro Social (impacto economico) [Cost-benefit analysis of the Mexican Social Security Institute's family planning programme (economic impact)]*. Mexico City, Academia Mexicana de Investigacion en Demografia Medica, 1987.

41. Belli PC, Appaix O. *The economic benefits of investing in child health*. Washington, DC, World Bank, 2003 (Health, Nutrition and Population Discussion Paper).

42. Karoly LA, Greenwood PW, Everingham SS, Houbé J, Kilburn MR, Rydell CP et al. *Investing in our children, what we know and don't know about the costs and benefits of early childhood interventions*. Santa Monica, CA, RAND Corporation, 1998.

43. Behrman JR. The economic rationale for investing in nutrition in developing countries. *World Development*, 1993, 21:1749–1771.

44. Behrman JR, Hoddinott J. *Evaluacion del impacto de progresa en la talla del nino en edad preescolar [An evaluation of the impact of PROGRESA on pre-school child height]*. Washington, DC, International Food Policy Research Institute, 2000.

45. Van der Gaag J, Tan JP. *The benefits of early child development programs: an economic analysis*. Washington, DC, World Bank, 1996.

46. Quisumbing AR, Haddad L, Pena C. Are women overrepresented among the poor? An analysis of poverty in 10 developing countries. *Journal of Developing Economics*, 2001, 66:225–269.

47. Borghi J, Hanson K, Acquah CA, Ekanmian G, Filippi V, Ronsmans C et al. Costs of near-miss obstetric complications for women and their families in Benin and Ghana. *Health, Policy and Planning*, 2003, 18:383–390.

48. Sen A. *Development as freedom*. New York, NY, Anchor Books, 1999.

49. *Millennium Report of the Secretary-General of the United Nations*. New York, NY, United Nations 2000 (http://www.un.org/millennium/sg/report/, accessed 22 November 2004).

50. *United Nations Millennium Declaration*. New York, NY, United Nations, 2000 (United Nations General Assembly resolution 55/2; http://www.un.org/millennium/declaration/ares552e.pdf, accessed 22 November 2004).

51. *Human development report 2004 – Cultural liberty in today's diverse world*. New York, NY, United Nations Development Programme, 2004.

52. de Onis M, Blossner M. The World Health Organization Global Database on Child Growth and Malnutrition: methodology and applications. *International Journal of Epidemiology*, 2003, 32:518–526.

53. Maternal and child health: regional estimates of perinatal mortality. *Weekly Epidemiological Record*, 1989, 24:184–186.

54. *Perinatal mortality. A listing of available information*. Geneva, World Health Organization, 1996 (WHO/FRH/MSM/96.7).

55. *State of the world's newborns: a report from Saving Newborn Lives*. Washington, DC, Save the Children Fund, 2004:1–28.

56. Hyder AA, Wali SA, McGuckin J. The burden of disease from neonatal mortality: a review of South Asia and Sub-Saharan Africa. *BJOG: an international journal of obstetrics and gynaecology*, 2003, 110:894–901.

57. Tinker A, Ransom E. Healthy mothers and healthy newborns: the vital link. Washington, DC, Save the Children/Population Reference Bureau, 2002 (Policy Perspectives on Newborn Health).

58. *Best practices: detecting and treating newborn asphyxia*. Baltimore, MD, JHPIEGO, 2004.

59. Katz J, West KP Jr., Khatry SK, Christian P, LeClerq SC, Pradhan EK et al. Risk factors for early infant mortality in Sarlahi district, Nepal. *Bulletin of the World Health Organization*, 2003, 81:717–725.

60. *Maternal mortality in 2000. Estimates developed by WHO, UNICEF and UNFPA*. Geneva, World Health Organization, 2004.

61. Graham W, Hussein J. The right to count, *Lancet*, 363:67-68.

62. Elkoff VA, Miller JE. Trends and differentials in infant mortality in the Soviet Union, 1970–90: how much is due to misreporting? *Population Studies*, 1995, 49:241–258.

63. Mugford M. A comparison of reported differences in definitions of vital events and statistics. *World Health Statistics Quarterly*, 1983, 36:201–212.

64. *Social Monitor, 2003. Special feature: infant mortality*. New York, NY, United Nations Children's Fund, 2003.

65. Bouvier Colle MH, Varnoux N, Costes P, Hatton F. Reasons for the under-reporting of maternal mortality in France, as indicated by a survey of all deaths among women of childbearing age. *International Journal of Epidemiology*, 1991, 20:717–721.

66. *The sisterhood method for estimating maternal mortality: guidance for potential users*. Geneva, World Health Organization, 1997 (WHO/RHT/97.28).

67. *Human development report 2003 – Millennium Development Goals: a compact among nations to end human poverty*. New York, NY, Oxford University Press for the United Nations Development Programme, 2003.

68. United Nations Population Division. *World population prospects: the 2002 revision population database* (http://esa.un.org/unpp/, accessed 28 December 2004).

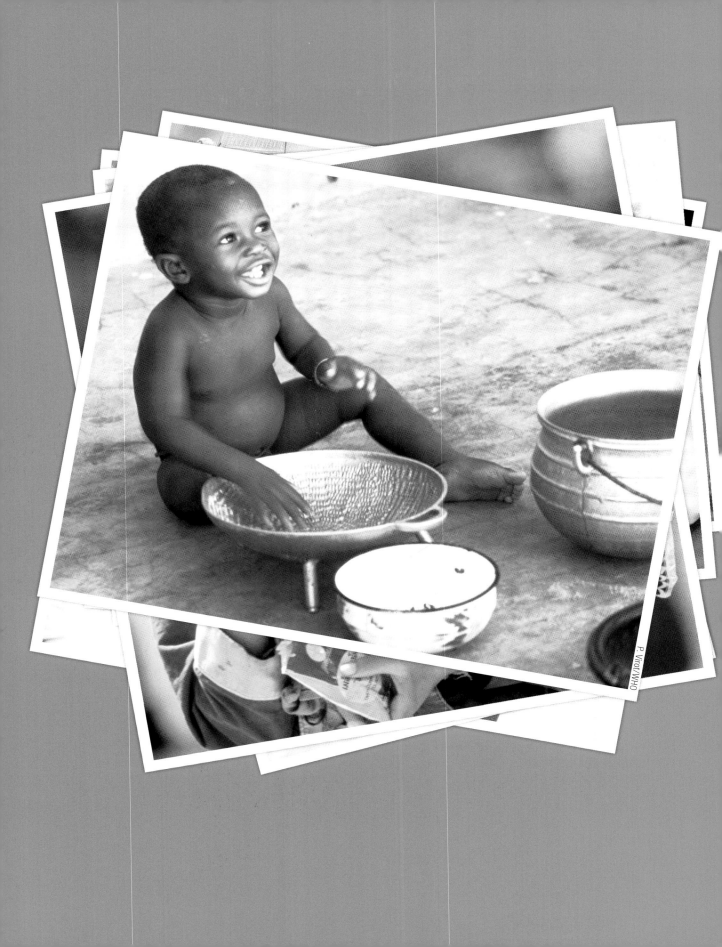

P. Virot/WHO

chapter two
obstacles to progress:
context or policy?

This chapter seeks to explain why progress in maternal and child health has apparently stumbled so badly in many countries. It shows in detail how stagnations, reversals and slow progress in some countries are clearly related to poverty, HIV/AIDS, and humanitarian crises, leading to exclusion from access to health care. In many countries, the strategies put in place to provide health services have not produced the hoped for results. While many countries have based their health care systems on health districts, with a backbone of health centres and a referral district hospital, there has often been a failure to implement this model successfully in an exceedingly resource-constrained context. The chapter argues that the health district model still stands as a rational way for governments to organize decentralized health care delivery.

Although there has been, for decades now, a global consensus that the health of mothers and children is a public priority, much still needs to be done. Most progress is being made by countries that were already in a relatively good position in the early 1990s, whereas those less favourably placed, particularly in sub-Saharan Africa, have been left behind. Much of this large and growing gap can be explained by the context in which health systems have developed. The stagnations, reversals and slow progress seen in some countries are clearly related to contexts of poverty, humanitarian crisis and the direct and indirect effects of HIV/AIDS (see Table 2.1). These lead to an increasingly visible gap between people who have access to health care and others who are excluded from such benefits. Exclusion from health benefits leads to even greater inequalities in survival for mothers and newborns than for children. Whatever the context, lack of progress is also due to failures of health systems to provide good-quality care and services to all mothers and children.

Moving towards universal access to health care must take account of the contextual barriers to progress, the reasons for exclusion from care, and the various patterns of exclusion. Many countries, and particularly those that face the biggest challenges, have based their health care systems on the health district model, with a backbone of health centres and a referral district hospital. This chapter argues that the disappointing situation in many countries often has more to do with the conditions under which this strategy has been implemented

Table 2.1 Factors hindering progress

Decline of child mortality	More than two years of humanitarian crisis since 1992	Adult HIV prevalence rate (weighted average)	GDP per capita (weighted average 1990–2002 in 1995 international dollars)
93 countries are on track[a]	3/93 countries	0.3	20 049 (OECD) 4179 (non-OECD)
51 countries are making slower progress[a]	10/51 countries	0.7	2657
14 countries are in reversal	8/14 countries	10.2	1627 (excluding South Africa)
29 countries have stagnating mortality	11/29 countries	4.1	896

[a] Towards Millennium Development Goal 4.

than with the failure of the strategy itself. A new commitment is needed to create the conditions for moving towards effective implementation.

CONTEXT MATTERS

Poverty undermines progress

Many of the countries whose child mortality rates are stagnating or reversing are poor in terms of gross domestic product; others are facing economic downturn. Conventional wisdom has it that income poverty is on its way out because the proportion and the total number of people around the world living on less than US$ 1 per day is decreasing (1). However, almost all of this progress has been made in Asia. Sub-Saharan Africa, where most of the countries whose child mortality rates have stagnated or reversed are to be found, has emerged as the region with the highest incidence of extreme poverty, and the greatest depth of poverty (2). Furthermore, the average income of poor people in Africa has been falling over time, in contrast with that of poor people in the rest of the developing world (3).

But poverty also influences maternal health. When women die in childbirth it is usually the result of a cascade of breakdowns in their interactions with the health system: delays in seeking care, inability to act on medical advice, and failure of the health system to provide adequate or timely care. These breakdowns are more likely to occur and to come together into a fateful combination when the macroeconomic and social contexts deteriorate. In Mongolia, for example, widespread social chaos and economic collapse followed the introduction of economic "shock therapy" in the early 1990s (4, 5), with a rapid increase in unemployment and widespread poverty. Government ex-

Box 2.1 Economic crisis and health system meltdown: a fatal cascade of events

Dashnyam, a 41-year-old housewife, was a very poor migrant from the countryside to a provincial capital of Mongolia. She and her husband were unemployed and often homeless, with six children. During her last pregnancy Dashnyam had oedema and pre-eclampsia and required manual extraction of the placenta. Afterwards, she said she wanted no more children and was given an intrauterine device (IUD). She had problems with the IUD and finally, in 2002 after six years of use, she asked to have it removed because of pelvic inflammatory disease and associated pain. The obstetrician who removed the IUD urged her to use another form of birth control, and her primary care physician gave her the same advice. For reasons that are unclear,

she did not follow their advice and was soon pregnant again. She did not seek prenatal care, but the family doctor discovered her pregnancy during an antenatal examination of her 18-year-old daughter. Because of Dashnyam's history and age, and because she said that she did not want the child, the family doctor urged her to go to the provincial hospital for an abortion. However, by the time she had collected sufficient funds, her pregnancy was too far advanced and abortion was no longer an option. She returned home and received antenatal care from the family doctor. As she came closer to term, she manifested symptoms of pre-eclampsia – high blood pressure and oedema. Because of her age, history of complications, and the presence

of these serious symptoms, the doctor urged her to go to the provincial hospital's maternity waiting home. However, her admission was delayed for over a week to solve bureaucratic issues, initially because she had no proof of having health insurance, and then because there were no beds available. Eventually, Dashnyam delivered via caesarean section, but suffered severe haemorrhage. After delay in finding the anaesthetist, the bleeding was eventually stopped by emergency surgery, but the hospital had no blood for transfusion. She died from haemorrhagic shock. (Names and places have been changed.)

Source: (7).

penditure halved, reflecting a widespread drop in investment in social services, health care and education. Hospitals, clinics and maternity homes closed or curtailed operations *(6)*. The health sector recovered eventually with the support of sizeable development loans, but not before the meltdown of services had led to a temporary reversal in maternal mortality (see Figure 2.1). The ways in which the dynamics of increasing poverty can create a fatal series of events are illustrated in Box 2.1.

The direct and indirect effects of HIV/AIDS

In a number of countries, particularly in sub-Saharan Africa, the effects of poverty and economic downturns on the environment in which people live, on their health and on the functioning of health systems are compounded by HIV/AIDS epidemics.

Figure 2.1 A temporary reversal in maternal mortality: Mongolia in the early 1990s

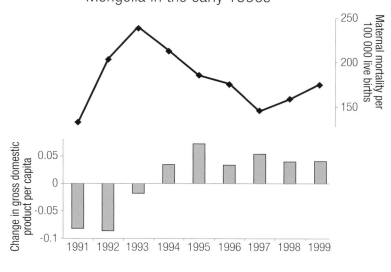

HIV/AIDS has direct and indirect effects. It directly affects the health of infected women and children (see Box 2.2). Globally, the direct contribution of HIV/AIDS to the number of children dying is limited, but it has been increasing steadily in sub-Saharan Africa. In 1990 HIV/AIDS accounted for around 2% of under-five mortality in that part of the world; 10 years later this had risen to 6.5%, although there are significant

Box 2.2 How HIV/AIDS directly affects the health of women and children

The HIV/AIDS pandemic takes an increasing toll of women and children, especially in sub-Saharan Africa. Some 39 million people are now living with HIV, of whom 2.2 million are children under 15 years of age and 18 million are women. In 2004, there were 4.9 million new cases of infection, including 640 000 children under 15 *(8)*. Almost 90% of paediatric infections occur in sub-Saharan Africa, where there are both high fertility rates and high HIV prevalence rates among women *(9)*. In 2004, 3.1 million people died of AIDS, 510 000 of whom were children *(8)*. HIV/AIDS has thus led to significant increases in mortality in many countries: it is a leading cause of death among women and children in the most severely affected countries in sub-Saharan Africa *(10)*.

Across the world, around 2.2 million women with HIV infection give birth each year *(11)*. HIV infection in pregnancy increases the risk of complications of pregnancy and childbirth

(miscarriage, anaemia, postpartum haemorrhage, puerperal sepsis and post-surgical complications). AIDS is also a major indirect cause of maternal mortality through increased rates of malaria and opportunistic infections such as tuberculosis *(12)*. The combined effect of these different mechanisms may overshadow progress made in reducing maternal mortality from other causes. In Rakai, Uganda, for example, maternal mortality was 1687 per 100 000 live births among HIV-infected women and 310 among non-infected women *(13)*. The maternal mortality ratio in the University Teaching Hospital in Lusaka, Zambia, has increased eightfold over the past two decades, mainly because of the increase in non-obstetric causes of death. While such causes were almost negligible in 1975, HIV-related tuberculosis and unspecified chronic respiratory illnesses accounted for 27% of all causes of maternal deaths in 1997 *(14)*.

Children of an HIV-positive mother have a higher mortality risk than children of HIV-negative mothers *(13)*. As parents die of AIDS, the number of orphans increases: 9% of children under 15 years of age in 40 countries in sub-Saharan Africa have lost one parent, and 1% have lost both *(15)*. Orphans are especially vulnerable to social and health risks: they are less likely to attend school and may live in households where conditions are less favourable for health and development than the average. HIV infection in children, almost always acquired through mother-to-child transmission, causes high mortality rates and some 60% die before their fifth birthday *(16)*. In Malawi, HIV/AIDS accounts for up to 10% of child deaths, and in one of the most affected countries, Botswana, child mortality doubled in the 1990s, and HIV/AIDS was responsible for more than 60% of child mortality in 2000 *(16)*.

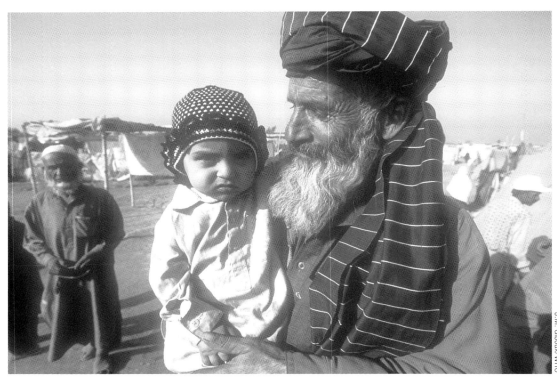

J.M. Giboux/WHO

In humanitarian crises, basic maternal and child health services are often disrupted
(New Jalozai refugee camp, Peshawar, Pakistan).

differences among countries. HIV prevalence rates are much higher in the countries in stagnation or reversal than in the others *(17)*; in 9 of the 10 African countries in reversal, HIV/AIDS was responsible for more than 10% of child deaths in 1999, a much higher proportion than in 1990 *(18)*. But HIV/AIDS as a direct cause of death cannot explain all of the slowing or reversal of trends in child mortality.

HIV/AIDS also affects the health of mothers and children in a more indirect way. Appropriate diagnosis and treatment of HIV/AIDS in women and children are rarely provided and pose particular challenges in resource-limited settings. HIV/AIDS puts an additional strain on fragile health systems. It generates demand for new services such as prevention of HIV transmission from mothers to infants, HIV testing and counselling, and complex diagnostic and investigative procedures *(19, 20)*. This calls for increased spending on infrastructure, equipment, drugs and human resources. Where increases in funding do not follow, maternal and child health services have to share their scarce resources and personnel. As health workers themselves fall ill, the workforce becomes overstretched *(21)*. Work performance is further reduced by fear, lack of knowledge about HIV/AIDS and protective practices, and the stress of caring for patients whose condition appears hopeless. As a result it is increasingly difficult to recruit young people into medical and nursing professions, particularly obstetrics.

Conflicts and emergencies set systems back

Of the 43 countries showing stagnation or reversal in child mortality, 19 have been the subject of a Consolidated Appeal Process for a humanitarian crisis with a duration of more than two years on their territory. Such situations, where local or national systems are disrupted or overwhelmed to the extent of being unable to meet the people's most basic needs, and that require an international response going beyond the mandate or capacity of any single agency, often involve a considerable breakdown of authority and a large amount of violence – against human beings, against the environment, infrastructure and property. In such situations women and children pay the heaviest price: they are the most vulnerable and also the most exposed (adult men tend to leave such areas, to fight or to look for work) *(22)*. Armed attacks often target key infrastructures and systems, such as roads, water supplies, communications and health facilities. The collapse of immunization and disease control programmes, referral systems and hospitals primarily affect women and children. Insecurity and military operations deny access to large areas of territory and constrain the delivery of and access to health services. Much, however, depends on the way health systems are organized to cope with such difficult situations, and well-structured health districts have proved to be remarkably resilient (see Box 2.3).

THE MANY FACES OF EXCLUSION FROM CARE

Many more mothers and children have access to reproductive, maternal and child care entitlements than ever before in history. In many countries, however, universal access to the goods, services and opportunities that improve or preserve health is still a distant goal. A varying but large proportion of mothers and children remain excluded from the health benefits that others in the same country enjoy. Exclusion is related to socioeconomic inequalities. In many countries it is a sign of increasing dualism in society: as growing middle classes in urban areas gain disproportionate access to public services, including education and health care, they effectively enter into competition with the poor for scarce resources, and easily come out on top *(24)*.

The result is that exclusion from access to health care is commonplace in poor countries. In the 42 countries that in 2000 accounted for 90% of all deaths of children under five years of age, 60% of children with pneumonia failed to get the antibiotic they needed, and 70% of children with malaria failed to receive treatment *(25)*. One third of children did not receive the vitamin A available to others in the same countries, and half had no safe water or sanitation. From 1999 to 2001, less than 2% of children from endemic malaria areas slept under insecticide-treated nets every night. Stagnation of progress in coverage for a number of interventions has meant that large parts

Box 2.3 Health districts can make progress, even in adverse circumstances

Since the 1980s, in North Kivu Province of the Democratic Republic of the Congo (formerly Zaire), the socioeconomic environment has been deteriorating. The province also faced an influx of Rwandan refugees in July 1994. In these difficult circumstances the Rutshuru Health District was nevertheless able to adjust and maintain its medical activities. For 11 years the health care network remained accessible and functional, although human and financial resources were extremely limited (external assistance fluctuated between US$ 1.5 and US$ 3 per inhabitant per year), especially when compared with those available in refugee camps in the same area through relief agencies. Utilization of curative services and preventive coverage rates has actually increased: vaccination coverage has tripled. Maternal health activities have been intensified both quantitatively and qualitatively, with 52% of deliveries taking place in health centres and the hospital, and a population-based caesarean section rate of 1.4%; case-fatality of caesarean sections dropped from 7.2% to 2.9%. The district was able to cope with a workload of 65 000 cases of various pathological conditions in Rwandan refugees settled outside the camps, a 400% increase in the curative workload. The district was under severe pressure but its services managed to respond efficiently to the repeated crisis situations, mainly by maintaining a solid district management structure rooted in ongoing communication and participation of the population *(23)*.

of the population have continued to be excluded *(26)*. Immunization coverage, for example, maintained its upward trend during the 1990s in the WHO European Region, the Region of the Americas and the Western Pacific Region, but in the other regions it has levelled off at a mere 50% to 70% (see Figure 2.2).

Sources of exclusion

In many of the countries experiencing stagnation and reversal (particularly in sub-Saharan Africa), barriers to the uptake of health benefits, and specifically the lack of an accessible supply of services, are a critical source of exclusion. For many people, services simply do not exist, or cannot be reached. For example, lack of access to hospitals where major obstetric interventions can be performed is the prime reason why large numbers of mothers in rural areas are excluded from life-saving care at childbirth (see Box 2.4).

But there are many other barriers to the uptake of health benefits: service use is often constrained because of women's lack of decision-making power, the low value placed on women's health and the negative or judgemental attitudes of family members *(28, 29)*. Gender is thus a frequent source of exclusion: in India, for example, a girl is 1.5 times less likely to be hospitalized than a boy *(30)* – and up to 50% more likely to die between her first and fifth birthdays *(31)*.

People excluded from health care benefits by such barriers to the uptake of services are also usually excluded from other services such as access to electricity, water supply, basic sanitation, education or information. Their exclusion from care is also reflected in inferior health indicators. In Kazakhstan, for example, children born to ethnic Kazakh parents have a 1.5 times higher risk of death than those born to parents of Russian ethnicity; in Nigeria, children of uneducated mothers have about a 2.5 times higher risk of death than those of mothers with secondary school or higher education.

As part of its work on extension of social protection in health, the Pan American Health Organization has started mapping exclusion from health benefits in a number of Latin American countries *(32)*. Nearly half of the population is excluded from some, and usually from most health care benefits. The relative importance of underlying reasons for exclusion varies from country to country.

"External" sources of exclusion, such as the ones described above, include geographical isolation, as well as barriers generated by poverty, race, language and culture – often in association with unemployment or informal employment. For many people the critical factor is the

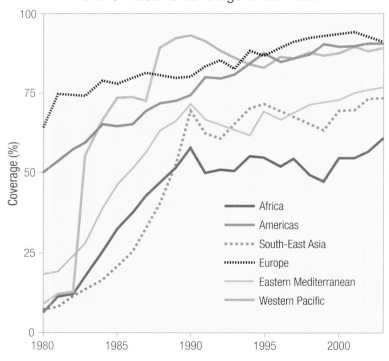

Figure 2.2 **Levelling off after remarkable progress: DTP3[a] vaccine coverage since 1980**

Coverage (%)

- Africa
- Americas
- South-East Asia
- Europe
- Eastern Mediterranean
- Western Pacific

[a] Third dose of diphtheria, tetanus and pertussis vaccine.

Box 2.4 Mapping exclusion from life-saving obstetric care

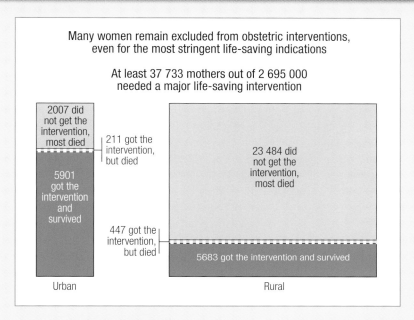

Many women remain excluded from obstetric interventions, even for the most stringent life-saving indications

At least 37 733 mothers out of 2 695 000 needed a major life-saving intervention

2007 did not get the intervention, most died

211 got the intervention, but died

5901 got the intervention and survived

23 484 did not get the intervention, most died

447 got the intervention, but died

5683 got the intervention and survived

Urban

Rural

The extent of exclusion from major life-saving obstetric interventions has been quantified in Burkina Faso, Mali and Niger, and in parts of Benin, Haiti, Pakistan and the United Republic of Tanzania, in a study of 2.7 million deliveries. The Unmet Obstetric Needs Network, a collaboration of ministries of health, clinicians and researchers, analysed this population over a one-year period. The network established a benchmark of 1.4% as a conservative estimate of the proportion of deliveries where a major obstetric intervention (caesarean section, hysterectomy, craniotomy, laparotomy, or version extraction) was required to prevent the mother from dying from a specified set of life-threatening complications. Interventions performed for other indications, including fetal conditions, were not included. The figure illustrates the results.

Only 1.1% of urban mothers and 0.3% of rural mothers benefited from these interventions. Between 80% (in Niger) and 98% (in Pakistan) of the interventions were caesarean sections. Among the 12 242 mothers who benefited from the interventions, 93.8–99.5% survived (in Burkina Faso and Pakistan, respectively), as did 7779 of the babies. None of these interventions was for a reason other than the identified life-threatening maternal indications. As such indications are present in at least 1.4% of births, the implication is that no less than 25% of urban and 79% of rural mothers in the study were excluded from access to the major obstetric intervention they needed.

Although there is, on average, at least one hospital for every 500 000 inhabitants in the areas of the study (except Niger), the extent of exclusion is clearly related to the availability and accessibility of the health care infrastructure. Indeed, the average distance women have to travel to reach a hospital varies from 9 km in Haiti to 43 km in Burkina Faso and 103 km in Niger.

The survey made it possible to map the number of mothers in need of a major life-saving intervention who failed to get it. Similar maps of unmet needs exist in a few other countries. They can be used as a planning tool and as a baseline against which to measure progress in coverage.

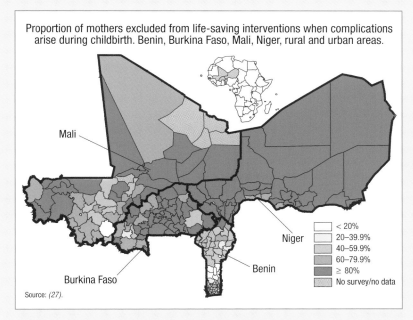

Proportion of mothers excluded from life-saving interventions when complications arise during childbirth. Benin, Burkina Faso, Mali, Niger, rural and urban areas.

Mali

Niger

Benin

Burkina Faso

< 20%
20–39.9%
40–59.9%
60–79.9%
≥ 80%
No survey/no data

Source: *(27)*.

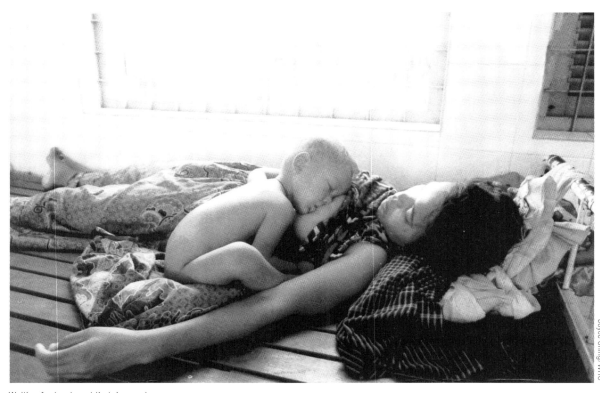

Joyce Ching/WHO

Waiting for treatment that does not come.

deterrent effect of uncertainty about the cost of care, or of the awareness that care will be unaffordable or catastrophically expensive. Such external factors affecting uptake of services are the most important source of exclusion in, for example, Peru and Paraguay *(32)*.

Other, "internal", sources of exclusion lie within the way the health system actually operates. Even for people who do use services, what is offered may be untimely, ineffective, unresponsive or discriminatory. Being poor or being a woman is often a reason for being discriminated against, and may result in abuse, neglect and poor treatment, poorly explained reasons for procedures, compounded by the view sometimes held by health workers that women are ignorant. When, for example, in a busy urban maternity hospital in India, the nurses in the labour ward do not complete patient case notes for low-caste women, that deprives them of the quality safeguards given to other women *(33)*. Poor and anonymous patients often have to wait longer, are examined more superficially, or are treated with disdain; they may get inferior treatment, especially when scarce resources are reserved for richer patients. In rural areas of the United Republic of Tanzania, for example, children from the poorest part of the population who sought care for probable pneumonia were less than half as likely to be given antibiotics as richer children *(34)*.

Such factors internal to health services can be important sources of exclusion; throughout the world, many mothers and children are excluded from what they are entitled to because of the failure of the health system to deliver the right services at the right time, to the right people, and in the right manner. In Ecuador and Honduras, for example, what happens within the health system, rather than failed uptake, is the dominant source of exclusion *(32)*.

Exclusion from "normal" treatment – what a patient can expect, based on what other people are given – does not go unnoticed by those concerned. In India, for example, 55% of poorer mothers said they had been made to wait too long (only half as many of the richer mothers had that impression), and only 50% were given clear information about their treatment, as against 89% of the richer patients. Other patients are also aware of such practices: 67% of the patients in Conakry, Guinea, are convinced that rich and well-dressed patients get better treatment *(34)*.

The – often justified – expectation of ill-treatment or discrimination in turn discourages uptake of services, completing a vicious circle of exclusion, compounded by the absence of adequate systems to protect mothers and children against catastrophic expenditure or financial exploitation.

Poverty, humanitarian crises, and the HIV/AIDS epidemics all directly affect the health and survival of mothers and children. But they also affect their health by creating barriers to the uptake of services. Furthermore, they influence the way services are provided to mothers and children who do use them, and thus add to sources of exclusion within the health system.

Patterns of exclusion

The extent and depth of exclusion vary from region to region within countries, but also between countries. At one extreme are the poorest countries where large parts of the population are deprived of care, even among the better off: only a small minority enjoys reasonable access to a reasonable range of health benefits, creating a pattern of massive deprivation. At the other extreme are countries where a large part of the population enjoys a wide range of benefits but a minority is excluded: a pattern of marginalization.

Looking at health care coverage by wealth group provides a crude illustration of these different patterns (see Figure 2.3). Between the extremes of massive deprivation (typical for countries with major problems of supply of services and low-density health care networks) and marginalization (typical for rich or middle-income countries with dense health care networks) are the countries where poor populations have to queue behind the better off, waiting to get access to health services and hoping that benefits will eventually trickle down.

As countries move from a pattern of massive deprivation towards one of marginalization, the poor-rich gap in coverage and uptake of services grows in size, to diminish only as the curves flatten out when universal access is within reach

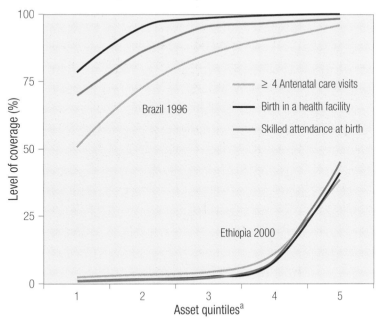

Figure 2.3 Different patterns of exclusion: massive deprivation at low levels of coverage and marginalization of the poorest at high levels

- ≥ 4 Antenatal care visits
- Birth in a health facility
- Skilled attendance at birth

Brazil 1996

Ethiopia 2000

Level of coverage (%)

Asset quintiles[a]

[a] Asset quintiles provide an index of socioeconomic status at the household level. They divide populations into five groups (in ascending order of wealth from 1 to 5), using a methodology that combines information on household head characteristics as well as household ownership of certain assets, availability of services, and housing characteristics *(35)*.

Data source: *(36)*.

(see Figure 2.4). Unless specific measures are taken to extend coverage and promote uptake in all population groups simultaneously, improvement of aggregate population coverage will go through a phase of increasing inequality.

These complex dynamics also affect the distribution of health outcomes. For a long time policy-makers used aggregate health indicators – particularly the under-five mortality rate – to monitor health policies. As more sophisticated analyses of health outcomes by asset quintile have become possible (37), attention has been drawn to the occurrence of increasing survival gaps between the poorest and the better off (38). The gaps in mortality rates between the children of rich and poor families have increased in the majority of 21 developing countries that had reduced their overall rate of mortality among children under five years of age (see Figure 2.5). Health and survival among the poorest actually deteriorated in eight of these countries, while the richest children in the same countries improved their chances of survival. As a result, national averages that show progress may conceal persisting or widening inequalities. Similar divergence appears to be occurring for maternal mortality in some countries (39).

DIFFERENT EXCLUSION PATTERNS, DIFFERENT CHALLENGES

The policy challenges differ between countries that are close to universal access (where exclusion is limited) and those where exclusion is pervasive. The countries where exclusion is limited to a small and marginalized part of the population are usually on track, or at least show slow progress in terms of reduction of child mortality. These are countries with well-extended health systems, although not always with an

Figure 2.4 From massive deprivation to marginal exclusion: moving up the coverage ladder

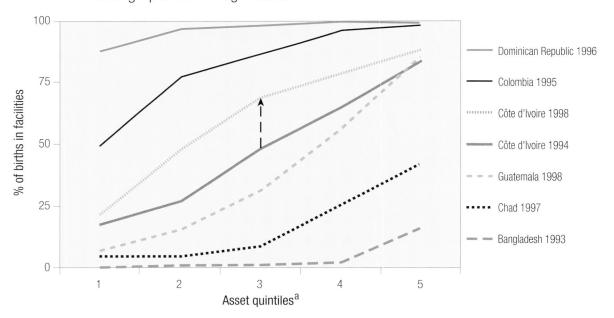

[a] Asset quintiles provide an index of socioeconomic status at the household level. They divide populations into five groups (in ascending order of wealth from 1 to 5), using a methodology that combines information on household head characteristics as well as household ownership of certain assets, availability of services, and housing characteristics (35).

Data source: (36).

optimal range of technical interventions. Examples of countries in this group include Brazil, Colombia and the Dominican Republic. Here, the challenge is one of targeting to give the mothers and children currently excluded the possibility of claiming their entitlements: tackling the roots of social exclusion, removing the barriers to the uptake of health benefits, responding appropriately to their needs, and offering them financial protection from the consequences of illness and obtaining care.

Most of the countries that stagnated or went into reversal, and many of those that showed slow progress in terms of child mortality reduction, show patterns of massive exclusion or queuing. Such countries include Bangladesh, Chad and Ethiopia. They typically have weak, low-density and fragile health systems; they also suffer from poverty, and sometimes HIV/AIDS and complex emergencies, additional constraints to health systems development. In this group the main challenge is to build and roll out primary health care as the vehicle for maternal, newborn and child health care.

The momentum created by the primary health care movement of the early 1980s focused attention on issues of equity and access, and resulted in the extension of basic health services to the rural poor. Maternal and child health programmes were integral to this extended coverage: antenatal clinics were intended to provide the first contact that would continue through childbirth and postnatal care for the mother and with clinics for children.

In the early 1990s, the view gained ground that primary health care had to be de-centralized and organized in "integrated health districts". Countries that had been

Figure 2.5 **Survival gap between rich and poor: widening in some countries, narrowing in others**

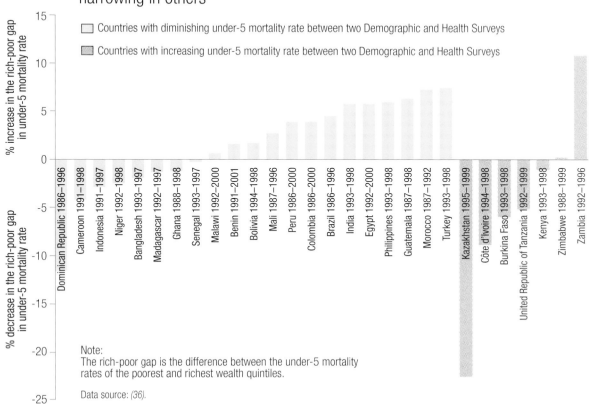

doing so for quite some time saw their earlier choices reinforced, and others, such as Cambodia and Niger, moved to adopt district policies. Many development agencies put districts at the core of their health development strategies, particularly for the countries that combined the poorest health status with the weakest health systems.

Are districts the right strategy for moving towards universal coverage?

Organizing the delivery of primary health care through health districts promised a fast-track response to the rising demand for health care. Apart from the frustration caused by the diminishing returns of the vertical approaches of the 1970s and 1980s, there were three good reasons for this.

The first was that the "health centre" – the heir of the dispensaries, but now the centrepiece of the whole system, and the equivalent of the family doctor or general practitioner – was the most viable alternative to village health workers, vertical programmes and commercial health care. It was also the only one that responded to the demand for care by the population. National decision-makers were alert to this argument, which was based on the experiences of a number of small and medium-scale field projects: Pahou in Benin, Danfa in Ghana, Machakos in Kenya, Pikine in Senegal, and Kasongo and Kinshasa in Zaire. These projects had shown that health centres were a feasible *(40, 41)*, affordable *(42–44)* and efficient *(45–47)* option for delivering care, and a realistic alternative to vertical disease control programmes.

Second, hospitals providing referral-level care were part and parcel of the district model. Although the referral system remained the weak point, it became possible to take on the maternal health agenda because of the hospital's ability to deal with obstetric complications. Moreover, the inclusion of hospitals brought a vital part of the public health infrastructure and personnel back on the scene. This was a relief for the administrative elite and the middle class, who had never considered the grassroots primary health care of the 1980s as something to aspire to for themselves.

Third, the health district fitted well with the movement towards decentralization, to which most countries were at least theoretically committed. Health districts seemed both manageable and sufficiently decentralized to be flexible and affordable *(40,48)*.

A strategy without resources

By the mid-1990s many countries were creating district systems, setting up drug procurement agencies and defining a minimum package of services. However, as in the years after Alma-Ata, money did not follow, particularly in sub-Saharan Africa, and results were slow to come. In the bleak economic environment, financing remained a real barrier to progress. With a decrease in gross domestic product per capita in real terms between 1990 and 2002, total health expenditure in many African countries stagnated or decreased, and public health expenditure remained below US$ 10 per person. External assistance did not make up for this, as per capita flows also stagnated up to 1999 *(49)*.

The real extent of the failure to increase financing of the health sector during the 1980s and 1990s appears in the detailed breakdown of what financing there was: in Cameroon, for example, recurrent public expenditure declined from US$ 5 per inhabitant in 1990 to US$ 3.5 in 1996. Of this, US$ 2.1 went on salaries and US$ 1.12 on other recurrent expenditures. The districts were left with a mere US$ 0.28 per person per year for non-salary recurrent expenditures.

There has been little flexibility to improve working conditions in the public sector, especially in terms of salaries and incentives, because of civil service regulations and structural adjustment policies. As a result many health workers have moved to the private sector. Data from Ghana, Zambia and Zimbabwe show that losses of health workers from the public health sector continued or accelerated during the 1990s *(50)*. The stringent budgetary measures under structural adjustment programmes also imposed ceilings on recruitment. Even in countries with unemployed health professionals such as Zambia, governments often were not able to enrol more staff *(50)*.

Absenteeism was another major issue that affected the already scarce human resources. In Burkina Faso, for example, absenteeism of health district doctors in seven rural districts in 1997 varied between 30% and more than 80% *(51)*. Vacancy rates for doctors in Ghana increased from 43% in 1998 to 47% in 2002. Over the same period vacancy rates for registered nurses rose from 26% to 57% *(52)*. Much of the absenteeism was related to inadequate working conditions, insufficient salaries and declining staff morale. In a number of countries, however, the HIV/AIDS epidemics aggravated what was becoming an acute human resource crisis. Data are scarce but suggest that besides contributing to absenteeism, HIV/AIDS may cost Africa's health systems one fifth of their employees over the next few years *(53)*. The absence of adequate measures to protect health workers against HIV/AIDS and the stress of caring for HIV/AIDS patients are additional factors motivating them to migrate.

The real wages of public servants continued their decline in the 1990s: in six years they dropped by 21% from their 1990 level in Togo, 34% in Burkina Faso, 35% in Guinea-Bissau, and 41% in Niger. Absenteeism continued – 35% for district doctors in 1997 in Burkina Faso – as did "seminaritis": in 1995 in Mali, regional health staff spent 34% of their total working time in workshops and supervision missions supported by international agencies; this figure rose to 48% for chief medical officers. Predatory behaviour *(54–57)* and moonlighting *(58, 59)* became the norm, contributing to the shortage of health workers in the public sector *(50)*.

The shortages of health personnel are the most visible aspect of the human resources crisis in sub-Saharan Africa. The figures are stark: in Zimbabwe, of the 1200 physicians trained during the 1990s, only 360 were still practising in the country in 2001 *(60)*. Ghana's loss of 328 nurses in 1999 was the equivalent of its annual output *(50)*. More than half of the health professionals in Zimbabwe, Ghana and South Africa are thinking of migrating to other countries *(61)*. At the same time, 35 000 South African nurses are not employed in the health sector and two thirds of the health workforce in Swaziland is working in the private sector *(62, 63)*.

Have districts failed the test?

The environment in which district health systems had to be set up has been decidedly unfavourable. Some countries, such as Mali, managed to expand health centre networks and services for mothers and children *(64)*. Overall expansion, however, has been slow. In 2000, for example, only 13 of Niger's hospitals had appropriate facilities to perform a caesarean section *(65)*. This was also the case for only 17 of the 53 district hospitals in Burkina Faso, nearly 10 years after districts had been established; moreover, only five of those 17 hospitals had the three doctors required to ensure continuity throughout the year *(66)*.

The slowness of rolling out health districts has been disappointing: it takes time to transform an administrative district into a functional health system (see Box 2.5). Nevertheless, where districts have reached the critical point of becoming stable and viable

Box 2.5 Building functional health districts: sustainable results require a long-term commitment

In the mid-1990s Ouallam, one of the poorest districts in Niger with 250 000 inhabitants living at an average distance of 74 km from the hospital, had seven dysfunctional health centres and an almost empty district hospital. Emergencies could not be referred to the hospital in an area with no means of communication. Several measures were, however, put in place to change the situation. Some were general measures to solve problems in the district and others were specifically aimed at improving the referral system. Making the changes took eight years (see table below).

This sustained investment of time and effort paid off: antenatal care coverage increased by 42%, coverage by clinics for children under five years of age tripled, and vaccination coverage doubled. In a year the number of new acceptors for modern family planning methods increased from 568 to 1444, and hospitalizations increased from 434 to 1420; surgical interventions and blood transfusions, not possible previously, totalled 219 and 86, respectively, in 2003. The number of emergency evacuations to the hospital increased markedly, mainly for obstetric causes. Over

distances averaging more than 50 km, these evacuations were carried out by the hospital's vehicle, partly subsidized and partly on a cost-recovery basis at US$ 23 per emergency evacuation (see figure below).

No single intervention alone explains the progress that has been made: the results came from the combined action on different aspects of the system, and investment in the capacities of the personnel *(65)*.

The combination of diverse initiatives undertaken to facilitate effective access to health services in Ouallam, Niger, 1996–2003

Initiatives aimed at increasing demand for services	Initiatives aimed at increasing uptake of services	Initiatives aimed at improving case management in the health centre	Initiatives aimed at facilitating emergency transfer to the hospital	Initiatives aimed at improving case management in the hospital
Established health committees	Established a health care coverage plan	Standardized diagnosis-treatment-referral procedures	Introduced solar energy radios and ambulance service	Rehabilitated physical infrastructure
Discussed and negotiated health care coverage plan	Created seven additional health centres	Introduced vitamin A distribution, stepped up vaccination coverage, introduced detection/treatment of malnutrition	Introduced cost-recovery mechanisms for ambulance	Introduced surgery and blood transfusion
Negotiated fees for emergency evacuation			Renegotiated emergency evacuation fees	Internal reorganization negotiated and implemented with staff
Built credibility of health centre through improved quality of care		Introduced outreach		Introduced system of patient records
Increased acceptability of referral to district hospital through discussion of referrals and emergency evacuations		Discussed referral results with health care nurses		Introduced nutritional rehabilitation unit
		Standardized referral criteria and procedures		Improved laboratory and X-ray services
				Introduced quality assurance

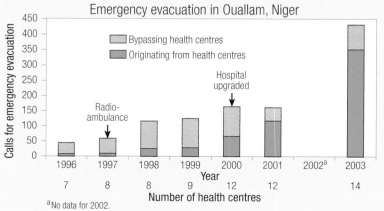

Emergency evacuation in Ouallam, Niger

a No data for 2002.

structures, they have shown credible and visible results, sometimes in very adverse circumstances, as in Guinea and the Democratic Republic of the Congo.

On balance, the experience of the last decade suggests that health districts still stand as a rational way for governments to roll out primary health care through networks of health centres, family practices or equivalent decentralized structures, backed up by referral hospitals. There are no real alternatives to serve as a vehicle for a continuum of integrated care for mothers, newborns and children. The challenge now is to scale up implementation in an adverse environment where exclusion is further fuelled by the rampant commercialization of the health sector, including within public and not-for-profit facilities. The second challenge is to tailor health care delivery strategies to the specific situation and exclusion patterns of each country. At the same time, it is no longer possible to experiment with district projects without looking at the wider context of cross-cutting, system-wide constraints. Without a real commitment to strengthening district health services, talking about the priority status of mothers and children is likely to remain mere lip service.

Part of the task ahead is political. Maternal, newborn and child health cannot be reduced to a set of programmes to be delivered to a target population. Rather, mothers and children must be in a position to claim a set of entitlements as their right. This implies an adjustment of macro-level health policies and resource mobilization, at country level and internationally. Three issues cry out for attention: the funding of the health sector, the human resource crisis, and the accountability of health systems and providers to their clients.

But the task ahead is also one of refocusing programme content. For too long attention has been directed towards the development of technologies, rather than towards embedding these in viable organizational strategies that organize and ensure a continuum of care. Given the complexity of expanding district health care systems, the temptation is to go back to vertical programmes built around disease control technologies. In the past this has led to a considerable amount of fragmentation, at the expense of ensuring the continuity of care from pregnancy throughout childhood. Much of the challenge, in fact, is to accommodate both programmatic and systemic concerns: an organizational rather than a technical problem. The next chapters relocate the technical strategies available for improving the health of mothers, newborns and children within health systems that are scaling up and facing an increasingly vocal demand for care.

References

1. *World development indicators 2004*. Washington, DC, World Bank, 2004.
2. *Human development report 2003 – Millennium Development Goals: a compact among nations to end human poverty*. New York, NY, Oxford University Press for the United Nations Development Programme, 2004.
3. Chen S, Ravaillon M. *How have the world's poorest fared since the early 1980s?* Washington, DC, World Bank, 2004.
4. Griffin K, Brenner MD, Kusago T, Ickowitz A, McKinley T. *A strategy for poverty reduction in Mongolia. Report of a UNDP mission on the integration of equity and poverty reduction concerns into development strategy*. Ulaanbaatar, United Nations Development Programme, 2001.
5. *Human development report Mongolia 2000*. Ulaanbaatar, Government of Mongolia/United Nations Development Programme, 2000.
6. Government of Mongolia/WHO. *Mongolia health sector review*. Ulaanbaatar, World Health Organization, 1999.
7. Janes CR, Chuluundorj O. Free markets and dead mothers: the social ecology of maternal mortality in post-socialist Mongolia. *Medical Anthropology Quarterly*, 2004, 18:230–257.
8. UNAIDS/WHO. *AIDS epidemic update, December 2004*. Geneva, Joint United Nations Programme on HIV/AIDS, 2004.
9. De Cock KM, Fowler MG, Mercier E, de Vincenzi I, Saba J, Hoff E et al. Prevention of mother-to-child HIV transmission in resource-poor countries: translating research into policy and practice. *JAMA*, 2000, 283:1175–1182.
10. Zaba B, Whiteside A, Boerma JT. Demographic and socioeconomic impact of AIDS: taking stock of the empirical evidence. *AIDS*, 2004, 18(Suppl. 2):S1–S7.
11. *The world health report 2004 – Changing history*. Geneva, World Health Organization, 2004.
12. McIntyre J. Mothers infected with HIV. *British Medical Bulletin*, 2003, 67:127–135.
13. Sewankambo NK, Gray RH, Ahmad S, Serwadda D, Wabwire-Mangen F, Nalugoda F et al. Mortality associated with HIV infection in rural Rakai District, Uganda. *AIDS*, 2000, 14:2391-2400.
14. Ahmed Y, Mwaba P, Chintu C, Grange JM, Ustianowski A, Zumla A. A study of maternal mortality at the University Teaching Hospital, Lusaka, Zambia: the emergence of tuberculosis as a major non-obstetric cause of maternal death. *International Journal of Tuberculosis and Lung Disease*, 1999, 3:675–680.
15. Monasch R, Boerma JT. Orphanhood and childcare patterns in sub-Saharan Africa: an analysis of national surveys from 40 countries. *AIDS*, 2004, 18(Suppl. 2):S55–S65.
16. Newell ML, Brahmbhatt H, Ghys PD. Child mortality and HIV infection in Africa: a review. *AIDS*, 2004, 18(Suppl. 2):S27–S34.
17. *Report on the global AIDS epidemic 2004*. Geneva, Joint United Nations Programme on HIV/AIDS, 2004.
18. Walker N, Schwartlander B, Bryce J. Meeting international goals in child survival and HIV/AIDS. *Lancet*, 2002, 360:284–289.
19. Tawfik L, Kinoti S. *Impact of HIV/AIDS on the health sector in sub-Saharan Africa: the issue of human resources*. Washington, DC, United States Agency for International Development, 2001.
20. *Evidence base for the impact of HIV upon health systems*. London, John Snow International UK and Health Systems Research Centre, 2003.
21. Dambisya YM. The fate and career destinations of doctors who qualified at Uganda's Makerere Medical School in 1984: retrospective cohort study. *BMJ*, 2004, 329:600–601.
22. Al Gasseer N, Dresden E, Keeney GB, Warren N. Status of women and infants in complex humanitarian emergencies. *Journal of Midwifery and Women's Health*, 2004, 49(Suppl. 1):7–13.
23. Porignon D, Soron'gane EM, Lokombe TE, Isu DK, Hennart P, Van Lerberghe W. How robust are district health systems? Coping with crisis and disasters in Rutshuru, Democratic Republic of Congo. *Tropical Medicine and International Health*, 1998, 3:559–565.
24. Pronk, J. Collateral damage or calculated default. The Millennium Development Goals and the politics of globalisation. The Hague, Institute of Social Studies, 2003.
25. Jones G, Steketee RW, Black R, Bhutta, ZA, Morris S and the Bellagio Child Survival Study Group. How many child deaths can we prevent this year? *Lancet*, 2003, 362: 65–71.

26. Bryce J, el Arifeen S, Pariyo G, Lanata C, Gwatkin D, Habicht JP. Reducing child mortality: can public health deliver? *Lancet*, 2003, 362:159–164.

27. *L'approche des besoins obstétricaux non couverts pour les interventions obstétricales majeures. Etude comparative Bénin, Burkina Faso, Haïti, Mali, Maroc, Niger, Pakistan et Tanzanie. [Tackling unmet needs for major obstetric interventions. Case studies in Benin, Burkina Faso, Haiti, Mali, Morocco, Niger, Pakistan and Tanzania]*. Antwerp, Unmet Obstetric Needs Network, 2002:1–47 (www.uonn.org).

28. Matthews Z, Ramasubban R, Rishyasringa B, Stones WR. *Autonomy and maternal health-seeking among slum populations of Mumbai*. Southampton, Southampton Statistical Sciences Research Institute, 2004.

29. *Reproductive health strategy to accelerate progress towards the attainment of international development goals and targets*. Geneva, World Health Organization, 2004.

30. Bhan G, Bhandari N, Taneja S, Mazumder S, Bahl R, and other members of the Zinc Study Group. The effect of maternal education on gender bias in care-seeking for common childhood illnesses. *Social Science and Medicine*, 2005, 60:715–724,

31. Claeson M, Bos ER, Mawji T, Pathmanathan I. Reducing child mortality in India in the new millennium. *Bulletin of the World Health Organization*, 2000, 78:1192–1199.

32. *Exclusion in health in Latin America and the Caribbean*. Washington, DC, Pan American Health Organization, 2004.

33. Hulton L, Matthews Z, Stones RW. *A framework for the evaluation of quality of care in maternal services*. Southampton, University of Southampton, 2000.

34. Jaffré Y, Olivier de Sardan JP. *Une médecine inhospitalière: les difficiles relations entre soignants et soignés dans cinq capitales d'Afrique de l'Ouest [Inhospitable medicine: difficult relations between carers and cared for in five West African capital cities]*. Paris, Karlhala, 2003.

35. Ferguson BD, Tandon A, Gakidou E, Murray CJL. *Estimating permanent income using indicator variables*. Geneva, World Health Organization, 2003 (Global Programme on Evidence for Health Policy Discussion Paper No. 42).

36. Demographic and Health Surveys. *Country statistics* (http://www.measuredhs.com/countries/start.cfm, accessed 16 December 2004).

37. Gwatkin D, Rutstein S, Johnson K, Pande R, Wagstaff A. *Socio-economic differences in health, nutrition and population*. Washington, DC, World Bank, 2000 (Health, Nutrition and Population Discussion Papers).

38. Gwatkin D. *Who would gain most from efforts to reach the MDGs for health? An enquiry into the possibility of progress that fails to reach the poor*. Washington, DC, World Bank, 2002.

39. Graham W, Fitzmaurice AE, Bell JS, Cairns JA. The familial technique for linking maternal death with poverty. *Lancet*, 2004, 363:23–27.

40. Pangu KA. *La santé pour tous d'ici l'an 2000: c'est possible; expérience de planification et d'implantation des centres de santé dans la zone de Kasongo au Zaïre [Health for all by the year 2000: it can be achieved; experience of planning and setting up health centres in the area of Kasongo in Zaire]*. Brussels, Université Libre de Bruxelles, Faculté de Médecine, Ecole de Santé Publique, 1988.

41. Equipe du Projet Kasongo, Darras C, Van Lerberghe W, Mercenier P. Le Projet Kasongo: une expérience d'organisation d'un système de soins de santé primaires [The Kasongo Project: experience of organizing a system of primary health care]. *Annales de la Société Belge de Médecine Tropicale*, 1981, 61(Suppl.):1–54.

42. Knippenberg R, Soucat A, Oyegbite K, Sene M, Bround D, Pangu K et al. Sustainability of primary health care including expanded program of immunizations in Bamako Initiative programs in West Africa: an assessment of 5 years' field experience in Benin and Guinea. *International Journal of Health Planning and Management*, 1997, 12(Suppl. 1):S9–S28.

43. Jancloes M, Seck B, Van de Velden L, Ndiaye B. Financing urban primary health services. Balancing community and government financial responsibilities, Pikine, Senegal, 1975–81. *Tropical Doctor*, 1985, 15:98–104.

44. Pangu KA, Van Lerberghe W. Self-financing and self-management of basic health services. *World Health Forum*, 1990, 11:451–454.

45. Van Lerberghe W, Pangu K. Comprehensive can be effective: the influence of coverage with a health centre network on the hospitalisation patterns in the rural area of Kasongo, Zaire. *Social Science and Medicine*, 1988, 26:949–955.

46. Van den Broek N, Van Lerberghe W, Pangu K. Caesarean sections for maternal indications in Kasongo (Zaire). *International Journal of Gynecology and Obstetrics*, 1989, 28:337–342.

47. Van Lerberghe W, Pangu KA, Van den Broek N. Obstetrical interventions and health centre coverage: a spatial analysis of routine data for evaluation. *Health Policy and Planning,* 1988, 3:308–314.

48. *Better health in Africa*. Washington, DC, World Bank, 1994.

49. Organisation for Economic Co-operation and Development. *International Development Statistics on line* (http://www.oecd.org/dataoecd/50/17/5037721.htm, accessed 15 December 2004).

50. *The health sector human resources crisis in Africa: an issue paper.* Washington, DC, United States Agency for International Development, Bureau for Africa, Office of Sustainable Development, SARA Project, 2003.

51. Bodart C, Servais G, Mohamed YL, Schmidt-Ehry B. The influence of health sector reform and external assistance in Burkina Faso. *Health Policy and Planning*, 2001, 16:74–86.

52. Dovlo D. *The brain drain and retention of health professionals in Africa. A case study.* Paper presented at: Regional Training Conference on Improving Tertiary Education in Sub-Saharan Africa: the things that work! Accra, 23–25 September 2003.

53. Tawfik L, Kinoti SN. *The impact of HIV/AIDS on the health sector in sub-Saharan Africa: the issue of human resources.* Washington, DC, United States Agency for International Development, Bureau for Africa, Office of Sustainable Development, SARA Project, 2001.

54. Lambert D. Study of unofficial health service charges in Angola in two health centers supported by MSF. *MSF Medical News*, 1996, 5:24–26.

55. Meesen B. *Corruption dans les services de santé: le cas de Cazenga [Corruption within the health services: the case of Cazenga]*. Brussels, Médecins Sans Frontières, 1997 (Repères: 1–20).

56. Parker D, Newbrander W. Tackling wastage and inefficiency in the health sector. *World Health Forum*, 1994, 15:107–113.

57. Asiimwe D, McPake B, Mwesigye F, Ofoumbi M, Ortenblad L, Streefland P, Turinde A. The private-sector activities of public-sector health workers in Uganda. In: Bennett S, McPake B, Mills A, eds. *Private health providers in developing countries: serving the public interest?* London, Zed Press, 1997.

58. Roenen C, Ferrinho P, Van Dormael M, Conceicao MC, Van Lerberghe W. How African doctors make ends meet: an exploration. *Tropical Medicine and International Health*, 1997, 2:127–135.

59. Macq J, Van Lerberghe W. Managing health services in developing countries: moonlighting to serve the public? In: Ferrinho P, Van Lerberghe W. *Providing health care under adverse conditions: health personnel performance & individual coping strategies*. Antwerp, ITG Press, 2000 (Studies in Health Services Organisation and Policy, 16:177-186).

60. Lowell G, Findlay A. *Migration of highly skilled persons from developing countries: impact and policy responses*. Geneva, International Labour Office, 2001.

61. Awases M, Nyoni J, Gbary A, Chatora R. *Migration of health professionals in six countries: a synthesis report*. Brazzaville, World Health Organization Regional Office for Africa, 2003.

62. *The international mobility of health professionals: an evaluation and analysis based on the case of South Africa*. Paris, Organisation for Economic Co-operation and Development, 2004 (Trends in International Migration Part III SOPEMI 2003).

63. World Health Organization/Ministry of Health and Social Welfare of the Government of Swaziland. *A situation analysis of the health workforce in Swaziland*. Geneva, World Health Organization, 2004.

64. Maiga Z, Nafo TF, El Abassi A. *La réforme du secteur santé au Mali, 1989–1996 [Reform of the health sector in Mali, 1989–1996]*. Antwerp, ITG Press, 1999 (Studies in Health Services Organisation & Policy, 12).

65. Bossyns P, Abache R, Abdoulaye MS, Van Lerberghe W. Unaffordable or cost-effective? Introducing an emergency referral system in rural Niger (submitted).

66. Bodart C, Servais G, Mohamed YL, Schmidt-Ehry B. The influence of health sector reform and external assistance in Burkina Faso. *Health Policy and Planning*, 2001, 16:74–86.

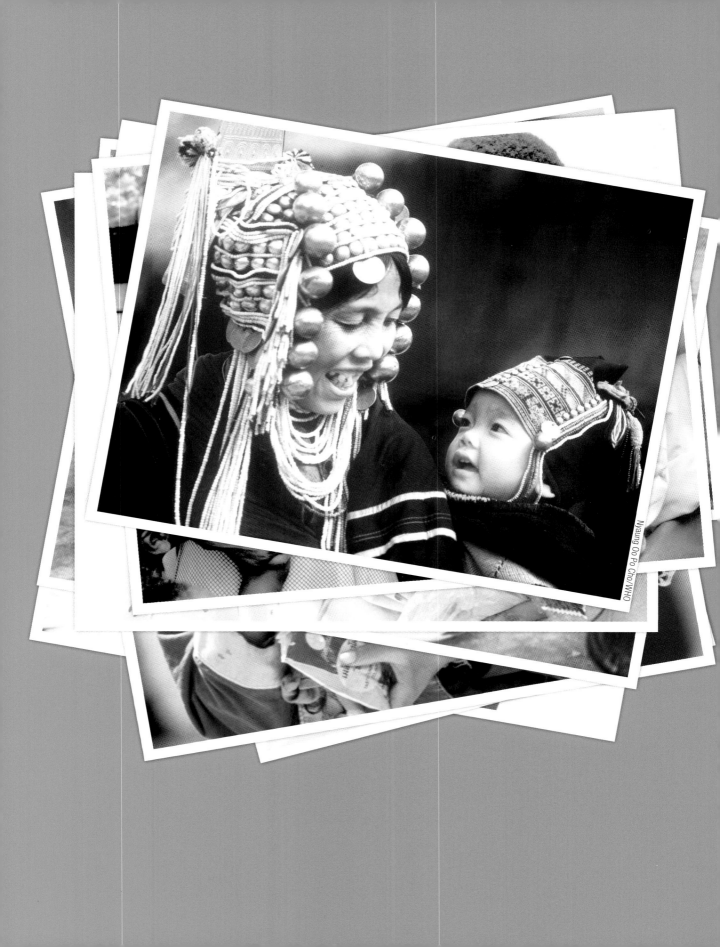

chapter three

great expectations:
making pregnancy safer

This chapter argues that the three most important components of care during pregnancy are first, providing good antenatal care, second, avoiding or coping with unwanted pregnancies, and third, building societies that support women who are pregnant. Despite increasing coverage in the last decade, antenatal care can only continue to realize its considerable potential by improving responsiveness, breaking down the barriers to access and refocusing on effective interventions. Given the extent of unintended pregnancy and the unacceptably high levels of unsafe abortion around the world, continuing efforts to provide family planning services, education, information and safe abortion services – to the extent allowed by law – are essential public health interventions. Tackling the low status of women, violence against women and lack of employment rights for pregnant women is vital in helping to build societies that support pregnant women.

Pregnancy is not just a matter of waiting to give birth. Often a defining phase in a woman's life, pregnancy can be a joyful and fulfilling period, for her both as an individual and as a member of society. It can also be one of misery and suffering, when the pregnancy is unwanted or mistimed, or when complications or adverse circumstances compromise the pregnancy, cause ill-health or even death. Pregnancy may be natural, but that does not mean it is problem-free.

Rarely is a pregnancy greeted with indifference. When a pregnancy occurs, women, their partners and families most often experience a mixture of joy, concern and hope that the outcome will be the best of all: a healthy mother and a healthy baby. All societies strive to ensure that pregnancy is indeed a happy event. They do so by providing appropriate antenatal care during pregnancy to promote health and cope with problems, by taking measures to avoid unwanted pregnancies, and by making sure that pregnancies take place in socially and environmentally favourable conditions. Women around the world face many inequities during pregnancy. At this crucial time women rely on care and help from health services, as well as on support systems in the home and community. Exclusion, marginalization and discrimination can severely affect the health of mothers and that of their babies.

REALIZING THE POTENTIAL OF ANTENATAL CARE

Meeting expectations in pregnancy

A pregnancy brings with it great hope for the future, and can give women a special and highly appreciated social status. It also brings great expectations of health care that is often willingly sought at this time. This explains, at least in part, the extraordinary success of antenatal care consultations. Women want confirmation that they are pregnant. At the same time they know that pregnancy can be dangerous, particularly in the developing world. In many countries pregnant women are likely to know of maternal deaths, stillbirths or newborn deaths among their own extended family or in their community. It is natural that demand is high for health care that can provide reassurance, solve problems that may arise and confirm the status conferred by pregnancy.

In high-income and middle-income countries today, use of antenatal care by pregnant women is almost universal – except among marginalized groups such as migrants, ethnic minorities, unmarried adolescents, the very poor and those living in isolated rural communities. Even in low-income settings, coverage rates for antenatal care – at least for one visit – are often quite high, certainly much higher than use of a skilled health care professional during childbirth.

There were noticeable increases in the use of antenatal care in developing countries during the 1990s. The greatest progress was seen in Asia, mainly as a result of rapid changes in a few large countries such as Indonesia (see Figure 3.1). Significant increases also took place in the Caribbean and Latin America, although countries in these areas already had relatively high levels of antenatal care. In sub-Saharan Africa, by contrast, antenatal care use increased only marginally over the decade (although levels in Africa are relatively high compared with those in Asia).

While antenatal care coverage has improved significantly in recent years, it is generally recognized that the antenatal care services currently provided in many parts of the world fail to meet the recommended standards. A huge potential thus

Figure 3.1 **Coverage of antenatal care is rising**

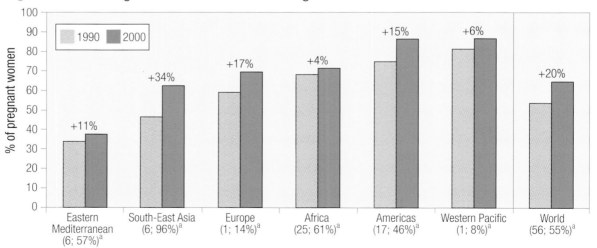

[a] Number of countries and percentage of the regional population included in the analysis.

Data source: Multiple Indicator Cluster Surveys (UNICEF) and Demographic and Health Surveys.

remains insufficiently exploited. Although progress has been made globally in terms of increasing access and use of one antenatal visit, the proportion of women who are obtaining the recommended minimum of four visits is too low *(1)*. The first consultation is often late in pregnancy, whereas maximum benefit requires an early initiation of antenatal care. Antenatal care is given by doctors, midwives and nurses and many other cadres of health workers *(2)*. Little is known about the capacities of non-professional workers such as traditional birth attendants to deliver the known effective interventions during pregnancy.

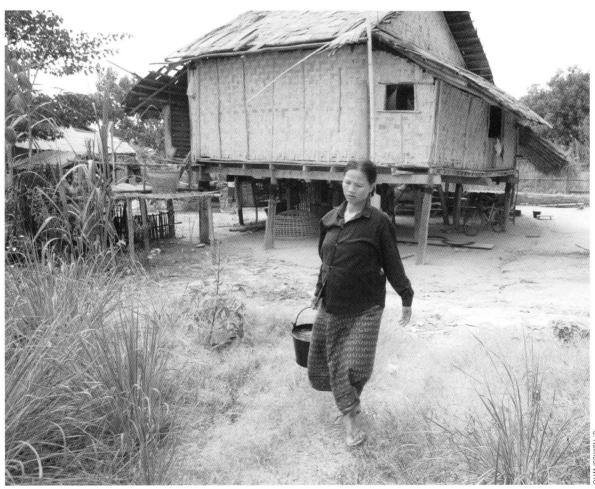

J. Holmes/WHO

It is October 2004 and Bounlid, from the Lao People's Democratic Republic, is seven months pregnant and feeling tired. She is finding it much harder to work and her family's income has slipped because of this. The rice-cropping season is starting and the rice needs to be brought in soon. When she goes to the fields she has to leave her children on their own, as she does not have the energy to deal with them and work at the same time.

"I've had no antenatal care and I don't expect to have any for the rest of my pregnancy. I plan to give birth at home, as I did with my other four children. It is too expensive for most people in my village to give birth with a skilled attendant at the clinic, which, in any case, has very basic facilities and no telephone or ambulance if there were complications."

Bounlid has not received any professional advice about the birth or nutrition concerning the baby.

Pregnancy – a time with its own dangers

Antenatal care is not just a way to identify women at risk of troublesome deliveries *(3, 4)*. While less prominent than the dangers that can occur during childbirth, those surrounding pregnancy are far from being negligible. Women expect that antenatal care will help them deal with the health problems that can occur during pregnancy itself. If left unchecked, some of these may threaten health and survival before the child is due to be born.

A substantial proportion of maternal deaths – perhaps as many as one in four – occur during pregnancy. Data on mortality during pregnancy, however, are very fragmentary *(5)*. The proportion of maternal deaths during pregnancy varies significantly from country to country according to the importance of unsafe abortion, violence, and disease conditions in the area *(6, 7)*. In Egypt 9% of all maternal deaths occur during the first six months of pregnancy and a further 16% during the last three months *(8)*.

Apart from complications of unsafe abortion, which can be prevented or dealt with by good post-abortion care, three types of health problems exist in pregnancy. First, the complications of pregnancy itself, second, diseases that happen to affect a pregnant woman and which may or may not be aggravated by pregnancy, and third, the negative effects of unhealthy lifestyles on the outcome of pregnancy. All have to be tackled by antenatal care.

Pregnancy has many complications that require care *(9)*. In Lusaka, Zambia, nearly 40% of pregnancy-related referrals to the university teaching hospital were related to problems of the pregnancy itself, rather than to childbirth: 27% for threatened abortion or abortion complications, 13% for illness not specific to pregnancy such as malaria and infections, and 9% for hypertensive disorders of pregnancy *(10)*. In a recent study of six west African countries, a third of all pregnant women were shown to experience some illness during pregnancy, (not including problems related to unsafe abortion) of whom 2.6% needed to be hospitalized *(11)*.

Box 3.1 Reducing the burden of malaria in pregnant women and their children

Each year, approximately 50 million women living in malaria-endemic countries throughout the world become pregnant. Around 10 000 of these women and 200 000 of their infants die as a result of malaria infection, severe malarial anaemia contributing to more than half of these deaths *(14,15)*. Malaria in pregnancy also increases the risk of stillbirth, spontaneous abortion, low birth weight and neonatal death. The risk of severe malaria is increased in pregnant women coinfected with HIV.

More than 90% of the one million annual deaths from malaria are among young African children, as are most cases of severe malarial anaemia *(16–18)*. Severe anaemia probably accounts for more than half of all childhood deaths from malaria in Africa, with case fatality rates of between 8% and 18% in hospitals *(16–22)* and probably more than that in the community.

Interventions against malaria and anaemia are well known, and though not perfect, can do a lot to reduce malaria morbidity and mortality. Maternal, neonatal and child health services are a prime vehicle for such interventions.

Apart from prompt treatment of malaria infections *(23)*, maternal, neonatal and child health services can contribute by increasing the use of insecticide-treated nets and providing intermittent preventive treatment.

Insecticide-treated nets limit the harm done by malaria: they reduce parasitaemia, the frequency of low birth weight, and anaemia *(24–26)*. These nets have been shown to reduce all-cause mortality in young children by around one fifth, saving an average of six lives for every 1000 children aged 1–59 months protected each year *(26)*. They represent a highly cost-effective use of scarce health care resources *(27)*.

Intermittent preventive treatment in pregnancy is the administration of a full therapeutic dose of an antimalarial drug (sulfadoxine-pyrimethamine) at specified intervals in the second and third trimesters, regardless of whether or not the woman is infected. This reduces maternal anaemia, placental malaria, and low birth weight by approximately 40% *(28–30)*. Intermittent preventive treatment is one of the most cost-effective strategies for preventing the morbidity and mortality associated with malaria *(31, 32)*, and recent evidence suggests that it may be a useful strategy for the control of malaria and anaemia in young infants *(33,34)*. An Intermittent Preventive Treatment in Infants Consortium, comprising WHO, UNICEF, and research groups in Africa, Europe and the USA, is tackling the outstanding research issues.

Classic complications of pregnancy include pre-eclampsia and eclampsia which affect 2.8% of pregnancies in developing countries and 0.4% in developed countries *(12)*, leading to many life-threatening cases and over 63 000 maternal deaths worldwide every year. Haemorrhage following placental abruption or placenta praevia affects about 4% of pregnant women *(13)*. Less common, but very serious complications include ectopic pregnancy and molar pregnancy.

Diseases and other health problems can often complicate, or become more severe during, pregnancy. Malaria worsens during pregnancy, for example, and together with anaemia is responsible for 10 000 maternal deaths and 200 000 infant deaths per year (see Boxes 3.1 and 3.2). Mortality from HIV/AIDS during pregnancy can be significant in areas where prevalence is high. Tuberculosis is frequently encountered among pregnant women and is responsible for 9% of all deaths of women of reproductive age. Maternal malnutrition is a huge global problem, both as protein-calorie deficiency and as micronutrient deficiency. Paradoxically, obesity is also increasingly becoming an issue and leads to diabetes and birthing difficulties *(45)*.

Mental ill-health in pregnancy appears to be more common than previously recognized. Although pregnancy has been regarded as a period of general psychological well-being for women *(46)*, high rates of psychiatric morbidity in pregnant women have been reported, for example in Uganda *(47)*. Pre-existing psychological disturbances can easily surface as depression, substance abuse or attempts at suicide, particularly when combined with a pregnancy that is unwanted. Rates of depression are at least as high, or higher, in late pregnancy than during the postpartum period *(48–51)*.

In addition, many pregnant women are exposed to risks that are directly related to their way of life. Unhealthy lifestyles, including consumption of alcohol, tobacco and drugs, are dangerous for both mother and fetus, as they may lead to problems such as premature detachment of the placenta, sudden infant death syndrome, fetal alcohol syndrome and childhood developmental problems *(52)*. Gender-based violence or exposure to hazards in the workplace may not be readily recognized by pregnant women as problems that health workers can help to resolve, but constitute major and underestimated public health problems (see Box 3.3).

Box 3.2   Anaemia – the silent killer

Anaemia is one of the world's leading causes of disability *(35)* and thus one of the most serious global public health problems. It affects nearly half of the pregnant women in the world: 52% in non-industrialized countries – compared with 23% in industrialized countries *(36)*. The commonest causes of anaemia are poor nutrition, iron and other micronutrient deficiencies, malaria, hookworm and schistosomiasis. HIV infection *(37)* and haemoglobinopathies make important additional contributions.

Anaemia during pregnancy has serious clinical consequences. It is associated with greater risk of maternal death, in particular from haemorrhage *(38)*. Severely anaemic pregnant women are less able to withstand blood loss *(39)* and may require blood transfusion which is not always available in poor countries and is not without risks. Anaemia during pregnancy is also associated with increased stillbirths, perinatal deaths, low-birth-weight babies and prematurity *(40)*. In malaria-endemic countries, anaemia is one of the commonest preventable causes of death in pregnant women and also in children under five years of age *(41)*. Reducing the burden of anaemia is essential to achieve the Millennium Development Goals relating to maternal and childhood mortality. The greatest burden of anaemia falls on the most "hard-to-reach" individuals. WHO has published clinical guidelines in its Integrated Management of Pregnancy and Childbirth series *(42–44)*.

The strategy for control of anaemia in pregnant women includes: detection and appropriate management; prophylaxis against parasitic diseases and supplementation with iron and folic acid; and improved obstetric care and management of women with severe anaemia.

Successful delivery of these cost-effective interventions requires the integrated efforts of several health programmes – particularly those targeted at pregnant women and young children – and the strengthening of health systems, increased community awareness, and financial investment.

Seizing the opportunities

Good antenatal care does more than just deal with the complications of pregnancy. Women are the largest group of health care users actively and willingly seeking care at clinics. This offers enormous opportunities to use antenatal care as a platform for programmes that tackle nutrition, HIV/AIDS, sexually transmitted infections, malaria and tuberculosis, among others. This and other opportunities have so far been insufficiently exploited. Three important opportunities during antenatal care should not be missed.

First, antenatal consultations offer an opportunity to promote healthy lifestyles that improve long-term health outcomes for the woman, her unborn child, and possibly her family. The promotion of family planning is the foremost example of this and can have a positive impact on contraceptive use after birth. Some women actually prefer to discuss family planning methods during pregnancy or as part of postnatal care *(64, 65)*. Another example of an opportunity for prenatal health promotion is that of smoking cessation programmes in pregnancy, which appear to be successful *(66)*. They reduce the risks of low birth weight and preterm birth, and improve the pregnant woman's health in the long term as well.

Second, antenatal care provides an opportunity to establish a birth plan *(67)*. Apart from planning the birth, making the plan is a chance to inform women and their families of the potential for unexpected events. Birth preparedness itself includes planning the desired place of birth, the preferred birth attendant and birth companion, and finding

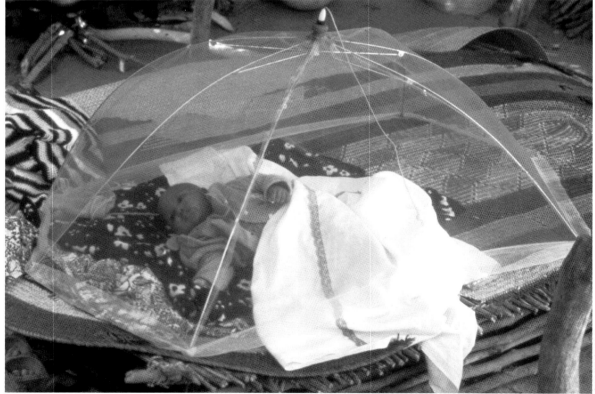

This young child in Niger is protected by an insecticide-treated bednet.

P. Carnevale/WHO

out the location of the closest appropriate care facility. It also involves securing funds for birth-related and emergency expenses, finding transport for facility-based birth and identifying compatible blood donors in case of emergency. Birth planning has been used in many developed countries for more than a decade with beneficial effects *(68–70)*, and has been introduced with success in developing countries as well, albeit on too limited a scale so far.

Third, the antenatal care consultation is an opportunity to prepare mothers for parenting and for what will happen after the birth. Women and their families can learn how to improve their health and seek help when appropriate, and, most importantly, how to take care of the newborn child. Advice on parenting skills is particularly important for pregnant adolescents and women with low self-esteem *(71)*, and can improve the care that newborns and children will receive in the future *(72)*. It helps to build a healthy family environment that is responsive to the child's needs.

Critical directions for the future

Antenatal care started out in the first half of the 20th century as a means to educate "ignorant" women with an emphasis on the welfare of the infant and child. This was a response to what had been identified as inadequate devotion to maternal duty resulting in the poor physical stock of nations *(73)*. In the 1950s it was used as an instrument for screening, so that women at higher risk of complications could be identified. Although antenatal care turned out to be a poor screening instrument, few people would deny that many pregnancy complications, concurrent illnesses and health problems can be dealt with in an antenatal care consultation that focuses on effective interventions.

Antenatal care has come a long way, but can go much further. Four directions are critical: to rationalize the rituals of care, to roll out antenatal care as a platform for a number of other key health programmes, to establish communication with women more effectively, and to avoid the overmedicalization that can do more harm than good. Most importantly, the unfinished agenda of reaching all women who are pregnant should be tackled.

All too often, antenatal care is still more a question of ritual than of effective interventions. Many of the tests and procedures carried out during a traditional antenatal consultation have very little scientific merit *(74)*. Many ineffective interventions, such

Box 3.3 Violence against women

Violence against women by a partner is a global public health problem and a human rights violation. This violence often persists and sometimes may start during pregnancy, with serious implications for the health of the mother and child. In studies from countries such as Egypt, Ethiopia, India, Mexico and Nicaragua, 14–32% of women report having been physically or sexually abused during pregnancy. The perpetrator is usually their partner *(53)*. In Peru, 15% of women in Lima and 28% in the Department of Cusco have experienced physical violence during pregnancy *(54)*. In Canada, Sweden, Switzerland and the United Kingdom,

rates of abuse during pregnancy are between 4% and 11%. Violence during pregnancy can kill: in Pune, India, 16% of all deaths during pregnancy in 400 villages and seven hospitals were attributed to partner violence *(55)*. Apart from physical trauma, violence increases the likelihood of premature labour, low birth weight, anaemia, sexually transmitted infections, urinary infections, substance use, depression and other mental health problems *(56)*.

Antenatal care provides an opportunity for the identification of instances of violence during pregnancy – a first step towards providing support to the expectant mother and help-

ing her to find solutions. Experience shows, however, that this identification is only useful when appropriate support and/or referral can be provided. Health workers must not only be sensitive to the subject, but also need to know how to deal with it. Physicians, nurses, midwives and others involved in the care of pregnant women have to be specifically trained to recognize and know how to ask about intimate partner violence, provide information in a confidential and non-judgemental way, and provide care and support, including through appropriate referral *(57–63)*.

as routine weighing of the woman at each consultation to assess maternal well-being and fetal growth, could be dispensed with *(75)*. They take up valuable time which could be more usefully dedicated to counselling women on healthy lifestyles and health problems such as the detection and management of existing diseases.

This interaction between antenatal care and coping with women's circumstances and pre-existing diseases is the most underestimated aspect of care in pregnancy. The potential for antenatal care to be much more far-reaching in this respect has not been fully exploited. As a platform for other health programmes such as HIV/AIDS and other sexually transmitted infections, malaria, TB and family planning, the resource of antenatal care is invaluable. WHO guidelines are readily available *(42)* to advise on care, prevention and treatment of diseases during pregnancy. Moreover, pregnancy is a time when a dialogue about health and relevant social issues can be established between women and health services staff. Establishing communication with women and linking up the medical and social worlds will make care more human, and ultimately more responsive.

A frequently forgotten issue is that of supply-driven overmedicalization of normal pregnancies, sometimes for reasons of financial gain. Overmedicalized care can needlessly damage the health of both mothers and babies and expose households to unnecessary expenditure. All too often, sophisticated investigations such as ultrasound scanning are performed without justification at every antenatal visit, while useful procedures such as blood pressure measurement are neglected and the establishment of birth plans and counselling on existing health problems are omitted. This has gone to extremes in some countries, where ultrasound is used to detect female fetuses for the purposes of sex-selective abortion.

In terms of coverage, there is some way to go to provide at least four care contacts during each pregnancy, starting early enough to ensure that effective interventions are used. Women need providers who are skilled enough to offer care that is linked into a health care system that has continuity with childbirth care. The barriers to extending coverage are twofold. First, in some areas no services are offered, implying the need for outreach or services that can be physically accessed. Second, services are often not responsive enough. Complaints of unhelpful and rude health personnel, unexpected and unfair costs, unfriendly opening hours and the lack of involvement of male partners are not uncommon. Relatively straightforward changes to the arrangements of how antenatal care sessions are run (for instance not limiting antenatal care to one session per week) can sometimes make significant improvements to uptake. Adolescent girls are particularly vulnerable in this respect. Services that are responsive to them and young women will make a great contribution to the expansion of antenatal care. The question should not be "why do women not accept the service that we offer?", but "why do we not offer a service that women will accept?" *(76)*.

NOT EVERY PREGNANCY IS WELCOME

Planning pregnancies before they even happen

Many women intend to get pregnant. Each year an estimated 123 million succeed. But a substantial additional number of women – around 87 million – become pregnant unintentionally. For some women and their partners this may be a pleasant surprise, but for others the pregnancy may be mistimed or simply unwanted *(77)*. Of the estimated 211 million pregnancies that occur each year, about 46 million end in induced abortion (see Figure 3.2) *(78)*.

Despite the large number of unintended pregnancies, many more women than ever before control their reproductive life by spacing their pregnancies more widely or limiting the number of pregnancies. Some 30 years of effort to bring contraceptive services within people's reach have not been in vain. In developing countries, contraceptive prevalence has risen from around 10% in the early 1960s to 59% at the turn of the millennium *(79)*. Despite falling international financial support, there has been a 1% annual increase in contraceptive prevalence over the last 10 years worldwide *(80)*. A corresponding global drop in fertility has been seen, with the current average number of children per woman standing at 2.69, compared with 4.97 in the early 1960s *(81)*.

Nevertheless, as more women than ever before reach reproductive age, millions who do not want a child or who want to postpone their next pregnancy are not using any contraception *(82)*. This growing unmet need may be due to the lack of access to contraceptives, an issue in particular for adolescents, or it may result from women not using them. The most commonly given reason – in about 45% of cases – for not using a contraceptive method is a perceived lack of exposure to pregnancy. Fear of side-effects and cost is a reason for non-use in about one third of cases. Opposition to use is a lesser but still significant reason for non-use, frequently attributed to the husband *(83)*. For all of these reasons, uptake of contraception is still very low in many parts of Africa, and patchy in other continents. According to recent survey data some countries are actually experiencing a reversal in family planning coverage.

Even if all the needs for contraception were met, there would still be many unwanted and mistimed pregnancies. Although most modern methods of contraception are highly effective if used consistently, advice and counselling on their correct use is often not available. If all users were to follow instructions perfectly, there would still be nearly 6 million accidental pregnancies per year. The fact is that with typical, real-life use of contraceptives, an estimated 26.5 million unintended pregnancies occur each year because of inappropriate use or method failure *(84)*. In addition, dissatisfaction with methods can lead to discontinuation, which is often associated with lack of choice, incorrect use or fear of side effects, all symptoms of poor quality family planning counselling and services.

What the research on unmet need for contraception and on contraceptive failure does not capture well is the role of unequal power relations between men and women. These contribute substantially to both unwanted sex and subsequent unwanted pregnancy *(85)*. Young women are at particular risk of unwanted sex, or sex in unwanted conditions, particularly when there are large age differences between them and their partners *(85)*. Between 7% and 48% of adolescent girls report that their first sexual experience was forced *(86, 87)*. Adolescent girls are more likely to be pressured into sexual activity at an

Figure 3.2 The outcomes of a year's pregnancies

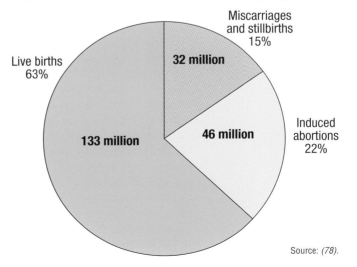

Live births 63% — 133 million

Miscarriages and stillbirths 15% — 32 million

Induced abortions 22% — 46 million

Source: *(78)*.

older man's request or by force, and often must rely on the man to prevent pregnancy. Women who are coerced into sex or who face abuse from partners are less likely to be in a position to use contraception, and are therefore more exposed to unintended pregnancy than others. Women who have experienced a sexual assault often fear pregnancy and delay medical examination or health care. There is increasing evidence that violence is associated with unintended pregnancies. Up to 40% of women attending for pregnancy termination have experienced sexual and/or physical abuse at some stage of their lives *(88, 89)*.

Unintended and unwanted pregnancies – owing to unmet need for contraception, to contraceptive failure, or to unwanted sex – if brought to term, carry at least the same risks as those that are desired and deliberate. It is estimated that up to 100 000 maternal deaths could be avoided each year if women who did not want children used effective contraception *(90)*. When maternal illnesses are also taken into account, preventing unwanted pregnancies could avert, each year, the loss of 4.5 million disability-adjusted life years *(91)*.

The implications of unwanted pregnancy are substantial enough, but there is also evidence to suggest that effective contraception can contribute to better maternal health – above and beyond averting these deaths and disabilities – in two ways. First, because unwanted pregnancies carry a greater risk than those that are wanted. By tackling unmet need for contraception for young girls and for older women and also for those who want to space their births, high-risk pregnancies that are unwanted can be avoided. Moreover, there are benefits for the child. Spacing pregnancies by at least two years increases the chance of child survival *(92)*. Second, there are some indications that women whose pregnancy is wanted take more care of their pregnancy than others: they are more likely to receive antenatal care early in pregnancy, to give birth under medical supervision, or to have their children fully vaccinated *(90)*. Finally, a major contribution of contraception to reducing maternal death and disability is through its potential to decrease unsafe abortions.

Unsafe abortion: a major public health problem

Of the 46 million pregnancies that are terminated each year around the world, approximately 60% are carried out under safe conditions. From a public health viewpoint the distinction between safe and unsafe abortion is important. When performed by trained health care providers with proper equipment, correct technique and sanitary standards, abortion carries little or no risk. The case fatality is no more than 1 per 100 000 procedures *(78, 84)*, which is less than the risk of a pregnancy carried to term in the best of circumstances.

However, more than 18 million induced abortions each year are performed by people lacking the necessary skills or in an environment lacking the minimal medical standards, or both, and are therefore unsafe *(93, 94)*. Almost all take place in the developing world. With 34 unsafe abortions per 1000 women, South America has the highest ratio, closely followed by eastern Africa (31 per 1000 women), western Africa (25 per 1000 women), central Africa (22 per 1000 women), and south Asia (22 per 1000 women) *(93)*. The fact that women seek to terminate their pregnancies by any means available in circumstances where abortion is unsafe, illegal or both, demonstrates how vital it is for them to be able to regulate their fertility. Women pay heavily for unsafe abortions, not only with their health and their lives but financially as well. In Phnom Penh, Cambodia, for example, the going rate for an abortion – legal, but most often unsafe – ranged between US$ 15 and US$ 55 in 2001: the equivalent of several months' salary for a public sector nurse *(95)*.

Unsafe abortion is particularly an issue for younger women. Two thirds of unsafe abortions occur among women aged between 15 and 30 years. Around 2.5 million, or almost 14% of all unsafe abortions in developing countries, are among women under 20 years of age. The age pattern of unsafe abortions differs markedly from region to region. The proportion of women aged 15–19 years in Africa who have had an unsafe abortion is higher than in any other region and almost 60% of unsafe abortions are among women aged less than 25 years. This contrasts with Asia where 30% of unsafe abortions are in women of this age group. In the Caribbean and Latin America, women aged 20–29 years account for more than half of all unsafe abortions *(93)*.

Everywhere, though, and in all age groups, the consequences are dramatic. The risk of dying from an unsafe abortion is around 350 per 100 000, and 68 000 women a year die in this way. In addition, the non-fatal complications and the sequelae contribute significantly to the global burden of disease *(96)*, not to mention the emotional turmoil that goes with so many unsafe abortions *(97)*. Unsafe abortions also result in high costs for the health system. In some developing countries, hospital admissions for complications of unsafe abortion represent up to 50% of obstetric intake *(98, 99)*. In Lusaka, Zambia, they represent 27% of non-delivery referrals to the obstetric-gynaecological services *(10)*. The mobilization of hospital beds, blood supplies, medication, operating theatres, anaesthesia and medical specialists is a serious drain on limited resources in many countries *(84)*. The daily cost of a patient hospitalized as a result of unsafe abortion can be more than 2500 times the daily per capita health budget *(100)*.

DEALING WITH THE COMPLICATIONS OF ABORTION

At the 1994 International Conference on Population and Development (ICPD) in Cairo, unsafe abortion was identified as a major public health concern and governments agreed to work for its elimination. The plan of action included better access to modern contraceptive methods, to high-quality post-abortion care (needed for treating the complications of miscarriages as well as those of unsafely induced abortions), and to safe abortion services to the full extent permitted by local laws. The United Nations General Assembly's special session in 1999 (ICPD+5) stated that "in circumstances where abortion is not against the law, health systems should train and equip health-service providers and should take other measures to ensure that such abortion is safe and accessible" *(101)*.

Safe and comprehensive post-abortion care for the complications of induced abortion, and the provision of abortion services to the extent permitted by law, remain severely restricted by the deficiencies of health systems and lack of access. Women, particularly adolescents, the poor and those living in rural areas, often do not know where to find services that are safe and legal. They may lack the resources, time or decision-making power to avail themselves of such services, or be deterred by lack of privacy and confidentiality and by the attitudes of health care providers *(102)*. The result is that many women, particularly in developing countries, may then resort to unqualified providers or "quacks" and put their lives in danger. A particularly dramatic case is that of refugees, in a context where systematic rape is increasingly used as a weapon of war. Most countries permit abortion in such circumstances, yet women as well as health care providers are often unaware of this, and humanitarian assistance, for example in refugee camps, tends to neglect this issue *(103)*.

Abortion is legal, on varying grounds, in many countries (see Figure 3.3), but even policy-makers and professionals are often only vaguely aware about what the law permits and what it does not. Where legislation is less restrictive, there are, in principle, more possibilities for women to terminate an unwanted pregnancy under safe conditions. Yet, services may be poorly equipped or health personnel inadequately trained, even though the training, equipment and policies needed to ensure that women eligible under law have access to safe care are neither complicated nor costly *(84)*. In India, for example, where a liberal abortion law has been in place since 1974, unsafe abortions still outnumbered safe abortions by a factor of 7 in the early 1990s, as a result of administrative barriers and lack of information, with deaths from unsafe abortion accounting for 20% of all maternal deaths. But where, to the extent permitted by law, measures are taken to train and equip professionals and facilitate access to safe services and information, as recommended by the United Nations General Assembly, women are less likely to resort to unsafe abortion.

Every year, many millions of women experience the distressing event of an unwanted pregnancy. Continued investment in education, information, and public provision of contraceptive services can go a long way to keep this to a minimum — although no family planning policy will prevent all unwanted pregnancies. But it is possible to avoid all of the 68 000 deaths as well as the disabilities and suffering that go with unsafe abortions. This is not only a question of how a country defines what is legal and what is not, but also of guaranteeing women access, to the fullest extent permitted by law, to good quality and responsive abortion and post-abortion care.

VALUING PREGNANCY: A MATTER OF LEGAL PROTECTION

Even in societies that value pregnancy highly, the position of a pregnant woman is not always enviable. A social environment that accords poor status to women generally also tends to marginalize pregnant women. An extreme expression of this is violence against women, a major public health challenge all over the world *(54)*. Women abused during pregnancy are at increased risk of miscarriage, murder and suicide, and their babies are prone to low birth weight and fetal distress *(105)*.

Figure 3.3 **Grounds on which abortion is permitted around the world**

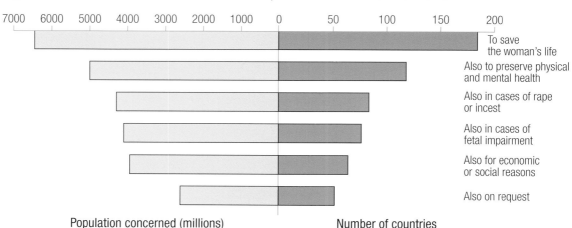

Population concerned (millions)   Number of countries

Data source: *(104)*.

Since the United Nations International Conference on Population and Development (ICPD) Programme of Action in 1994, many countries have elaborated or refined their laws to support the ICPD goals. For instance, many countries have passed laws criminalizing violence against women, and several have passed legislation outlawing female genital mutilation. As these laws are gradually implemented, they serve to protect girls and women who are pregnant, but also to promote their overall health.

Protection for women who are pregnant cannot be provided without the support of a legal and policy framework. Some of the most obvious laws and policies include establishing a minimum age for marriage, criminalizing violence against women, prohibiting harmful practices such as female genital mutilation, and enforcing birth registration. All countries have ratified at least one (and many have ratified all) of the international human rights treaties. These place the legal obligation on countries to take measures to ensure that their citizens' rights are protected and fulfilled, and provide a starting point for effective protection.

Based on such frameworks, a wide range of specific legal and regulatory measures can be taken to improve the protection of women who are pregnant. These rights include the provision of information on sexual and reproductive health, establishing mandatory routine audits and reviews of maternal, perinatal and neonatal deaths, and legal measures for the financial protection and support of pregnant women. The latter concern coverage of medical expenses as well as measures to guarantee their income.

The International Labour Organization's Maternity Protection Convention (adopted in 1919 and last revised in 2000) sets a minimum standard for what should be included in national legislation in this regard *(106)*. The Convention provides for protection against dismissal of women during pregnancy, maternity leave and the breastfeeding period, and also for cash benefits. It encompasses coverage of antenatal, childbirth and postnatal care and hospitalization care when necessary, and working hours and tasks that are not detrimental to mother or child. It calls for 14 weeks of maternity leave, of which six weeks must be postnatal leave to safeguard the health of mother and child. This aspect of the Convention covers all married and unmarried employed women, including those in unusual forms of dependent work. This can be interpreted broadly to cover women in all sectors of the economy, including the informal sector, but in practice legislation usually covers only women who are employed in the formal sector. With increasing urbanization and the development of the formal economy, compliance with these minimum standards is increasingly becoming an issue, in developing as well as developed countries.

On the other hand, existing laws, policies and regulations that limit access to health services for unmarried women or for those under a certain age, effectively screen out many women in need. The same is true for services that require up-front payment and exclude those too poor to pay. There are still health services that require third-party authorization (usually by a husband) for treating a woman, pregnant or not, even if no such requirement exists in the national law. If all women who are pregnant are to be protected, these kinds of situations need urgent attention, which often requires the revision of policies and regulations. Environmental, social and legal circumstances can be unfavourable for pregnant women. Referring to the overarching human rights frameworks can do much to eliminate sources of social exclusion, and is as important as providing antenatal care.

References

1. Carroli G, Villar J, Piaggio G, Khan-Neelofur D, Gulmezoglu M, Mugford M et al. WHO systematic review of randomised controlled trials of routine antenatal care. *Lancet*, 2001, 357:1565–1570.
2. WHO/UNICEF. *Antenatal care in developing countries. Promises, achievements, and missed opportunities. An analysis of trends, levels, and differentials 1990–2001.* Geneva, World Health Organization, 2003.
3. Backe B, Nakling J. Effectiveness of antenatal care: a population based study. *British Journal of Obstetrics and Gynaecology*, 1993, 100:727–732.
4. Hall MH, Chang PK, MacGillivary I. Is routine antenatal care worth while? *Lancet*, 1980, 2:78–80.
5. Fortney J, Smith J. Measuring maternal mortality. In: Bere M, Ravindran T, eds. *Safe motherhood initiatives: critical issues.* Oxford, Blackwell Science for Reproductive Health Matters, 1999.
6. Li X, Fortney J, Kotelchuck M, Glover L. The postpartum period: the key to maternal mortality. *International Journal of Gynecology and Obstetrics*, 1996, 54:1–10.
7. Hieu D, Hanenber R, Vach T, Vinh D, Sokal D. Maternal mortality in Vietnam. *Studies in Family Planning*, 1999, 30:329–338.
8. *Egypt national maternal mortality study 2000.* Cairo, Ministry of Health and Population, 2000.
9. Franks AL, Kendrick JS, Olson DR, Atrash HK, Saftlas AF, Moien M. Hospitalization for pregnancy complications, United States, 1986 and 1987. *American Journal of Obstetrics and Gynecology*, 1992, 166:1339–1344.
10. Murray SF, Davies S, Kumwenda Phiri R, Ahmed Y. Tools for monitoring the effectiveness of district maternity referral systems. *Health Policy and Planning*, 2001, 16:353–361.
11. de Bernis L, Dumont A, Bouillin D, Gueye A, Dompnier JP, Bouvier-Colle MH. Maternal morbidity and mortality in two different populations of Senegal: a prospective study (MOMA survey). *BJOG*, 2000, 107:68–74.
12. Magpie Trial Collaborative Group. Do women with pre-eclampsia, and their babies, benefit from magnesium sulphate? The Magpie Trial: a randomised placebo-controlled trial. *Lancet*, 2002, 359:1877–1890.
13. Fraser S, Watson R. Bleeding during the latter half of pregnancy. In: Chalmers I, Enkin M., Keirse MJNC, eds. *Effective care in pregnancy and childbirth.* Oxford, Oxford University Press, 1989.
14. Steketee RW, Nahlen BL, Parise ME, Menendez C. The burden of malaria in pregnancy in malaria-endemic areas. *American Journal of Tropical Medicine and Hygiene*, 2001, 64(1–2 Suppl.):28–35.
15. Murphy SC, Breman JG. Gaps in the childhood malaria burden in Africa: cerebral malaria, neurological sequelae, anemia, respiratory distress, hypoglycemia, and complications of pregnancy. *American Journal of Tropical Medicine and Hygiene,* 2001, 64(1–2 Suppl.): 57–67.
16. Schellenberg D, Menendez C, Kahigwa E, Font F, Galindo C, Acosta C et al. African children with malaria in an area of intense Plasmodium falciparum transmission: features on admission to the hospital and risk factors for death. *American Journal of Tropical Medicine and Hygiene*, 1999, 61:431–438.
17. Bojang KA, Van Hensbroek MB, Palmer A, Banya WA, Jaffar S, Greenwood BM. Predictors of mortality in Gambian children with severe malaria anaemia. *Annals of Tropical Paediatrics*, 1997, 17:355–359.
18. Newton CR, Warn PA, Winstanley PA, Peshu N, Snow RW, Pasvol G et al. Severe anaemia in children living in a malaria endemic area of Kenya. *Tropical Medicine and International Health*, 1997, 2:165–178.
19. Slutsker L, Taylor TE, Wirima JJ, Steketee RW. In-hospital morbidity and mortality due to malaria-associated severe anaemia in two areas of Malawi with different patterns of malaria infection. *Transactions of the Royal Society of Tropical Medicine and Hygiene*, 1994, 88:548–551.
20. Biemba G, Dolmans D, Thuma PE, Weiss G, Gordeuk VR. Severe anaemia in Zambian children with Plasmodium falciparum malaria. *Tropical Medicine and International Health*, 2000, 5:9–16.

21. Lackritz EM, Campbell CC, Ruebush TK, 2nd, Hightower AW, Wakube W, Steketee RW et al. Effect of blood transfusion on survival among children in a Kenyan hospital. *Lancet*, 1992, 340:524–528.

22. Marsh K, Forster D, Waruiru C, Mwangi I, Winstanley M, Marsh V et al. Indicators of life-threatening malaria in African children. *New England Journal of Medicine*, 1995, 332:1399–1404.

23. *Antimalarial drug combination therapy. Report of a WHO Technical Consultation.* Geneva, World Health Organization, 2001

24. ter Kuile FO, Terlouw DJ, Phillips-Howard PA, Hawley WA, Friedman JF, Kariuki SK et al. Reduction of malaria during pregnancy by permethrin-treated bed nets in an area of intense perennial malaria transmission in western Kenya. *American Journal of Tropical Medicine and Hygiene*, 2003, 68(4 Suppl.):50–60.

25. Lengeler C. Insecticide-treated bednets and curtains for preventing malaria (Cochrane Review). Oxford, Cochrane Library – Update Software, 2002.

26. ter Kuile FO, Terlouw DJ, Kariuki SK, Phillips-Howard PA, Mirel LB, Hawley WA et al. Impact of permethrin-treated bed nets on malaria, anemia, and growth in infants in an area of intense perennial malaria transmission in western Kenya. *American Journal of Tropical Medicine and Hygiene*, 2003, 68(4 Suppl.):68–77.

27. Wiseman V, Hawley WA, ter Kuile FO, Phillips-Howard PA, Vulule JM, Nahlen BL et al. The cost-effectiveness of permethrin-treated bed nets in an area of intense malaria transmission in western Kenya. *American Journal of Tropical Medicine and Hygiene*, 2003, 68(4 Suppl.):161–167.

28. Shulman CE, Dorman EK, Cutts F, Kawuondo K, Bulmer JN, Misore A et al. Intermittent sulphadoxine-pyrimethamine to prevent severe anaemia secondary to malaria in pregnancy: a randomised placebo-controlled trial. *Lancet*, 1999, 353:632–636.

29. Rogerson SJ, Chaluluka E, Kanjala M, Mkundika P, Mhango C, Molyneux ME. Intermittent sulfadoxine-pyrimethamine in pregnancy: effectiveness against malaria morbidity in Blantyre, Malawi, in 1997–99. *Transactions of the Royal Society of Tropical Medicine and Hygiene*, 2000, 94:549–553.

30. Parise ME, Ayisi JG, Nahlen BL, Schultz LJ, Roberts JM, Misore A et al. Efficacy of sulfadoxine-pyrimethamine for prevention of placental malaria in an area of Kenya with a high prevalence of malaria and human immunodeficiency virus infection. *American Journal of Tropical Medicine and Hygiene*, 1998, 59:813–822.

31. Goodman CA, Coleman PG, Mills A. Cost-effectiveness of malaria control in sub-Saharan Africa. *Lancet*, 1999, 354:378–385.

32. Schellenberg D, Menendez C, Kahigwa E, Aponte J, Vidal J, Tanner M et al. Intermittent treatment for malaria and anaemia control at time of routine vaccinations in Tanzanian infants: a randomised, placebo-controlled trial. *Lancet*, 2001, 357:1471–1477.

33. Massaga JJ, Kitua AY, Lemnge MM, Akida JA, Malle LN, Ronn AM et al. Effect of intermittent treatment with amodiaquine on anaemia and malarial fevers in infants in Tanzania: a randomised placebo-controlled trial. *Lancet*, 2003, 361:1853–1860.

34. Ekvall H, Premji Z, Bjorkman A. Chloroquine treatment for uncomplicated childhood malaria in an area with drug resistance: early treatment failure aggravates anaemia. *Transactions of the Royal Society of Tropical Medecine and Hygiene*, 1998, 92:556–560.

35. Murray C. *The global burden of disease*. Cambridge, MA, Harvard University Press, 1996.

36. UNICEF/UNU/WHO. *Iron deficiency anemia: assessment, prevention, and control.* Geneva, World Health Organization, 2001.

37. V an den Broek NR, White SA, Neilson JP. The relationship between asymptomatic human immunodeficiency virus infection and the prevalence and severity of anemia in pregnant Malawian women. *American Journal of Tropical Medicine and Hygiene*,1998, 59:1004–1007.

38. Rush D. Nutrition and maternal mortality in the developing world. *American Journal of Clinical Nutrition*, 2000, 72(Suppl.):212S–240S.

39. *Surgical care at the district hospital.* Geneva, World Health Organization, 2003.

40. Schorr TO, Hediger M. Anemia and iron-deficiency anemia: compilation of data on pregnancy outcome. *American Journal of Clinical Nutrition*, 1994, 59(Suppl.):492S–501S.

41. McDermott JM, Slutsker L, Steketee RW, Wirima JJ, Breman JG, Heymann DL. Prospective assessment of mortality among a cohort of pregnant women in rural Malawi. *American Journal of Tropical Medicine and Hygiene*, 1996, 55(1 Suppl-):66–70.

42. *Pregnancy, childbirth, postpartum, and newborn care (PCPNC). A guide for essential practice.* Geneva, World Health Organization, 2004.

43. *Managing complications in pregnancy and childbirth.* Geneva, World Health Organization, 2003.

44. *Managing newborn problems: a guide for doctors, nurses, and midwives.* Geneva, World Health Organization, 2003.

45. Morin KH. Perinatal outcomes of obese women: a review of the literature. *Journal of Obstetric, Gynecologic, and Neonatal Nursing*, 1998, 27:431–440.

46. Kendell RE, Chalmers JC, Platz C. Epidemiology of puerperal psychoses. *British Journal of Psychiatry*, 1987, 150:662–673.

47. Cox, JL. Psychiatric morbidity and pregnancy: a controlled study of 263 semi-rural Ugandan women. *British Journal of Psychiatry*, 1979, 134, 401–405.

48. Evans J, Heron J, Francomb H, Oke S, Golding J. Cohort study of depressed mood during pregnancy and after childbirth. *BMJ*, 2001, 323:257–260.

49. Josefsson A, Berg G, Nordin C, Sydsjo G. Prevalence of depressive symptoms in late pregnancy and postpartum. *Acta Obstetricia et Gynecologica Scandinavica*, 2001, 80:251–255.

50. Zuckerman B, Amaro H, Bauchner H, Cabral H. Depressive symptoms during pregnancy: relationship to poor health behaviors. *American Journal of Obstetrics and Gynecology*, 1989, 160(5 Pt. 1):1107–1111.

51. Da Costa D, Larouche J, Dritsa M, Brender W. Psychosocial correlates of prepartum and postpartum depressed mood. *Journal of Affective Disorders*, 2000, 59:31–40.

52. DiFranza JR, Aligne CA, Weitzman M. Prenatal and postnatal environmental tobacco smoke exposure and children's health. *Pediatrics*, 2004, 113(4 Suppl.):1007–1015.

53. Campbell J, Garcia-Moreno C and Sharps P. Abuse during pregnancy in industrialized and developing countries. *Violence Against Women*, 2004, 10: 770–789.

54. *World report on violence and health.* Geneva, World Health Organization, 2002.

55. Guezmes A, Palomino N. and Ramos M. *Violencia sexual y física contra las mujeres en el Perú: estudio multi céntrico de la OMS sobre la violencia de pareja y la salud de las mujeres, OMS [Sexual and physical violence against women in Peru: WHO multicentre study on violence inflicted by partners and women's health].* Universidad Peruana Cayetano Heredia, 2002

56. Ganatra BR, Coyaji KJ, Rao VN. Too far, too little, too late: a community-based case control study of maternal mortality in rural west Maharashtra, India. *Bulletin of the World Health Organization*, 1998, 76:591–598.

57. Covington DL, Hage M, Hall T, Mathis M. Preterm delivery and the severity of violence during pregnancy. *Journal of Reproductive Medicine*, 2001, 46:1031–1039.

58. Valladares E, Ellsberg M, Pena R, Hogberg U, Persson LA. Physical partner abuse during pregnancy: a risk factor for low birth weight in Nicaragua. *Obstetrics & Gynecology*, 2002, 100:700–705.

59. Huth-Bocks AC, Levendosky AA, Bogat GA. The effects of domestic violence during pregnancy on maternal and infant health. *Violence and Victims*, 2002, 17:169–185.

60. Neggers Y, Goldenberg R, Cliver S, Hauth J. Effects of domestic violence on preterm birth and low birth weight. *Acta Obstetricia et Gynecologica Scandinavica*, 2004, 83:455–460.

61. Campbell JC. Health consequences of intimate partner violence. *Lancet*, 2002, 359: 1331–1336.

62. Parker B, McFarlane J, Soeken K. Abuse during pregnancy: effects on maternal complications and birth weight in adult and teenage women. *Obstetrics & Gynecology*, 1994, 84:323–328.

63. Velzeboer M, Ellsberg M, Clavel Arcas C, Garcia-Moreno C. *Violence against women: the health sector responds.* Washington, DC, Pan American Health Organization, 2003.

64. Glasier AF, Logan J, McGlew TJ. Who gives advice about postpartum contraception? *Contraception*, 1996, 53:217–220.

65. Ozvaris S, Akin A, Yildiran M. Acceptability of postpartum contraception in Turkey. *Advances in Contraceptive Delivery Systems*, 1997, 13:63–71.

66. Lumley J, Oliver S, Waters E. Interventions for promoting smoking cessation during pregnancy (Cochrane Review). *The Cochrane Library*, Issue 3. Chichester, John Wiley & Sons, 2004

67. *WHO Antenatal Care Randomized Trial: manual for for the implementation of the new model*. Geneva, World Health Organization, 2002.

68. Whitford HM, Hillan EM. Women's perceptions of birth plans. *Midwifery*, 1998, 14:248–253.

69. Moore M, Hopper U. Do birth plans empower women? Evaluation of a hospital birth plan. *Birth*, 1995, 22:29–36.

70. Moore, M. Safer motherhood 2000: toward a framework for behavior change to reduce maternal deaths. *The Communication Initiative*, 2000 (http://www.comminit.com/strategicthinking/st2001/thinking-467.html, accessed 13 January 2005).

71. Pasinlioglu T. Health education for pregnant women: the role of background characteristics. *Patient Education and Counseling*, 2004, 53:101–106.

72. Zuniga de Nuncio ML, Nader PR, Sawyer MH, De Guire M, Prislin R, Elder JP. A prenatal intervention study to improve timeliness of immunization initiation in Latino infants. *Journal of Community Health*, 2003, 28:151–165.

73. Oakley A. *The captured womb. A history of the medical care of pregnant women*. Oxford, Basil Blackwell, 1986.

74. Villar J, Bergsjo P. Scientific basis for the content of routine antenatal care. I. Philosophy, recent studies, and power to eliminate or alleviate adverse maternal outcomes. *Acta Obstetricia et Gynecologica Scandinavica*, 1997, 76:1–14.

75. Altman D, Hytten F. Assessment of fetal size and fetal growth. In: Chalmers I, Enkin M, Keirse MJNC, eds. *Effective care in pregnancy and childbirth*. Oxford, Oxford University Press, 2004:411–418.

76. Fathalla M. Preface. *Paediatric and Perinatal Epidemiology*, 1988, 12(Suppl. 2):vii–viii.

77. Adetunji JA *Unintended childbearing in developing countries: levels, trends and determinants*. Calverton, MD, Macro International, 1998 (Demographic and Health Surveys Analytical Report, No. 8).

78. *Sharing responsibility: women, society and abortion worldwide*. New York, NY, Alan Guttmacher Institute, 1999.

79. *World contraceptive use 2001*. New York, NY, United Nations Department of Economic and Social Affairs, 2002.

80. *World contraceptive use 2003*. New York, NY, United Nations Department of Economic and Social Affairs, 2003.

81. *World population prospects, 2002 revision*. New York, NY, United Nations Development Programme, 2002.

82. Ross JA, Winfrey WL. Unmet need for contraception in the developing world and the former Soviet Union. *International Family Planning Perspectives*, 2002, 28:138–143.

83. Westoff CF. *Unmet need at the end of the century*. Calverton, MD, ORC Macro, 2001 (DHS Comparative Reports, No. 1).

84. *Safe abortion: technical and policy guidance for health systems*. Geneva, World Health Organization, 2003.

85. Bott S. Unwanted pregnancy and induced abortion among adolescents in developing countries: results of WHO case studies. In: Puri CP, Van Look PFA, eds. *Sexual and reproductive health: recent advances, future directions*. New Delhi, New Age International Limited, 2001:351–366.

86. Ganju D, Finger W, Jejeebhoy S, Nidadavoluand V, Santhya KG, Shah I et al. *The adverse health and social outcomes of sexual coercion: experiences of young women in developing countries*. New Delhi, Population Council, 2004.

87. Jewkes R, Sen P, Garcia-Moreno C. Sexual violence. In: Krug E, Dahlberg LL, Mercy JA, Zwi AB, Lozano R, eds. *World report on violence and health*. Geneva, World Health Organization, 2002.

88. Glander A, Moore M, Michielutte R, Parsons L. The prevalence of domestic violence among women seeking abortion. *Obstetrics and Gynecology*, 1998, 91:1002–1006.

89. Allanson S, Astbury J. Attachment style and broken attachments: violence, pregnancy and abortion. *Australian Journal of Psychology*, 2001, 53:146–151.

90. Marston C, Cleland JC. Do unintended pregnancies carried to term lead to adverse outcomes for mother and child? An assessment in five developing countries, *Population Studies*, 2003, 57:77–93.

91. Collumbien M, Gerressu M, Cleland J, Non-use and use of effective methods of contraception. In: Ezzati M, Lopez AD, Rodgers A, Murray CJL. *Comparative quantification of health risks: global and regional burden of disease attributable to selected major risk factors*, Vol 2. Geneva, World Health Organization, 2004.

92. Setty-Venugopal V, Upadhyay UD. *Birth spacing: three to five saves lives* (Population Reports, Series L, Number 13). Baltimore, MD, Johns Hopkins Bloomberg School of Public Health, Population Information Program, 2002.

93. *Unsafe abortion: global and regional estimates of the incidence of unsafe abortion and associated mortality in 2000*, 4th ed. Geneva, World Health Organization, 2004.

94. *The prevention and management of unsafe abortion. Report of a Technical Working Group.* Geneva, World Health Organization, 1992.

95. Van Lerberghe W. *Safer motherhood in Cambodia. Health sector support programme.* London, Cambodia JSI, DFID Resource Centre for Sexual and Reproductive Health, 2001.

96. AbouZahr C, Åhman E. Unsafe abortion and ectopic pregnancy. In: Murray CJL, Lopez AD, eds. *Health dimensions of sex and reproduction: the global burden of sexually transmitted diseases, HIV, maternal conditions, perinatal disorders, and congenital anomalies.* Cambridge, MA, Harvard University Press, 1998.

97. Huntington D, Nawar L, Abdel-Hady D. Women's perceptions of abortion in Egypt. *Reproductive Health Matters*, 1997, 9:101–107.

98. *Priority ranking of diseases based on scoring system.* Yangon, Department of Health, Ministry of Health, 1993.

99. Murray SF, Davies S, Phiri RK, Ahmed Y. Tools for monitoring the effectiveness of district maternity referral systems. *Health Policy and Planning.* 2001;16(4):353–361.

100. Mpangile GS, Leshabari MT, Kihwele DJ. Induced abortion in Dar es Salaam. In: Mundigo AI, Indriso C, eds. *Abortion in the developing world.* New Delhi, Vistaar Publications for the World Health Organization, 1999:387–406.

101. *ICPD + 5: Key actions for the further implementation of the programme of action* (http://www.un.org/esa/population/publications/POPaspects/ICPD+5%20Key%20Actions.pdf, accessed 13 January 2005).

102. Mundigo AI, Indriso C, eds. *Abortion in the developing world.* New Delhi, Vistaar Publications for the World Health Organization, 1999.

103. Vekemans M, Hurwitz M. Access to safe abortion services to the fullest extent permitted by law. *IPPF Medical Bulletin*, 2004, 38.

104. *World abortion policies 1999.* New York, NY, United Nations Populations Division, 1999.

105. Campbell J, Garcia-Moreno C, Sharps P. Abuse during pregnancy in industrialized and developing countries. *Violence Against Women*, 10:770–789, 2004.

106. International Labour Organization. *Maternity Protection Convention, 2000* (http://www.ilo.org/ilolex/cgi-lex/convde.pl?C183, accessed 13 January 2005).

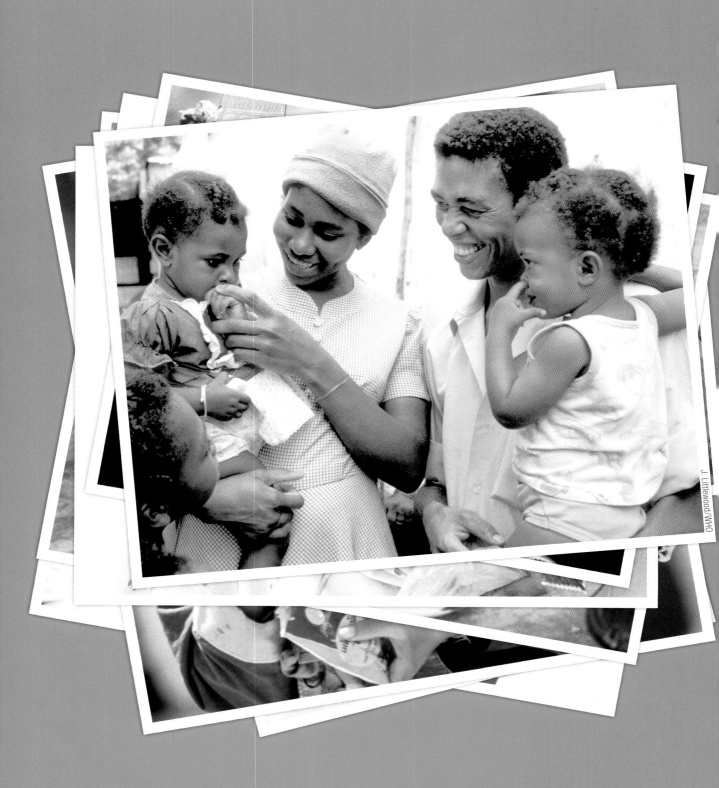

chapter four

attending to 136 million births, every year

For both mother and baby, childbirth can be the most dangerous moment in life. This chapter examines the main complications of childbirth, which claim an estimated 529 000 maternal deaths per year – almost all of them in developing countries. Most of the deaths and disabilities attributable to childbirth are avoidable, because the medical solutions are well known. Immediate and effective professional care during and after labour and delivery can make the difference between life and death for both women and their newborns. Each and every mother and each and every newborn needs skilled maternal and neonatal care provided by professionals at and after birth – care that is close to where and how people live, close to their birthing culture, but at the same time safe, with a skilled professional able to act immediately when largely unpredictable complications occur. The challenge that remains is therefore not technological, but strategic and organizational.

RISKING DEATH TO GIVE LIFE

For anyone who has been through the experience, or seen someone else go through it, there is no doubt that childbirth is a life-changing event. Unfortunately, as wonderful and joyful experience as it is for many, it can also be a difficult period, bringing with it new problems as well as the potential for suffering. In the most extreme cases the mother, or the baby, or both, may die; these deaths are only the tip of the iceberg. Many health problems are laid down in the critical hours of childbirth – both for mother and for child. Many more continue to unfold in the days and weeks after the birth. The suffering related to childbirth adds up to a significant portion of the world's overall tally of ill-health and death *(1)*. Most of the deaths and disabilities attributable to childbirth are avoidable, because the medical solutions are

well known. The challenge that remains is therefore not technological, but strategic and organizational.

Maternal mortality is currently estimated at 529 000 deaths per year *(2)*, a global ratio of 400 maternal deaths per 100 000 live births. Where nothing is done to avert maternal death, "natural" mortality is around 1000–1500 per 100 000 births, an estimate based on historical studies and data from contemporary religious groups who do not intervene in childbirth *(3)*. If women were still experiencing "natural" maternal mortality rates today – if health services were discontinued, for example – then the maternal death toll would be four times its current size, totalling over two million maternal deaths per year worldwide. The truth is that three quarters of these deaths are currently avoided throughout the world: nearly all the "natural" maternal mortality in developed countries, but only two thirds in the South-East Asia and Eastern Mediterranean Regions and only one third in African countries.

There are immense variations in death rates in different parts of the world. Maternal deaths are even more inequitably spread than newborn or child deaths. A tiny 1% of maternal deaths occur in the developed world. Maternal mortality ratios range from 830 per 100 000 births in African countries to 24 per 100 000 births in European countries. Of the 20 countries with the highest maternal mortality ratios, 19 are in sub-Saharan Africa. Regional rates mask very large disparities between countries. Regions with low overall mortality rates, such as the European Region, contain countries with high rates. Within one single country there can be striking differences between subgroups of the population. Rural populations suffer higher mortality than urban dwellers, rates can vary widely by ethnicity or by wealth status, and remote areas bear a heavy burden of deaths.

Maternal deaths are deaths from pregnancy-related complications occurring throughout pregnancy, labour, childbirth and in the postpartum period (up to the 42nd day after the birth). Such deaths often occur suddenly and unpredictably. Between 11% and 17% of maternal deaths happen during childbirth itself and between 50% and 71% in the postpartum period (4–8). The fact that a high level of risk is concentrated during childbirth itself, and that many postpartum deaths are also a result of what happened during birth, focuses attention on the hours and sometimes days that are spent in labour and giving birth, the critical hours when a joyful event can suddenly turn into an unforeseen crisis. The postpartum period – despite its heavy toll of deaths – is often neglected (4, 9). Within this period, the first week is the most prone to risk. About 45% of postpartum maternal deaths occur during the first 24 hours, and more than two thirds during the first week (4). The global toll of postpartum maternal deaths is accompanied by the great and often overlooked number of early newborn deaths and stillbirths.

Maternal deaths result from a wide range of indirect and direct causes. Maternal deaths due to indirect causes represent 20% of the global total. They are caused by diseases (pre-existing or concurrent) that are not complications of pregnancy, but complicate pregnancy or are aggravated by it. These include malaria, anaemia, HIV/AIDS and cardiovascular disease. Their role in maternal mortality varies from country to country, according to the epidemiological context and the health system's effectiveness in responding (10).

The lion's share of maternal deaths is attributable to direct causes. Direct

Figure 4.1 Causes of maternal death[a]

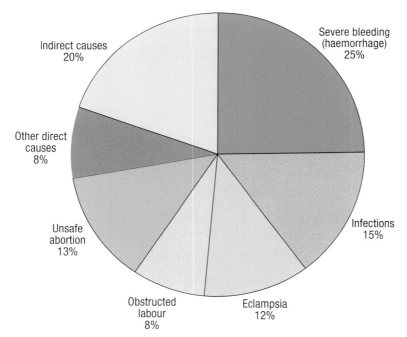

- Indirect causes 20%
- Other direct causes 8%
- Unsafe abortion 13%
- Obstructed labour 8%
- Eclampsia 12%
- Infections 15%
- Severe bleeding (haemorrhage) 25%

[a] Total is more than 100% due to rounding.

maternal deaths follow complications of pregnancy and childbirth, or are caused by any interventions, omissions, incorrect treatment or events that result from these complications, including complications from (unsafe) abortion. The four other major direct causes are haemorrhage, infection, eclampsia and obstructed labour (see Figure 4.1). The levels of maternal mortality depend on whether these complications are dealt with adequately and in a timely manner *(10)*.

The most common cause of maternal death is severe bleeding, a major cause of death in both developing and developed countries *(11, 12)*. Postpartum bleeding can kill even a healthy woman within two hours, if unattended. It is the quickest of maternal killers. An injection of oxytocin given immediately after childbirth is very effective in reducing the risk of bleeding. In some cases a fairly simple – but urgent – intervention such as manual removal of the placenta may solve the problem. Other women may need a surgical intervention or a blood transfusion, both of which require hospitalization with appropriate staff, equipment and supplies. The proportion needing hospital care depends, to some extent, on the quality of the first-level care provided to women; for example, active management of the third stage of labour reduces postpartum bleeding. The proportion that dies depends on whether appropriate care is provided rapidly. The situation with regard to postpartum bleeding could improve if the promising potentialities of the drug misoprostil are realized. Misoprostil is less effective than oxytocin, but it is cheaper, easier to store safely and does not require an injection. Therefore it remains attractive where women do not have access to professional care at birth. If further research can demonstrate its effectiveness in the many cases where oxytocin is not an option, misoprostil could save many lives and reduce the number of women who suffer anaemia as a result of a postpartum haemorrhage – currently 1.6 million every year.

The second most frequent direct cause of death is sepsis, responsible for most late postpartum deaths. During the 19th century puerperal sepsis took on epidemic proportions, particularly in lying-in hospitals. The introduction of aseptic techniques brought a spectacular reduction of its importance in the developed world *(13)*. However, sepsis is still a significant threat in many developing countries. One out of 20 women giving

Table 4.1 Incidence of major complications of childbirth, worldwide

Complication	Incidence (% of live births)	Number of cases per year	Case-fatality rate (%)	Maternal deaths in 2000	Main sequelae for survivors	DALYs lost (000)
Postpartum haemorrhage	10.5	13 795 000	1	132 000	Severe anaemia	4 418
Sepsis	4.4	5 768 000	1.3	79 000	Infertility	6 901
Pre-eclampsia and eclampsia	3.2	4 152 000	1.7	63 000	Not well evaluated	2 231
Obstructed labour	4.6	6 038 000	0.7	42 000	Fistula, incontinence	2 951

Source: *(12)*.

birth develops an infection, which needs prompt treatment so as not to become fatal or leave sequelae *(14)*. Puerperal sepsis leads to tubal occlusion and infertility in 450 000 women per year.

Hypertensive disorders of pregnancy (pre-eclampsia and eclampsia) – which are associated with high blood pressure and convulsions – are the cause of 12% of maternal deaths. They usually occur during pregnancy but also during childbirth *(15)*. Mild pre-eclampsia can be monitored in pregnancy, but the transition to severe pre-eclampsia or eclampsia requires care in a hospital environment.

Obstructed labour – owing to disproportion between the fetal head and the mother's pelvis, or to malposition or malpresentation of the fetus during labour – varies in incidence: as low as 1% in some populations but up to 20% in others. It accounts for around 8% of maternal deaths globally, while the baby may be stillborn, suffer asphyxia and brain damage or die soon after birth. Skilled practitioners, such as midwives, can deal with many of these problems before labour becomes obstructed, or recognize slow progress and refer for caesarean section or instrumental delivery. Disabilities associated with obstructed labour that is dealt with late or inadequately can be very significant both for mother and child *(12)*. For the mother the most distressing potential long-term conditions following obstructed labour are obstetric fistulae (see Box 4.1).

Of the 136 million women who give birth each year, some 20 million experience pregnancy-related illness after birth *(30)*. The list of morbidities is very diverse, ranging from fever to psychosis, and the range of care responses needed is correspondingly varied. For those women who have almost died in childbirth, recovery from organ failure, uterine rupture, fistulas and other severe complications can be long, painful and leave lasting sequelae. Other, non-life-threatening illnesses are frequent as well: in India, for example, 23% of women report health problems in the first months after delivery *(31)*. Some of these problems are temporary but others become chronic. They include urinary incontinence, uterine prolapse, pain following poor repair of episiotomy

Box 4.1 Obstetric fistula: surviving with dignity

An obstetric fistula is a devastating yet often neglected injury that occurs as a result of prolonged or obstructed labour (usually resulting in a stillbirth as well). Trauma to the vaginal wall results in an opening between the vagina and the bladder, the vagina and the rectum, or both; this leaves the woman leaking urine and/or faeces continuously from the vagina *(16)*. Without surgical repair, the physical consequences of fistula are severe, and include vaginal incontinence, a fetid odour, frequent pelvic and/or urinary infections, pain, infertility and often early mortality *(16–18)*. The social consequences of fistula are immense: women with fistula are ostracized and frequently abandoned by their husbands, families and communities; they often become destitute and must struggle to survive *(19, 20)*. To make matters worse, many women are so embarrassed by this condition that they suffer in silence, rather than seek medical help, even if such help were available.

This devastating condition affects more than two million women worldwide *(21)*. There are an estimated 50 000 to 100 000 additional cases each year *(22)*, a figure some believe to be an underestimate *(23, 24)*. Most are young women or adolescents. Early marriage, early or repeated childbearing, along with poverty and lack of access to quality health care in pregnancy and at birth, are the main determinants *(25)*. Fistulae occur in areas where access to care at childbirth is limited, or of poor quality, mainly in sub-Saharan Africa and parts of southern Asia *(26)*. In the areas where fistulae are most often seen, few hospitals offer the necessary corrective surgery, which is not profitable and for which surgeons and nurses are often poorly trained. In 2003, the United Nations Population Fund along with WHO and other partners launched a Global Campaign for the Elimination of Fistula *(27)*.

Good-quality first-level and back-up care at childbirth prevents fistula. Once the condition has occurred it is treatable *(28)*. The plight of women living with fistula is a powerful reminder that programmatic concerns should go beyond simply preventing maternal deaths. Decision-makers and professionals should be aware that the problem is not infrequent, that the girls and women who suffer from it need support to get access to treatment, that enough trained doctors and nurses need to be available to provide surgical repair, and that further support is necessary for women who return home after treatment. Collective action can eliminate fistula and ensure that girls and women who suffer this devastating condition are treated so that they can live in dignity *(29)*.

and perineal tears, nutritional deficiencies, depression and puerperal psychosis, and mastitis *(32)* (see Box 4.2). Even less is known about these morbidities than about maternal deaths. They are difficult to quantify, owing to problems with definitions and inadequate records *(33)*. More and more reliable information on the whole range of morbidities would be an important step towards better planning of services and improved care around childbirth.

SKILLED PROFESSIONAL CARE: AT BIRTH AND AFTERWARDS

Immediate and effective professional care during and after labour and delivery can make the difference between life and death for both women and their newborns, as complications are largely unpredictable and may rapidly become life-threatening *(34, 35)*. Both maternal and neonatal mortality are lower in countries where mothers giving birth get skilled professional care, with the equipment, drugs and other supplies needed for the effective and timely management of complications *(10, 34)*. The history of successes and failures in reducing maternal mortality (including in industrialized countries) shows that this is not a spurious statistical association *(3, 36)*. Reversals in maternal and neonatal mortality in countries where health systems have broken down provide further confirmation that care matters.

Successes and reversals: a matter of building health systems

Industrialized countries halved their maternal mortality in the early 20th century by providing professional midwifery care at childbirth; they further reduced it to current historical lows by improving access to hospitals after the Second World War *(37)*. Quite a number of developing countries have gone the same way over the last few decades *(3)*. One of the earliest and best-documented examples is Sri Lanka, where maternal

Box 4.2 Maternal depression affects both mothers and children

Women are between two and three times more likely to experience depression and anxiety than men. Mothers who are pregnant or caring for infants and young children are more vulnerable. Depression in women during pregnancy and in the year after birth has been reported in all cultures. Rates vary considerably, but average about 10–15% in industrialized countries. Contrary to what was previously thought, even higher rates are reported from developing countries. This contributes substantially to maternal mortality and morbidity. Parasuicide – thoughts of suicide or actual self-harm – occurs in up to 20% of mothers in developing countries. It is associated with entrapment in intolerable situations such as unwanted pregnancy (particularly in young single women), forced displacement as a refugee, or intractable poverty. Suicide is a leading cause of maternal mortality in countries as diverse as the United Kingdom and Vietnam.

Many factors contribute to maternal depression during pregnancy and after birth, including:

- unwanted pregnancy;
- poor relationship with a partner, including his being unavailable during the baby's birth, providing insufficient practical or emotional support, having little involvement in infant care, holding traditional rigid sex role expectations, or being coercive or violent;
- lack of practical and emotional support, or criticism from mother or mother-in-law;
- insufficient social support, including absence of attachment to a peer group, few confiding relationships and lack of assistance in crises;
- poverty and social adversity, including crowded living conditions and lack of employment;
- previous personal history of depression or past psychiatric hospitalization;
- persistent poor physical health;
- coincidental adverse life events, such as the loss of a partner.

Maternal depression has serious physical and psychological consequences for children. Independent of other risk factors, the infants and children of mothers who are depressed, especially those experiencing social disadvantage, have significantly lower birth weight, are more than twice as likely to be underweight at age six months, are three times more likely to be short for age at six months, have significantly poorer long-term cognitive development, have higher rates of antisocial behaviour, hyperactivity and attention difficulties, and more frequently experience emotional problems.

Effective psychological and pharmacological treatment strategies for depression exist. In industrialized countries less than half of the mothers who would benefit from such treatment receive it. The situation is much worse in the developing countries where care may be available to only 5% of women. It is important that maternal, newborn and child health programmes recognize the importance of these problems and provide support and training to health workers for recognizing, assessing and treating mothers with depression.

mortality levels, compounded by malaria, had remained well above 1500 per 100 000 births in the first half of the 20th century – despite 20 years of antenatal care. In this period midwifery was professionalized, but access remained limited. From around 1947 mortality ratios started to drop, closely following improved access and the development of health care facilities in the country *(38)*. This brought mortality ratios down to between 80 and 100 per 100 000 births by 1975. Improved management and quality then further lowered them to below 30 in the 1990s, according to Ministry of Health time series *(36)*.

Malaysia also has a long-standing tradition of professional midwifery – since 1923. Maternal mortality was reduced from more than 500 per 100 000 births in the early 1950s to around 250 in 1960. The country then gradually improved survival of mothers and newborns further by introducing a maternal and child health programme. A district health care system was introduced and midwifery care was stepped up through a network of "low-risk delivery centres", backed up by high-quality referral care, all with close and intensive quality assurance and on the initiative of the public sector authorities. This brought maternal mortality to below 100 per 100 000 by around 1975, and then to below 50 per 100 000 by the 1980s *(36, 39, 40)*.

Until the 1960s Thailand had maternal mortality levels well above 400 per 100 000 births, the equivalent of those in the United Kingdom in 1900 or the USA in 1939. During the 1960s traditional birth attendants were gradually substituted by certified village midwives, 7191 of whom were newly registered within a 10-year period: mortality came down to between 200 and 250 per 100 000 births. During the 1970s

Figure 4.2 Maternal mortality since the 1960s in Malaysia, Sri Lanka and Thailand

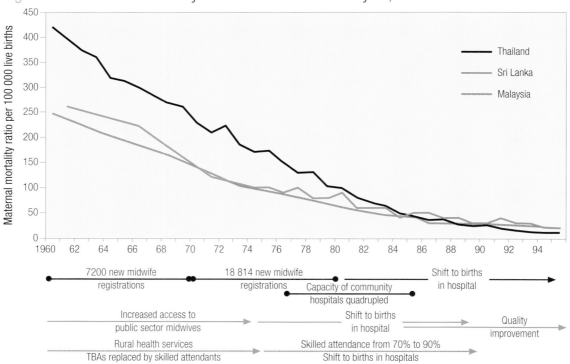

Source: *(3)*.

the registration of midwives was stepped up with 18 314 new registrations. Midwives became key figures in many villages, proud of their professional and social status. Mortality dropped steadily and caught up with Sri Lanka by 1980. The main effort then went into strengthening and equipping district hospitals. Within 10 years, from 1977 to 1987, the number of beds in small community hospitals quadrupled, from 2540 to 10 800, and the number of doctors in these districts rose from a few hundred to 1339. By 1990 the maternal mortality ratio was below 50 per 100 000 births (see Figure 4.2).

More recently, Egypt reduced its maternal mortality by more than 50% in eight years, from 174 in 1993 to 84 per 100 000 live births in 2000: major efforts to promote safer motherhood doubled the proportion of births attended by a doctor or nurse and improved access to emergency obstetric care *(41)*. Honduras brought maternal deaths down from 182 to 108 per 100 000 between 1990 and 1997 by opening and staffing seven referral hospitals and 226 rural health centres and by increasing the number of health personnel and skilled attendants *(42)*.

These examples illustrate that long-term initiatives and efforts to provide skilled professional care at birth produce results; unfortunately, the converse is true as well. Breakdowns of access to skilled care may rapidly result in an increase of unfavourable outcomes, as in Malawi or Mongolia (see Chapter 1). In Tajikistan too, economic upheaval following the break-up of the Soviet Union and newly won independence in 1991, compounded by civil war, led to a startling erosion of the capacity of the health care system to provide accessible care and a dramatic tenfold increase in the proportion of women giving birth at home with no skilled assistance *(43)*. Maternal

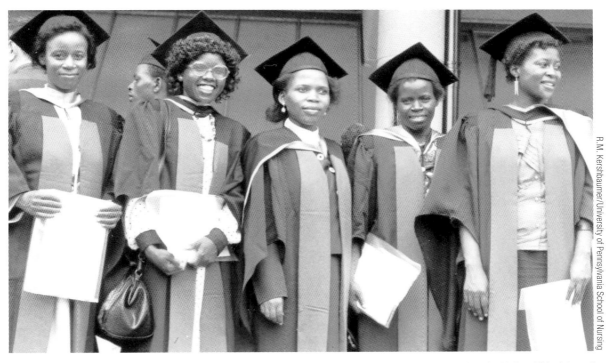

R.M. Kershbaumer/University of Pennsylvania School of Nursing

Some countries are trying to make good the shortfall in the number of midwives. This picture of nurse-midwifery graduates was taken on the day of their graduation from the University of Malawi Kamuzu College of Nursing.

mortality ratios rose as a result. Similarly, in Iraq, sanctions during the 1990s severely disrupted previously well-functioning health care services, and maternal mortality ratios increased from 50 per 100 000 in 1989 to 117 per 100 000 in 1997, and were as high as 294 per 100 000 in central and southern parts of the country *(44)*. Iraq also experienced a massive increase in neonatal mortality during this period: from 25 to 59 per 1000 between 1995 and 2000.

The good news is that countries that make a deliberate effort to provide professional childbirth care with midwives and other skilled attendants, backed up by hospitals, can improve maternal survival dramatically. As Figure 4.3 shows, it does take time, and, particularly at high levels, difficulties in measuring the evolution of maternal mortality may make it difficult to sustain the commitment that is needed.

Skilled care: rethinking the division of labour

The countries that have successfully managed to make motherhood safer have three things in common. First, policy-makers and managers were informed: they were aware that they had a problem, knew that it could be tackled, and decided to act upon that information. Second, they chose a common-sense strategy that proved to be the right one: not just antenatal care, but also professional care at and after childbirth for all mothers, by skilled midwives, nurse-midwives or doctors, backed up by hospital care. Third, they made sure that access to these services – financial and geographical – would be guaranteed for the entire population *(3)*. Where information is lacking and commitment is hesitant, where strategies other than that of professionalization of delivery care are chosen (see Box 4.4), or where universal access is not achieved, positive results are delayed. This explains why the USA lagged so far behind a number of northern European countries in the 1930s, and why many developing countries today still have appallingly high levels of maternal mortality *(3)*.

To provide skilled care at and after childbirth and to deal with complications is a matter of common sense – it is also what mothers and their families ask for. Putting it into practice is a challenge that many countries have not yet been able to meet. They have not been helped by the confusing technical terminology used by the international community: BEOC, CEOC, BEmOC, CEmOC, EOC[1], etc., to be provided by "skilled attendants" (who may be doctors, nurses or midwives), for whom the division

Figure 4.3 Number of years to halve maternal mortality, selected countries

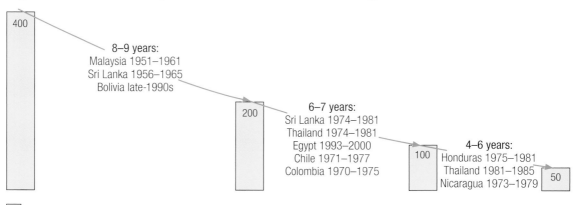

8–9 years:
Malaysia 1951–1961
Sri Lanka 1956–1965
Bolivia late-1990s

6–7 years:
Sri Lanka 1974–1981
Thailand 1974–1981
Egypt 1993–2000
Chile 1971–1977
Colombia 1970–1975

4–6 years:
Honduras 1975–1981
Thailand 1981–1985
Nicaragua 1973–1979

Maternal mortality ratio per 100 000 live births.

of tasks across these various acronyms is often unclear. Part of the confusion lies in the distinction between "basic" and "comprehensive" care, which was originally conceived as a device to monitor facilities, and not as a description of who can give care to whom in any given situation. The acronyms are even more bewildering because of the difference, still disputed, between "essential" and "emergency" care. It is time to clarify the issues.

Care that is close to women – and safe

All mothers and newborns, not just those considered to be at particular risk of developing complications, need skilled maternal and neonatal care provided by professionals at and after birth. There is a value in the rituals surrounding birth, and in keeping these as a central feature of family life. There is a consequent need and demand for care that is close to where and how people live, close to their birthing culture, but at the same time safe, with a skilled professional able to act immediately when largely unpredictable complications occur. The defining features of the type of care that is required is that it should be responsive, accessible in all ways, and that a midwife, or a person with equivalent skills, is there to provide it competently to all mothers, with the necessary means and in the right environment. This level of care is appropriately referred to as "first-level" care. Labelling it as "basic", "primary" or "routine" undervalues the complexity and skill-base required to attend to situations that can suddenly and unexpectedly become life-threatening. Table 4.2 summarizes the key features of first-level and back-up maternal and newborn care.

Recommended packages, the result of an international consensus, are extensively described in published guidelines (see Table 4.2). Most interventions, such as surveillance of the progress of labour, psycho-logical support, initiation of breastfeeding and others, have to be implemented for all mothers and newborns in all circumstances. Other elements in the package – such as manual removal of the placenta or resuscita-

---

[1] Basic Essential Obstetric Care, Comprehensive Essential Obstetric Care, Basic Emergency Obstetric Care, Comprehensive Emergency Obstetric Care, Emergency Obstetric Care.

Box 4.3 Screening for high-risk childbirth: a disappointment

Antenatal screening has a long history, dating back to the first WHO expert committee on motherhood in the early 1950s *(45)*. The idea was beguiling in its simplicity. If all women could be persuaded to attend antenatal care, screening tests could be carried out to determine which women were at high risk of developing complications; they could then be offered additional care. Although there had been evidence, from as early as 1932, that screening was not very effective *(46, 47)*, risk scoring systems were exported to developing countries. They soon became common wisdom *(48–51)* and, during the 1970s and 1980s, a mainstream doctrine under the label "risk approach" *(52, 53)*. This approach was a core component of safe motherhood strategies

for many years. International development agencies poured resources and efforts into information, education and communication campaigns to mobilize communities around a minimum of one antenatal visit for all pregnant women to identify those at risk, and those not at risk. The first group was told they should give birth in a health facility; for the others nothing further needed to be done.

In the early 1980s, the first evidence surfaced that questioned the cost-effectiveness of antenatal screening as a way to reduce maternal mortality *(52)*. The accepted wisdom began to be challenged *(54)*, with a growing view that the ineffectiveness of antenatal care "as an overall screening programme not only renders it less than what it claimed to be; it does not

even then say what it is" *(55)*. Six years later, it could be clearly stated that "no amount of screening will separate those women who will from those who will not need emergency medical care" *(56)*. Indeed, most women who eventually experience complications have few or no risk factors, and most of the women with risk factors go on to have uneventful pregnancies and deliveries. The Rooney report of 1992 formally changed the balance to scepticism *(57)*. Antenatal care is important to further maternal and newborn health – but not as a stand-alone strategy and not as a screening instrument. To ensure safe childbirth, on the other hand, skilled professional care needs to be available for all births, even the ones not at risk, according to the criteria of the 1980s.

tion of the newborn – are only needed when the situation demands it. However, it is crucial that the whole package be available and on offer to all, immediately, at every childbirth.

These interventions can only be provided by professionals with a variety of integrated skills and competences for whom the shortcut label is "skilled attendants". It is vital that a threshold of skills and competences is reached: it is not enough to be partially skilled, for example only able to carry out a so-called normal delivery. *"Any fool can catch a baby"*, as long as nothing goes wrong; as soon as a complication occurs, a situation which is difficult to predict, the level of skills and competence required to recognize the problem and decide on the right action is of a very high order. Choosing the wrong intervention or hesitating for too long to intervene or to refer the woman at the right time and in the right way can have disastrous consequences.

The prototype for a skilled attendant is the licensed midwife. Less cost-effective options include nurse-midwives and doctors, assuming they have been specifically prepared to do this kind of work (most are not – or not sufficiently). Gynaecologists-obstetricians – of whom there is a large deficit in stagnating and reversal countries – are, as a rule, perfectly able to provide first-level care, although they are less cost-effective and more appropriate for back-up referral care. There is no evidence that

Box 4.4 Traditional birth attendants: another disappointment

In the 1970s, training traditional birth attendants (TBAs) to improve obstetric services became widespread in settings where there was a lack of professional health personnel to provide maternity care, and where there were not enough beds or staff at hospital level to give all women access to hospital for their confinement. TBAs already existed and performed deliveries (for the most part in rural areas), they were accessible and culturally acceptable and they influenced women's decisions on using health services. Training them in modern methods of delivery was seen as a new way forward. In fact, this analysis was not new. In some countries such efforts had begun many years before: in 1921 in Sudan, and in the early 1950s in India, Thailand and the Philippines (58, 59).

In 1970, an interregional seminar in Malaysia, organized by WHO, recommended a wide-ranging international study of patterns of care for pregnancy and childbirth – including TBAs – in order to improve the planning of maternal health programmes (60). The study recommended the preparation of guidelines for countries regarding the training and use of TBAs. Mobilization of the community was at the core of the primary health care strategy of the late 1970s, and this idea fitted into the movement's goals (61). Tens of thousands of TBAs were trained, principally in Asia and Latin America but also in Africa (62). It was even hoped that they might conduct antenatal

clinics (63–65) and be integrated into the health system as health personnel (66, 67).

While WHO continued to encourage this strategy until the mid-1980s, some specialists began to express their doubts about its effectiveness. Evidence emerged that training TBAs has had little impact on maternal mortality. It may improve "knowledge" and "attitude", and be associated with small but significant decreases in perinatal mortality and birth asphyxia, but there are no elements to demonstrate that this training is cost-effective (68). Instead, it has become clear that the most effective measure is to provide professional skilled care, including the possibility to reach a well-equipped hospital if needed (69–73).

In most settings, it is unrealistic to suppose that a training course can have any effect on maternal mortality. Some important factors have been underestimated. First, the function, knowledge and experience of TBAs vary widely between one region and another, and even within the same country. It is not, therefore, technically valid to frame a general training strategy without taking account of these variations. Advocates, in response, claim that the fault lies not in the strategy itself but in the lack of supervision and support which has reduced its effectiveness (59, 74). However, because TBAs are in much greater need of supervision than obstetric specialists or professional midwives, this supervision would

not be sustainable in a situation in which health professionals have neither the time nor the resources for it.

A second problem is qualitative: it is not clear what TBAs ought to be taught. To change their behaviour it is necessary to understand it. This has seldom been proposed (75). Even if it were possible to alter some of the components of traditional knowledge, this can "destabilize" the whole. The social role of a TBA, like that of a traditional healer, is profoundly rooted in the local culture. It is not confined to the care to be provided for a particular pathology: it is all-embracing, and reinterprets the patient's suffering in its cultural context (76). The proponents of the TBA strategy have not appreciated the immense cultural gap between modern methods of care and the activities of TBAs.

Finally, while some specialists hope that TBAs will at least help to persuade women with complications to go to hospital (63, 65, 77), others observe the exact opposite – that they tend to delay or even deliberately discourage women from doing so (78, 79).

The strategy is now increasingly seen as a failure. It will have taken more than 20 years to realize this, and the money spent would perhaps, in the end, have been better used to train professional midwives.

Table 4.2 Key features of first-level and back-up maternal and newborn care

	First-level **maternal and newborn care**	**Back-up** **maternal and newborn care**
Defining feature	Close to client: demedicalized, but professional	Referral level technical platform
For whom?	For all mothers and newborns	For mothers and newborns who present problems that cannot be solved by first-level care
By whom?	Best by midwives; alternatively, by doctors or by doctors or nurses if correctly trained and skilled	Best by a team that includes gynaecologists-obstetricians and paediatricians; alternatively, appropriately trained doctors or mid-level technicians
Where?	Preferably in midwife-led facilities; also in all hospitals with maternity wards	In all hospitals

Note: For recommended interventions, see: *Pregnancy, childbirth, postpartum and newborn care: a guide for essential practice*. Geneva, World Health Organization, 2003; *Managing complications in pregnancy and childbirth: a guide for midwives and doctors*. Geneva, World Health Organization, 2003; *Managing newborn problems: a guide for doctors, nurses and midwives*. Geneva, World Health Organization, 2003.

lower level staff or non-professionals can deal with the complex decision-making required when complications occur at birth (see Box 4.5).

Providing close-to-client first-level maternal and newborn care is not just a matter of "carrying out normal deliveries". Such care has three functions. The first is to make sure that the birth takes place in the best of circumstances, by building a personal relationship between the pregnant woman and the professional. The second function is to resolve complications as they arise, making sure that they do not degenerate into life-threatening emergencies. The third is to respond to life-threatening emergencies when they do occur, either directly or by calling on referral-level care that has to be available as a back-up.

Contrary to what the current emphasis on life-saving emergency hospital care suggests, first-level maternal and newborn care is thus not only uneventful routine care. First-level care does save lives and manage emergencies. It does so by controlling conditions before they become life threatening (by treating anaemia, for example), or by avoiding complications (through active management of the third stage of labour, for example). A midwife or other professional with midwifery skills also actually deals with a range of emergencies on the spot, such as by administering vacuum extraction in case of fetal distress or by arranging emergency referral for caesarean section or other back-up care. What is specific about first-level care is that it takes place in an environment where a woman is comfortable with her surroundings, and where the fear and pain that go with giving birth are managed positively.

Maternal and newborn care at first level thus provides a whole package of care that can go a long way towards improving maternal and newborn outcomes. Experience shows that even in the absence of hospitals, first-level maternal and newborn care can bring maternal mortality below 200 per 100 000 – in optimal circumstances it may actually reduce maternal mortality to levels of 90 per 100 000 *(37)*. Clearly the contrasting of routine, normal deliveries with life-saving emergency hospital care is not helpful.

First-level maternal and newborn care should preferably be organized in midwife-led birthing centres, combining cultural proximity in a non-medicalized setting, with professional skilled care, the necessary equipment, and the potential for emergency evacuation. Decentralization for easy access obviously has to be balanced by the need to concentrate the staff and equipment necessary to be available 24 hours a day, something more easily done in birthing centres with a team of several skilled attendants than in solo practices. Any hospital with a maternity unit naturally also has to provide such first-level care to all the mothers and babies it admits, alongside the back-up care that is the added value of the hospital. Even within the walls of a hospital, however, first-level care should maintain the demedicalized and close-to-client characteristics of midwifery-led birthing homes.

A back-up in case of complications

In an ideal world, first-level maternal and newborn care would include all the useful interventions, including all the life-saving ones. That is obviously not possible – it would require an operating theatre in each village. That is where the back-up provided by hospitals comes in: to assist the minority of women and newborns who have problems requiring more complex care. Health workers who provide first-level care need back-up when a problem occurs that they are unable to deal with as it goes beyond their competence or beyond the means they have at their disposal. Mothers need the back-up to solve their problem, midwives (or their equivalent) need to be able rely on a back-up for their clients and to maintain credibility. Any pregnant woman has to be sure that if things go wrong, her midwife will either solve the problem or get her to a place where it can be solved.

Back-up maternal and newborn care encompasses emergencies (such as a hysterectomy for a ruptured uterus or treatment of neonatal tetanus or meningitis) as well as non-emergency interventions (such as treatment of congenital syphilis). The criterion to consider an intervention as part of back-up rather than first-level care is

Box 4.5 Preparing practitioners for safe and effective practice

There is little evidence on the best methods or models of pre-service training to prepare professionals for their future roles and responsibilities. There is more material on in-practice training that tackles what is known as the "knowledge-skills gap". Even in the latter case, however, there is little evidence that the millions of dollars spent on updating and improving skills result in improved outcomes.

Pre-service education and training is often a continuation of past local practice, and varies considerably from place to place. In the South-East Asia Region for example, all the pre-service programmes for nurses, nurse-midwives and midwives who provide maternal care, give similar skills outcomes as their objective. Nonetheless, the length of training varies considerably, from as short as three months to as long as 48 months (the median length is 24 months). There is considerable variation in

other regions as well. Experience shows that revisions to training curricula rarely result in major alterations to the entry criteria or the balance between practice and theory. Revisions to pre-service education programmes are usually incremental, adding content and prolonging training because of concerns about academic status or shifting responsibilities between ministries of health and of education.

The evidence is too weak to make specific recommendations on the optimal duration and content of pre-service training. There are, however, no examples yet of satisfactory results with models based on the inclusion of midwifery subjects in a three-year general nursing curriculum, even when the entry level is more than 10 years' education. There are no examples either of satisfactory results with curricula for which the entry level is 10 years of general education or less, even when this is

followed by three years of basic nursing and one year of midwifery training. There are two formulas for which satisfactory results have been documented in some contexts. The first is the training of nurse-midwives, with an entry level of more than 10 years' education, three years of nursing training and one to two years of midwifery. This formula has shown good results in Australia, Botswana, Kenya, Senegal, Sweden and the United Kingdom. The second formula is direct-entry midwife training: three years' combined theoretical and practical specialist midwifery training after more than 10 years of general education. This has been successful in Canada, Indonesia and the United Kingdom. The provisional conclusion is that reaching the skills threshold where a midwife or nurse-midwife can work autonomously requires a considerable investment in high-level basic training.

not whether the complication is dangerous, life-threatening or an emergency: it is its complexity. If it is technically feasible to carry out an intervention at first level, then it should be part of the first-level maternal and newborn care package.

Back-up is ideally provided in a hospital where doctors – specialists, skilled general practitioners or mid-level technicians with the appropriate skills – can deal with mothers whose problems are too complex for first-level providers. To make the difference between life and death, the required staff and equipment must be available 24 hours a day, and the links between the two levels of care should be strong. To reduce the risks and costs inherent in medical interventions and at the same time provide a responsive, humanized environment for care, overmedicalization, so often seen as part of commercialized care, should be discouraged.

Rolling out services simultaneously

First-level maternal and newborn care and the referral hospital services that should provide back-up have to be rolled out in parallel. In industrialized countries, and also in countries such as Malaysia, Sri Lanka and Thailand, first-level midwifery care has preceded reliance on back-up by hospitals. To replicate this sequence would not be acceptable today, not for authorities, not for the medical establishment, and, most importantly, not for the clients. However, reversing the sequence – that is, developing emergency hospital services only, without a network of first-level care – is not an option either. This happens now in many countries and means that a number of problems and complications are needlessly allowed to degenerate into emergency life-threatening situations.

The challenge of simultaneous roll-out has striking similarities to the one that led the primary health care movement to opt for the health districts, with both health centres and a district hospital, linked by referral mechanisms, and organized to ensure a continuum of care. More than for any other programme, the extension of coverage with maternal and newborn care depends on the development of district health care.

Postpartum care is just as important

While the need for immediate postpartum care is widely acknowledged, later postpartum care is often completely forgotten or neglected. In many low-income countries, even where the proportion of institutional deliveries is already quite high or is increasing, women are often discharged less than 24 hours after a birth *(34)*, but more than half of maternal deaths occur after this period, as do many of the newborn deaths. Despite the burden of morbidity during this period, uptake of postpartum care in developing countries is usually extremely low, typically less than half the level of uptake for antenatal or delivery care *(80)*.

Women do not, and probably often cannot, embark on care-seeking paths even when they know that they have a life-threatening condition. For many women, poverty combines with cultural constraints to construct a "social curtain" around them which health services do not penetrate *(81)*. In places where the majority of births take place at home, postpartum care may be unavailable or women may not know that services exist. Many service providers and families focus on the well-being of the new baby and may not be aware or able to assess the importance of women's complications such as postpartum bleeding *(82)*.

Where childbirth is under professional supervision, be it at home or in a health facility, women are usually expected to attend at a health facility for a postpartum checkup six weeks after delivery. This is clearly not sufficient to be effective. Moreover, these check-ups are often provided by different people, in a different location from childbirth services. Women may not attend because they do not know that the service is available to them, they may not perceive any benefit in attending, or the opportunity costs of attending may be too great *(83–85)*. Health staff themselves may not feel empowered or skilled in providing postpartum interventions *(86)*. Apart from some countries, such as Sri Lanka, rates of postnatal visits among women are low and inequitably spread. The structures that exist are often not fully suited to the needs of poor women who require better first-level care as well as easy-to-reach back-up facilities for complications. In most areas, there are severe shortages of trained health workers with adequate capability to diagnose, refer and treat these problems.

Guidelines for postpartum care exist *(87)*. They can be implemented by midwives, but also by multipurpose professionals, who may be less scarce. The need now is for a pragmatic approach to implementation in resource-poor settings, and for more attention to be paid to the handover between those who care for the mother and the baby at childbirth and those who ensure continuity afterwards.

References

1. Murray CJL, Lopez AD. Quantifying the health risks of sex and reproduction: implications of alternative definitions. In: Murray CJL, Lopez AD, eds. *Health dimensions of sex and reproduction: the global burden of sexually transmitted diseases, HIV, maternal conditions, perinatal disorders, and congenital anomalies*. Cambridge, MA, Harvard School of Public Health on behalf of the World Health Organization and the World Bank, 1998 (Global Burden of Disease and Injury Series, No. III):1–17.
2. *Maternal mortality in 2000: estimates developed by WHO, UNICEF and UNFPA*. Geneva, World Health Organization, 2004.
3. Van Lerberghe W, De Brouwere V. Of blind alleys and things that have worked: history's lessons on reducing maternal mortality. In: De Brouwere V, Van Lerberghe W, eds. *Safe motherhood strategies: a review of the evidence*. Antwerp, ITG Press, 2001 (Studies in Health Services Organisation and Policy, 17:7–33).
4. Li XF, Fortney JA, Kotelchuck M, Glover LH. The postpartum period: the key to maternal mortality. *International Journal of Gynecology and Obstetrics*, 1996, 54:1–10.
5. Alauddin M. Maternal mortality in rural Bangladesh: the Tangail District. *Studies in Family Planning*, 1986, 17:13–21.
6. Bhatia JC. Levels and causes of maternal mortality in southern India. *Studies in Family Planning*, 1993, 24:310–318.
7. Koenig MA, Fauveau V, Chowdhury AI, Chakraborty J, Khan MA. Maternal mortality in Matlab, Bangladesh: 1976–85. *Studies in Family Planning*, 1988, 19:69–80.
8. MacLeod J, Rhode R. Retrospective follow-up of maternal deaths and their associated risk factors in a rural district of Tanzania. *Tropical Medicine and International Health*, 1998, 3:130–137.
9. Kilaru A, Matthews Z, Mahendra S, Ramakrishna J, Ganapathy S. 'She has a tender body': postpartum care and care-seeking in rural south India. In: Unnithan M, ed. *Reproductive agency, medicine, and the state*. Oxford, Berghahn Press, 2004.
10. *Reduction of maternal mortality: a joint WHO/UNFPA/UNICEF/World Bank Statement*. Geneva, World Health Organization, 1999.
11. AbouZahr C. Antepartum and postpartum haemorrhage. In: Murray CJL, Lopez AD, eds. *Health dimensions of sex and reproduction: the global burden of sexually transmitted diseases, HIV, maternal conditions, perinatal disorders, and congenital anomalies*. Cambridge, MA, Harvard School of Public Health on behalf of the World Health Organization and the World Bank, 1998 (Global Burden of Disease and Injury Series, No. III):165–189.
12. AbouZahr C. Global burden of maternal death and disability. In: Rodeck C, ed. *Reducing maternal death and disability in pregnancy*. Oxford, Oxford University Press, 2003:1–11.
13. Adriaanse AH, Pel M, Bleker OP. Semmelweis: the combat against puerperal fever. *European Journal of Obstetrics & Gynecology and Reproductive Biology*, 2000, 90:153–158.

14. AbouZahr C, Aahman E, Guidotti R. Puerperal sepsis and other puerperal infections. In: Murray CJL, Lopez AD, eds. *Health dimensions of sex and reproduction: the global burden of sexually transmitted diseases, HIV, maternal conditions, perinatal disorders, and congenital anomalies*. Cambridge, MA, Harvard School of Public Health on behalf of the World Health Organization and the World Bank, 1998 (Global Burden of Disease and Injury Series, No. III):191–217.

15. AbouZahr C, Guidotti R. Hypertensive disorders of pregnancy. In: Murray CJL, Lopez AD, eds. *Health dimensions of sex and reproduction: the global burden of sexually transmitted diseases, HIV, maternal conditions, perinatal disorders, and congenital anomalies*. Cambridge, MA, Harvard School of Public Health on behalf of the World Health Organization and the World Bank, 1998 (Global Burden of Disease and Injury Series, No. III):219–241.

16. Arrowsmith SD, Hamlin EC, Wall LL. Obstructed labour injury complex: obstetric fistula formation and the multifaceted morbidity of maternal birth trauma in the developing world. *Obstetrical and Gynecological Survey*, 1996, 51:568–574.

17. Wall LL, Dead mothers and injured wives: the social context of maternal morbidity and mortality among the Hausa of northern Nigeria. *Studies in Family Planning*, 1998, 29: 341–359.

18. Faces of dignity: seven stories of girls and women with fistula. Dar es Salaam, Women's Dignity Project, 2003.

19. Murphy M. Social consequences of vesicovaginal fistulae in northern Nigeria. *Journal of Biosocial Science*, 1981, 13:139–150.

20. Kelly J, Kwast BE. Epidemiological study of vesicovaginal fistulas in Ethiopia. *International Urogynecology Journal*, 1993, 4:278–281.

21. Murray CJL, Lopez AD, eds. *Health dimensions of sex and reproduction: the global burden of sexually transmitted diseases, HIV, maternal conditions, perinatal disorders, and congenital anomalies*. Cambridge MA, Harvard School of Public Health on behalf of the World Health Organization and the World Bank, 1998 (Global Burden of Disease and Injury Series, No. III).

22. *Obstetric fistula needs assessment report: findings from nine African countries*. New York, NY, United Nations Population Fund/EngenderHealth, 2003.

23. Vangeenderhuysen C, Prual A, Ould el Joud D. Obstetric fistulae: incidence estimates for sub-Saharan Africa. *International Journal of Gynecology and Obstetrics*, 2001, 73:65–66.

24. Donney F, Weil L. Obstetric fistula: the international response. Lancet, 2004, 363:6161.

25. Wall LL, Karshima J, Kirschner C, Arrowsmith SD. The obstetric vesicovaginal fistula: characteristics of 899 patients from Jos, Nigeria. *American Journal of Obstetrics and Gynecology*, 2004, 190:1011–1019.

26. Rasheed AH. *Journeys and voices: a collection of excerpts. Obstetric fistula: a sociomedical problem in Morocco 1988–1993. Journey and voices*. International Development Research Centre, 2004 (http://web.idrc.ca/en/ev-67414-201-1-DO_TOPIC.html, accessed 20 January 2005).

27. *Campaign to end fistula*. United Nations Population Fund, 2004 (http://www.endfistula.org, accessed 20 January 2005).

28. Cook RJ, Dickens BM, Syed S. Obstetric fistula: the challenge to human rights. *International Journal of Gynecology and Obstetrics*, 2004, 87:72–77.

29. *Women's dignity project* (http://www.womensdignity.org, accessed 20 january 2005).

30. Neilson JP, Lavender T, Quenby S, Wray S. Obstructed labour. *British Medical Bulletin*, 2003, 67:191–204.

31. Bhatia JC, Cleland J. Obstetric morbidity in South India: results from a community survey. *Social Science and Medicine*, 1996, 43:1507–1516.

32. *Postpartum care of the mother and the newborn: a practical guide*. Geneva, World Health Organization, 1998.

33. Fortney JA, Smith JB. Measuring maternal morbidity. In: Berer M, Ravindran TKS, eds. *Safe motherhood initiatives: critical issues*. Oxford, Blackwell Science, 1999:43–50.

34. Graham W, Bell J, Bullough CH. Can skilled attendance at delivery reduce maternal morbidity in developing countries? In: De Brouwere V, Van Lerberghe W, eds. *Safe motherhood strategies: a review of the evidence*, ITG Press, 2001 (Studies in Health Services Organisation and Policy, 17:91–131).

35. Kowalewski M, Jahn A. *Health professionals for maternity services: experiences on covering the population with quality maternal care.* In: De Brouwere V, Van Lerberghe W, eds. *Safe motherhood strategies: a review of the evidence.* Antwerp, ITG Press, 2001 (Studies in Health Services Organisation and Policy, 17:131–150).

36. Pathmanathan I, Liljestrand J, Martins JM, Rajapaksa LC, Lissner C, de Silva A et al. *Investing in maternal health: learning from Malaysia and Sri Lanka.* Washington, DC, World Bank, 2003.

37. Loudon I. *Death in childbirth: an international study of maternal care and maternal mortality, 1800–1950.* Oxford, Clarendon Press, 1992.

38. Seneviratne HR, Rajapaksa LC. Safe motherhood in Sri Lanka: a 100-year march. *International Journal of Gynecology and Obstetrics*, 2000, 70:113–124.

39. Koblinsky MA, Campbell O, Heichelheim J. Organizing delivery care: what works for safe motherhood? *Bulletin of the World Health Organization*, 1999, 77:399–406.

40. Suleiman AB, Mathews A, Jegasothy R, Ali R, Kandiah N. A strategy for reducing maternal mortality. *Bulletin of the World Health Organization*, 1999, 77:190–193.

41. *Maternal Mortality Study 2000.* Cairo, Ministry of Health and Population., 2001.

42. Danel I. *Maternal mortality reduction, Honduras, 1990–1997: a case-study.* Atlanta, GA, Centers for Disease Control and Prevention, 1998.

43. Falkingham J. Inequality and changes in women's use of maternal health-care services in Tajikistan. *Studies in Family Planning*, 2003, 34:32–43.

44. *Situation analysis of children and women in Iraq.* New York, NY, United Nations Children's Fund, 1998.

45. *Expert Committee on Maternity Care: first report. A preliminary survey.* Geneva, World Health Organization, 1952 (WHO Technical Report Series, No. 51).

46. Browne FJ, Antenatal care and maternal mortality. *Lancet,* 1932, 220:1–4.

47. Reynolds F. Maternal mortality. *Lancet*, 1934, 224:1474–1476.

48. Lawson B, Stewart DB. *Obstetrics and gynaecology in the tropics and developing countries.* London, Edward Arnold, 1967.

49. King M. Medical care in developing countries. *A primer on the medicine of poverty and a symposium from Makerere.* Oxford, Oxford University Press, 1966.

50. Van der Does C, Haspels A. *Antenatal care. Obstetrical and gynaecological hints for the tropical doctor.* Utrecht, Costhoek, 1972.

51. Cranch G. *The role of nursing/midwifery in maternal and infant care. Nursing-midwifery aspects of maternal and child health and family planning.* Washington, DC, Pan American Health Organization, 1974:30–34.

52. Backett EM, Davies AM, Petros-Barvazian A. *The risk approach in health care. With special reference to maternal and child health, including family planning.* Geneva, World Health Organization, 1984 (Public Health Papers, No. 76).

53. *Risk approach for maternal and child health care.* Geneva, World Health Organization, 1978 (WHO Offset Publication, No. 39).

54. Smith JS, Janowitz B. Antenatal monitoring. In: Janowitz B, Lewis J, Burton N, Lamptey P. *Reproductive health in Africa: issues and options.* Research Triangle Park, NC, Family Health International, 1984:19–22.

55. Oakley A. *The captured womb. A history of the medical care of pregnant women.* Oxford, Blackwell, 1986.

56. Maine D, Rosenfield A, McCarthy J, Kamara A, Lucas A. *Safe motherhood programs: options and issues.* New York, NY, Columbia University, 1991.

57. Rooney C. *Antenatal care and maternal health: how effective is it? A review of the evidence.* Geneva, World Health Organization, 1992.

58. Bayoumi A. The training and activity of village midwives in the Sudan. *Tropical Doctor*, 1976, 6:118–125.

59. Mangay-Maglacas A. Traditional birth attendants. In: Wallace HM, Giri K, eds. *Health care for women and children in developing countries.* Oakland, CA, Third Party Publishing Company, 1990.

60. de Lourdes Verdese M, Turnbull LM. *The traditional birth attendant in maternal and child health and family planning: a guide to her training and utilization.* Geneva, World Health Organization, 1975.

61. Araujo JG, Oliveira FC. The place of caesarean section and choice of method. In: Philpott RH, ed. *Obstetric problems in the developing world.* London, W.B. saunders, 1982:757–772.

62. Chen PCY. Social background, customs and traditions. In: Wallace HM, Ebrahim GJ, eds. *Maternal and child health around the world.* London, Macmillan, 1981:71–75.

63. Estrada RA. Training and supervision of traditional birth attendants at the primary health care center level. In: del Mundo F, Ines-Cuyegkeng E, Aviado DM, eds. *Primary maternal and neonatal health: a global concern*. New York, NY, Plenum, 1983:483–493.

64. Favin M, Bradford B, Cebula D. *Improving maternal health in developing countries*. Geneva, World Federation of Public Health Associations, 1984.

65. Viegas OA, Singh K, Ratman SS. Antenatal care: when, where, how and how much. In: Omran AR, Martin J, Aviado DM, eds. *High risk mothers and newborns: detection, management and prevention*. Thun, Ott, 1987:287–302.

66. Hyppolito SB. Delegated health activity in rural areas: an experience in North Brazil. In: Omran AR, Martin J, Aviado DM, eds. *High risk mothers and newborns: detection, management and prevention*. Thun, Ott, 1987:325–339.

67. Awan AK. Mobilizing TBAs for the control of maternal and neonatal mortality. In: Omran AR, Martin J, Aviado DM, eds. *High risk mothers and newborns: detection, management and prevention*. Thun, Ott, 1987:340–346.

68. Sibley LM, Sipe TA. What can meta-analysis tell us about traditional birth attendant training and pregnancy outcomes? *Midwifery*, 2004, 20:51–60.

69. Greenwood AM, Bradley AK, Byass P, Greenwood BM, Snow RW, Barnett S et al. Evaluation of a primary health care programme in the Gambia. I. The impact of trained traditional birth attendants on the outcome of pregnancy. *Journal of Tropical Medicine and Hygiene*, 1990, 93:58–66.

70. Maine D, Rosenfield A, McCarthy J, Kamara A, Lucas AO. *Safe motherhood programs: options and issues*. New York, NY, Columbia University, 1991.

71. Koblinsky M, Tinker A, Daly P. Programming for safe motherhood: a guide to action. *Health Policy and Planning*, 1994, 9:252–266.

72. Fauveau V, Chakraborty J. Women's health and maternity care in Matlab. In: Fauveau V, ed. *Matlab, women, children and health*. Dhaka, International Centre for Diarrhoeal research:109–138.

73. Türmen T, AbouZahr C. Safe motherhood. *International Journal of Gynecology and Obstetrics*, 1994, 46:145–153.

74. Sai FT, Measham DM. Safe motherhood initiative: getting our priorities straight. *Lancet*, 1992, 339:478–480.

75. Williams CD, Baumslag N, Jelliffe DB. *Mother and child health: delivering the services*. London, Oxford University Press, 1985.

76. Singleton M. Du leurre de la douleur [The delusion of pain] . *Autrement*, 1994, 142:152–162.

77. Caflish A. Prevention of obstetric mortality in high risk pregnancy. In: Omran AR, Martin J, Aviado DM, eds. *High risk mothers and newborns: detection, management and prevention*. Thun, Ott, 1987:311–320.

78. Lawson JB, Stewart DB. *Obstetrics and gynaecology in the tropics and developing countries*. London, Edward Arnold, 1967.

79. Okafor CB, Rizzuto RR. Women's and health-care providers' views of maternal practices and services in rural Nigeria. *Studies in Family Planning*, 1994, 25:353–361.

80. AbouZahr C, Berer, When pregnancy is over: preventing post-partum deaths and morbidity. In: Berer M, Ravindran TKS, eds. *Safe motherhood initiatives: critical issues*. Oxford, Reproductive Health Matters, Blackwell Science.

81. Chatterjee M. *Indian women, their health and economic productivity*. Washington, DC, World Bank, 1990 (World Bank Discussion Papers, No. 109).

82. Thaddeus S, Nangalia R, Vivio D. Perceptions matter: barriers to treatment of postpartum hemorrhage. *Journal of Midwifery and Women's Health*, 2004, 49:293–297.

83. Lagro M, Liche A, Mumba T, Ntebeka R, van Roosmalen J. Postpartum health among rural Zimbabwean women. *African Journal of Reproductive Health*, 2003, 7:41–48.

84. Yassin K, Laaser U, Kraemer A. Maternal morbidity in rural upper Egypt: levels, determinants and care seeking. *Health care for Women International*, 2003, 24:452–467.

85. Mesko N, Osrin D, Tamang S, Shrestha B, Manandhar D, Manandhar M et al. Care for perinatal illness in rural Nepal: a descriptive study with cross-sectional and qualitative components. *LBMC International Health and Human Rights*, 2003, 3:3.

86. Lugna HI, Johansson E, Lindmark G, Christensson K. Developing a theoretical framework on postpartum care from Tanzanian midwives' views on their role. *Midwifery*, 2002, 18:12–20.

87. *Pregnancy, childbirth, postpartum and newborn care: a guide for essential practice*. Geneva, World Health Organization, 2003.

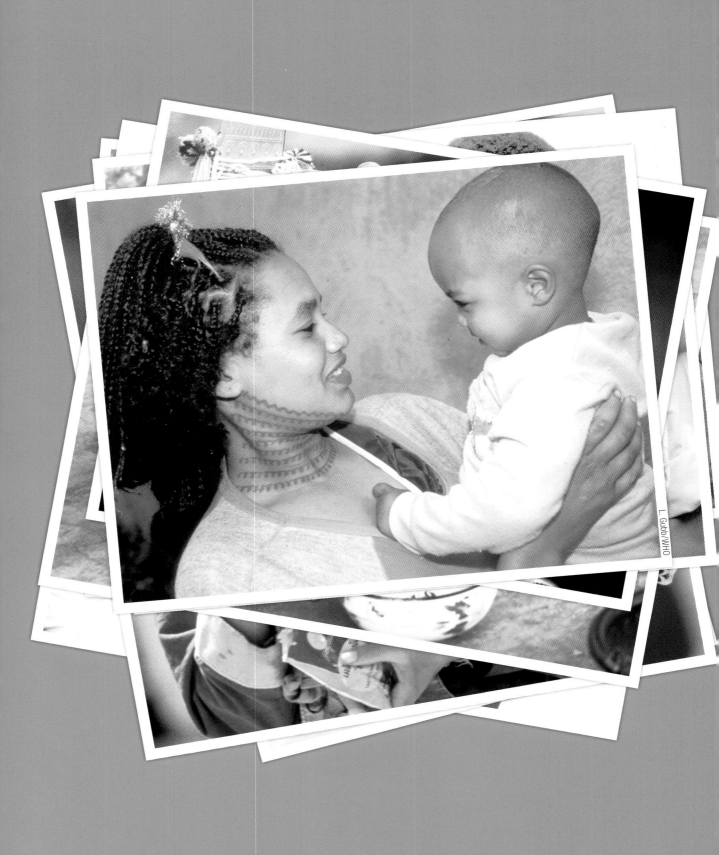

chapter five

newborns:
no longer going unnoticed

Each year nearly 3.3 million babies are stillborn, and more than 4 million others die within 28 days of coming into the world. Deaths of babies during this neonatal period are as numerous as those in the next 11 months or those among children aged 1–4 years. Until recently there has been little real effort to tackle the specific health problems of newborns systematically; the care of the newborn has fallen through the cracks, as the continuity between maternal and child health programmes is often inadequate. Improving the health of newborns, however, does not just mean inserting a new programme: rather, it means adapting the efforts of maternal and child programmes so as to scale up services in a seamless continuum of care. This chapter ends by presenting a set of benchmarks and scenarios for scaling up access to both maternal and newborn care, with estimates of the costs that such scenarios would entail.

THE GREATEST RISKS TO LIFE ARE IN ITS BEGINNING

Although a good start in life begins well before birth, it is just before, during, and in the very first hours and days after birth that life is most at risk. Babies continue to be very vulnerable throughout their first week of life, after which their chances of survival improve markedly (see Figure 5.1).

Globally, the largest numbers of babies die in the South-East Asia Region: 1.4 million newborn deaths and a further 1.3 million stillbirths each year. But while the actual number of deaths is highest in Asia, the rates for both neonatal deaths and stillbirths are greatest in sub-Saharan Africa. Of the 20 countries with the highest neonatal mortality rates, 16 are in this part of the world.

The conditions causing newborn deaths can also result in severe and lifelong disability in babies who survive. While data are limited, it is estimated that each year over a million children who survive birth asphyxia develop problems such as cerebral palsy, learning difficulties and other disabilities (1). Babies born prematurely or with low birth weight are more vulnerable to illnesses in later childhood (2) and often experience impaired cognitive development (3). There are indications that poor fetal growth during pregnancy may trigger the development of diabetes, high blood pressure and cardiovascular disease, consequences that become apparent only at a much later age (4). Rubella virus infection dur-

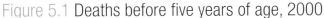

Figure 5.1 Deaths before five years of age, 2000

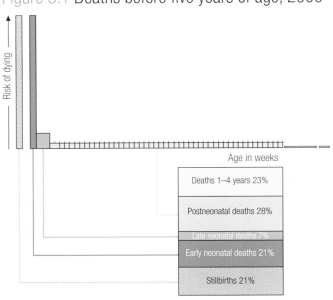

Risk of dying

Age in weeks

Deaths 1–4 years 23%

Postneonatal deaths 28%

Late neonatal deaths 7%

Early neonatal deaths 21%

Stillbirths 21%

ing pregnancy can lead to miscarriage and stillbirth, but also to congenital defects, including deafness, cataract, mental retardation and heart disease. About 100 000 babies each year are born with congenital rubella syndrome, which is avoidable through widespread introduction of rubella vaccine.

Newborns die from different causes than older children; only pneumonia and respiratory tract infections are common to both. Older infants and children in developing countries generally die of infectious diseases such as acute respiratory infections, diarrhoea, measles and malaria. These diseases are responsible for a much smaller proportion of deaths in newborns: deaths from diarrhoea are much less common, and measles and malaria are extremely rare. The interventions designed to prevent and treat these conditions in older infants and children have less impact on deaths within the first month of life.

Prematurity and congenital anomalies account for more than one third of newborn deaths, and these often occur in the first week of life. A further quarter of neonatal deaths are attributable to asphyxia – also mainly in the first week of life. In the late neonatal period, that is, after the first week, deaths attributable to infection (including

Figure 5.2 Number of neonatal deaths by cause, 2000–2003

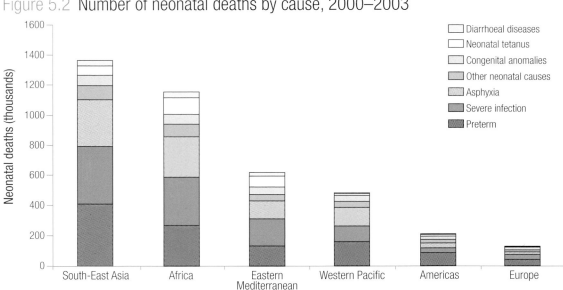

diarrhoea and tetanus) predominate; together, these causes are responsible for more than one third of newborn deaths. The importance of tetanus as a cause of neonatal death, however, has diminished sharply, thanks to intensified immunization efforts.

Direct causes of newborn death vary from region to region (see Figure 5.2). In general, the proportions of deaths attributed to prematurity and congenital disorders increase as the neonatal mortality rate decreases, while the proportions caused by infections, asphyxia, diarrhoea and tetanus decline as care improves. Patterns of low birth weight vary considerably between countries (5). Babies with a low birth weight are especially vulnerable to the hazards of the first hours and days of life, particularly if they are premature. The majority of low-birth-weight babies are not actually premature but have suffered from in utero growth restriction, usually because of the mother's poor health. These babies too are at increased risk of death.

The main causes of neonatal mortality are intrinsically linked to the health of the mother and the care she receives before, during and immediately after giving birth. Asphyxia and birth injuries usually result from poorly managed labour and delivery and lack of access to obstetric services. Many neonatal infections, such as tetanus and congenital syphilis, can be prevented by care during pregnancy and childbirth. Inadequate calorie or micronutrient intake also results in poorer pregnancy outcomes (6). It has been argued that nearly three quarters of all neonatal deaths could be prevented if women were adequately nourished and received appropriate care during pregnancy, childbirth and the postnatal period (7).

Figure 5.3 **Changes in neonatal mortality rates between 1995 and 2000**[a]

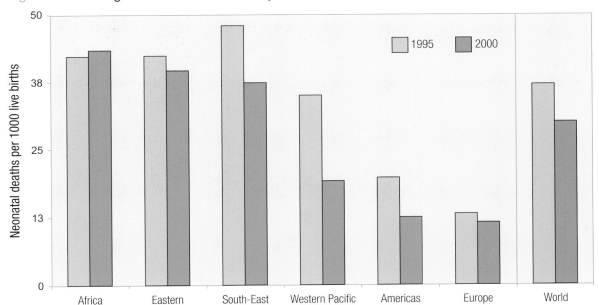

[a] Methods of calculation differed slightly in 1995 and 2000.

PROGRESS AND SOME REVERSALS

Neonatal mortality has not been measured for long enough to reach reliable conclusions on trends, but WHO estimates from 1995 to 2000 suggest that most countries in the Region of the Americas, and the South-East Asia, European and Western Pacific Regions have made some progress in reducing the mortality rate among newborns (see Figure 5.3). Improvements may have been less marked in the Eastern Mediterranean Region (but regional averages mask variations between countries), and the African Region may actually have experienced an increase in its neonatal mortality rate.

Consecutive household surveys from 34 developing countries show that most experienced a decrease in neonatal mortality over recent decades. Much of the progress in survival has been made in the late neonatal period, with little improvement in the first week of life *(8)*. This echoes the historical experience of many developed countries, where neonatal mortality (and particularly early neonatal mortality) did not begin to fall substantially until some years after a decline in post-neonatal and childhood mortality had been achieved *(9)*. In many countries, neonatal mortality has fallen at a lower rate than either post-neonatal or early childhood mortality *(10–12)*.

Household surveys also suggest that there has been reversal and stagnation in newborn mortality across sub-Saharan Africa since the beginning of the 1990s (see Figure 5.4). Indeed, the actual number of deaths has increased substantially in the African Region. In only five years, the dramatic drop in deaths in South-East Asia has meant that this region no longer has the highest neonatal mortality rate in the world; this place has been taken by Africa, where almost 30% of newborn deaths now occur.

Figure 5.4 **Neonatal mortality in African countries shows stagnation and some unusual reversals**

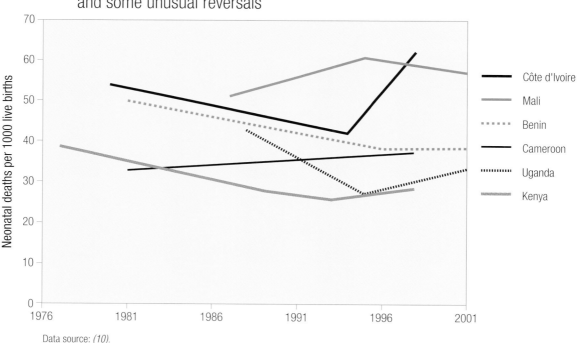

Data source: *(10)*.

Box 5.1 Explaining variations in maternal, neonatal and child mortality: care or context?

The debate over the contribution of maternal, newborn and child health programmes to saving lives is not new. Historical analyses have often indicated the important role of contextual factors such as a healthy environment, women's empowerment, education and poverty in reducing mortality levels. It can be difficult to disentangle these contextual effects from the contribution of the care provided through health systems. Poverty, for example, is often part and parcel of poorly functioning health systems as well as being part of the context in which mothers and children live. The current consensus is that both health systems and the environment – care and context – play their part, but that the balance may be different for the health of mothers from that of their children, maternal mortality depending more on health systems' efforts and less on contextual factors than child mortality.

One way to disentangle the relative contribution of care and context to mortality is to relate mortality levels across countries with various contextual or health systems indicators (21–24). There are 67 developing countries for which reliable estimates are available of the levels of maternal, neonatal, postneonatal and child mortality in 2000. For each of these countries a care score can be constructed through principal components analysis, reflecting financial inputs (total and government expenditure on health per inhabitant), human resource density (midwives and doctors per head of population) and responsiveness (determined through individual satisfaction ratings). Using the same technique it is also possible to construct a context score for each country, using the following indicators: income per inhabitant, female income, female literacy, sanitation and access to safe water (25).

Variations in country context scores explain between 10% and 15% of the differences between countries in maternal, neonatal and postneonatal mortality in a series of multiple regressions. They explain 24% of the differences in child mortality. Care scores explain around 50% of the differences in maternal and neonatal mortality, 37% of those in postneonatal mortality, and 50% of those in child mortality, with human resource density the main single explanatory factor within the care score. This suggests that care, and particularly human resources, plays a larger role in explaining the inter-country differences in mortality than differences in context.

A significant proportion of the variability in mortality levels is explained by the interaction between care and context. More detailed analysis suggests that where the context is particularly challenging even strong health systems can have only a limited effect on mortality; conversely, where there is an enabling context for health in terms of education, wealth, environment and women's empowerment, then a poor health system could hold back mortality reduction substantially. On the whole, the analysis confirms the importance of investing in health systems to reduce mortality.

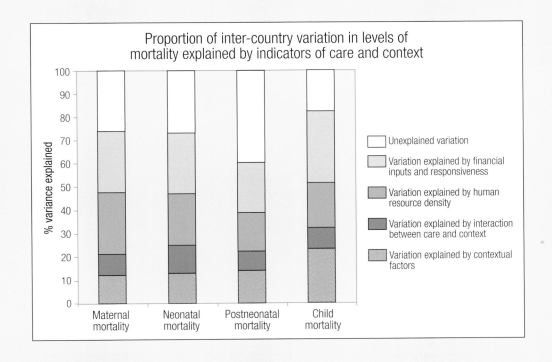

Proportion of inter-country variation in levels of mortality explained by indicators of care and context

The reversal of progress in neonatal health in sub-Saharan Africa is both concerning and unusual. Historically, declines in child mortality have often reversed when the social context deteriorated. Within Europe, these reversals mostly affected older children, while remaining modest for neonatal mortality *(13)*. The causes of the poor progress in reducing both neonatal and later childhood deaths in sub-Saharan Africa are likely to be many and complex. Economic decline and conflict are likely to have played significant roles through their disruptive effect on access to health services *(14–16)*. The impact of the HIV/AIDS epidemic on mortality is less well established for newborns than for the post-neonatal period, but infants born to HIV-positive mothers are more likely to be stillborn or premature; they are also likely to have low APGAR scores[1] and very low birth weights *(17, 18)*.

Reductions in child mortality in many countries are at least partly driven by socio-economic development: improvements in women's education and literacy, household income, environmental conditions (safe water supply, sanitation and housing), along with improvements in health services and child nutrition *(19, 20)*. While neonatal mortality is affected by these factors, they may have a greater impact in the post-neonatal and early childhood periods than for newborns (see Box 5.1). Historical data further support this hypothesis. There is little evidence that the often dramatic reductions in infant and child mortality in Europe during the first few decades of the 20th century

---

[1] The APGAR test evaluates a newborn's physical condition.

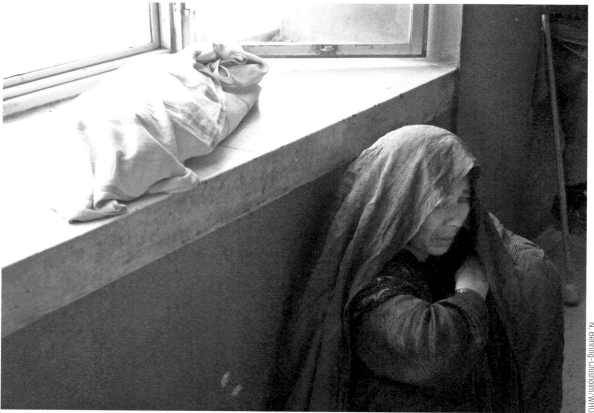

N. Behring-Chisholm/WHO

Each year more than 4 million babies die within 28 days of coming into the world, and nearly 3.3 million babies are stillborn.

were fuelled by improvements in health care provision, and most studies argue that they resulted from a number of factors including rising standards of living and nutrition, reduced fertility, safer water, better sanitation, and improved housing (26, 27). During this time, progress in reducing neonatal mortality was limited and was confined to the late neonatal period. Progress did not accelerate until around the time of the Second World War (28), which coincided with greater provision and use of maternal health care, improved quality of professional midwifery and obstetric services, and access to antibiotics. This suggests that, while some limited progress can be made in the late neonatal period as a result of general improvements in standards of living, progress will not accelerate and spread to the early neonatal period until appropriate maternal and neonatal health care is available and widely used.

NO LONGER FALLING BETWEEN THE CRACKS

It is often argued that a radical reduction of the number of newborn deaths is possible only where very high expenditure on health allows for large investments in sophisticated technology. But in actual fact, nurses and doctors can easily acquire the necessary skills without needing to become specialists. Countries such as Colombia and Sri Lanka, with fewer than 15 neonatal deaths per 1000 live births, have demonstrated that expensive technology is not a prerequisite for success. So have Nicaragua and Viet Nam, which lowered their neonatal mortality rates to 17 and 15 per 1000 births, respectively, while their spending on health in the 1990s was only US$ 45 and US$ 20 per capita, respectively. In northern European countries, well-coordinated antenatal, intrapartum and postnatal care for mothers and newborns coincided with reduced rates of mortality before the introduction of neonatal intensive care in the early 1980s (8). Intensive care facilities, specialists and expensive equipment are useful to reduce neonatal mortality even further only after very low levels have already been achieved. Rather than deploying high-tech instrumentation, the challenge is to find a

Box 5.2 Sex selection

The low value given to women and girls in some countries is reflected in a marked preference for boy children. Over the decades, this has translated into many practices that heavily discriminate against girls, such as neglect in feeding, education and health care. The practice of female infanticide has also been documented in some places.

Rapidly declining fertility and the trend to limit families to one or two children has increased the desire of couples to have a boy. The emergence and increased availability of ultrasound equipment, which can detect the sex of a fetus early in pregnancy, has opened up the opportunity for the commercial use of medical technology to pre-select and terminate pregnancies of female fetuses, thus reinforcing the devaluation of girls and women.

Over the last decade, the ratio of girls to boys in the 0–6 year age group has become increasingly skewed in a number of countries. For instance, India's census revealed that the

juvenile (0–6 years) sex ratio declined from 945 girls per 1000 boys in 1991 to 927 in 2001, with some of the steepest declines occurring among the better educated and in economically better-off districts that also have greater access to commercial health services. National records on sex ratio at birth in China and South Korea have shown similar rapid changes that are unlikely to be sustainable in the long term. The demographic impact of these adverse sex ratios is beginning to be felt in the form of a dearth of young women in some communities, thereby making women in general more vulnerable to violence, including sexual coercion and sale of brides.

Many women's rights organizations and others, in India and elsewhere, have seen prenatal sex selection as another form of discrimination against women, and have been active in moves to have such selection banned. On the other hand, in societies where giving birth to sons defines women's status and rights as wives,

daughters-in-law and mothers, sex determination and sex selective abortion allow women to gain control over at least one aspect of their lives.

This is a conundrum which cannot be resolved by focusing only on medical technology. The most severely affected countries such as China, India and South Korea have all banned prenatal sex determination through the use of ultrasound or pre-conception techniques; other measures taken include registration and regulation of genetic laboratories and ultrasound machines and self-regulation by the medical profession. Such policies have so far been largely ineffective because demand continues to be high. Various nongovernmental organizations and civil society organizations are currently involved in large-scale awareness and sensitization campaigns and in organizing a broader social debate on the devaluation of females and the consequences of sex preference.

better way of setting up the health care system with continuity between care during pregnancy, skilled care at birth, and the care given when the mother is at home with her newborn.

Care during pregnancy

Many things can, and must, be done during pregnancy. One of the most cost-effective and simple antenatal interventions is immunization against tetanus. In areas where malaria is endemic, intermittent presumptive treatment of malaria can reduce incidence of low birth weight, stillbirths, and neonatal and maternal mortality. Rubella vaccination reduces stillbirths and avoids congenital rubella syndrome. Diagnosis and treatment of reproductive tract infections reduce the risk of premature labour, as well as the direct perinatal deaths caused by syphilis. The antenatal period also presents an important opportunity for identifying threats to the unborn baby's health, as well as for counselling on nutrition, birth preparedness, parenting skills, and family planning options after the birth. Understanding the need for information and services for women who desire birth spacing methods has the potential to reduce neonatal mortality, as closely spaced births have been shown to be detrimental to the survival of the subsequent child *(29)*.

These interventions are at the core of an effective antenatal health care package. Ideally, the package of interventions should be provided by the same health worker – the midwife – who will attend the mother during childbirth; this is the best way to ensure seamless care through pregnancy and childbirth. Technically, however, antenatal care can be delegated to other health workers who would not necessarily qualify as having the required skills for attending childbirth. As multipurpose health workers are not in such short supply as midwives, they can help to increase coverage. In such cases, it is imperative, however, to establish links with those who will be in charge of mother and baby at birth: the mother needs to prepare for the birth, and the health services have to be ready to respond.

Professional care at birth

Skilled professional care at birth is as critical for the newborn baby as it is for the mother. For example, effective midwifery ensures non-traumatic birth and reduces mortality and morbidity from birth asphyxia, while at the same time strict asepsis at delivery and cord care reduce the risk of infection. Skilled care makes it possible to resuscitate babies who cannot breathe at birth and to deal with or refer unpredictable complications as they happen to mother or baby. When the birth is appropriately managed by a skilled health worker, it is safer for both mother and newborn. What, then, are the problems?

First, less than two thirds of women in less developed countries and only one third in the least developed countries have their babies delivered by a skilled attendant. Despite recent improvements in some countries, the development of effective maternal health services in many parts of the world has often been hampered by limited resources, lack of political will, and poorly defined strategies *(30)*: services have not kept up with the need for care at birth and not even with the expansion of antenatal care. Even when services do exist, quality is often poor, or social and financial barriers prevent women from making use of them. Some countries have shown high-level commitment to improving maternal health services and impressive progress in the uptake of professional care at birth (e.g. Bolivia, Egypt, Indonesia, Morocco and Togo). The general picture in Africa, however, where newborn mortality is high, is less positive.

The improvement of coverage to underserved communities is likely to prove a major challenge to many resource-poor countries for years to come.

The second problem is that the training of professional health workers who attend childbirth and the focus of their work have often been directed almost exclusively towards the safety of the mother at the moment of childbirth itself, to the neglect of the newborn and the critical week after the birth *(31)*. Newborn care is part of the curriculum and responsibility of midwives, nurse-midwives and the doctors who function as their equivalents, but in practice many of these professionals do not get the training or experience to ensure that they are competent to carry out all of the key procedures for newborns. In Benin, Ecuador, Jamaica and Rwanda, for example, only 57% of all doctors, midwives, nurses and medical interns who routinely assist at births were able to resuscitate a newborn adequately when their skills were tested *(32)*. Although the technology that is needed is actually quite simple and inexpensive, health workers can be unsure of how to deal with the sudden complications that may become life-threatening in a couple of hours, and essential drugs and equipment are usually even less readily available than they are for the care a mother may need in case of complications.

Even within a hospital, the back-up services for maternal and neonatal care that should be triggered when a complication arises are often not organized quickly enough; hospitals may not be set up to care for newborns in terms of staff training and equipment. Giving birth in a health facility (not necessarily a hospital) with professional staff is safer by far than doing so at home. But the same environment that makes for a safer birth also may put newborns at increased risk of iatrogenic infections, overmedicalization and inappropriate hospital practices. In all too many hospitals, mother and baby may be separated, which makes it difficult for mothers to bond with and provide warmth to their newborns. Babies born in hospitals in some settings are actually less likely to be breastfed than those born elsewhere *(33)*.

Maximizing synergies between maternal and neonatal health will require birthing facilities to give special attention to appropriate training of staff and the organization of care that takes account of the needs of the newborn. Facilities will also need to improve infection control, keep medical interventions to a minimum, and

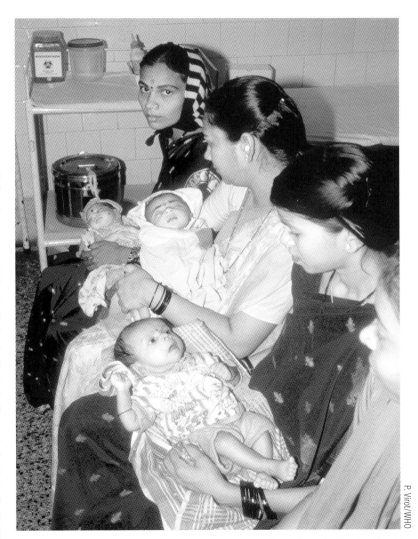

P. Virot/WHO

Professional care for newborns is often hard to get.

actively promote breastfeeding. Where quality is satisfactory, such places are much safer for mother and child than a home birth without professional assistance.

Universal access to professional, skilled care at birth for all mothers has, in combination with antenatal care, an enormous potential for reducing the burden of stillbirths and early neonatal deaths that form the majority of fetal and neonatal mortality. In most countries, the mortality of babies whose mothers benefit from antenatal care and skilled care at childbirth tends to be less than half that of babies whose mothers do not benefit from such care (see Figure 5.5). The consistency of these differences across a wide range of countries suggests that it is access to a continuum of skilled care that makes the difference.

Caring for the baby at home

Professional care at birth has less effect, however, on later neonatal deaths, which occur when the mother and newborn are at home, without professional support. Care within the household is very important for the newborn's health. If the mother has good parenting skills (which can be enhanced during the antenatal care consultations) and if she can breastfeed and keep the baby warm, it will be mostly fine: being a newborn is not a disease. In societies where women have extensive social networks, mobility, and the autonomy to control resources as well as access to good health care and information, mothers are in a better position to care for their babies. To move in that direction it helps to mobilize communities, for example through women's groups *(34)*. In Bolivia, encouraging women to participate in groups involved in promoting the health of the newborn contributed to a reduction in perinatal mortality from 117 to 44 per 1000 live births *(35)*. In Nepal, the development of a network of women's groups led to a 30% reduction in neonatal mortality rates, mainly through better uptake of services *(36)*.

Figure 5.5 Neonatal mortality is lower when mothers have received professional care

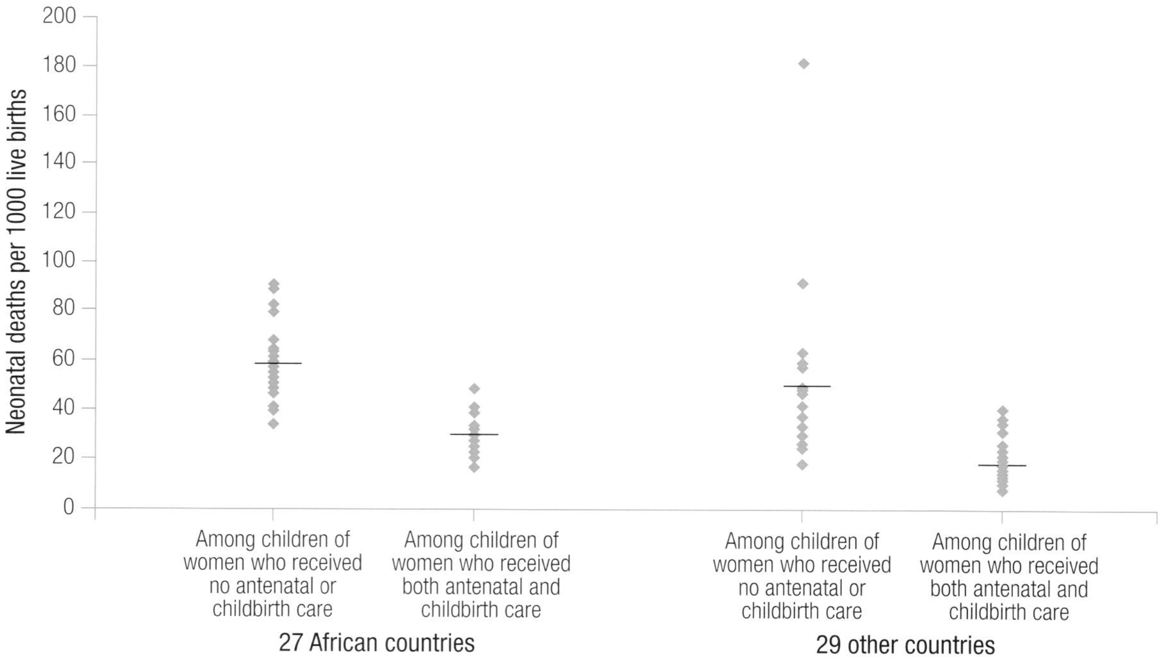

Data source: Demographic and Health Surveys.

An important aspect of caring for newborns is to seek help when problems occur. Even newborns who are not especially at risk may become ill in the days after birth: it is then important to seek professional care immediately. All high-risk babies, such as those with low birth weight, require professional care, and advice must be available to their mothers. The early weeks of life are particularly problematic because there is often no clear delineation of professional responsibilities to provide assistance to newborns in need of extra care.

Ensuring continuity of care

The handover of responsibilities of the newborn to child health services – typically from the midwife to the health centre – is a critical stage in the continuum of care. Newborn care often falls between the cracks. Maternal health services consider that their responsibility ends after childbirth or when the mother is discharged from hospital with her baby. Child health programmes, on the other hand, have been primarily aimed at preventing mortality in older children, focusing on vaccine-preventable diseases, diarrhoea and acute respiratory tract infections and less on the problems of newborns. The health workers in these programmes often tend to wait until the mother presents her child at the health centre for vaccination. Even when newborns are taken to facilities, health staff often lack confidence or have been inadequately trained to treat very young babies. Where mother and baby are confined to the home after birth, which is the case in many parts of the world, care is inaccessible unless the health worker is willing to make a home visit. In many settings there are no mechanisms for establishing communication and handover between maternal and child programmes.

There is a pressing need to develop and evaluate effective strategies for establishing a continuum of care that bridges the critical first weeks of life. In many countries – particularly in the industrialized world – there is a long tradition of home visits by health staff to check up on mother and newborn in the immediate postpartum period. In some countries this is part of the work of the midwife; in others, paediatric nurses or health visitors have the responsibility. The relative advantages of each solution are unclear, and probably depend on the local and historical contexts; all pose problems of coordination to prevent care of the newborn from slipping between fragmented services. The current shortages of professional skilled attendants mean that much of the postnatal follow-up of mothers and babies, and particularly the postnatal follow-up at home, will most often be shifted from birthing centres to health centre staff – nurses, general practitioners or paediatricians. This creates a need for attention to skills, job descriptions and mechanisms to ensure continuity of care.

Many countries today face a dilemma: either invest in the continuum of care and in access to skilled care at birth or, given the present unavailability of skilled professionals, go part of the way by investing in lay workers who could provide some of the care newborns need that mothers cannot provide themselves. Activities through which lay workers help to improve living conditions, enable women and their families to provide good care in the home, and promote uptake of services have been clearly shown to supplement professional care effectively *(36)*. Evidence for the usefulness of non-professional community workers providing treatment for newborns under routine circumstances is scantier and is subject to debate. Strategically, the question is whether this brings an added value and whether the opportunity cost is not too high, compared to focusing on expanding professional care and improving care within the home.

In countries and areas where professional skilled attendance at birth is high and increasing, developing a strategy that promotes lay community health workers would have little popular or political support compared to one that aims for universal access. It makes more sense, in such countries, to concentrate on speeding up coverage further, improving quality of professional newborn care by maternal and child health services, and establishing continuity with care at home.

The dilemma is real, however, in areas where present levels of professional skilled attendance coverage are very low. Betting on non-professional care has the appeal of doing something immediately. Ultimately, though, the objective is to roll out networks of effective professional services, to catch up with countries that started to do so in earlier decades. The existence of such professional services is in itself a precondition for lay workers to be effective. Care should be taken to avoid the mistake made in the 1980s, when a strategy of scaling up professional birthing services was replaced rather than complemented by working with traditional birth attendants (see Box 4.4). Likewise, local community health workers can complement professional services in caring for newborns, but they are not an alternative to building up professional services: the opportunity cost would be too high.

The weakest link in the care chain today is skilled attendance at birth. The main thrust of strategies aimed at improving the health of newborns should be to improve access to and uptake of professional care at birth by all pregnant women. It will be necessary to refocus care at birth to make sure that the interests of the newborn are given due attention. This needs to be done at first level and for the back-up services: timely referral here is just as important as it is in dealing with unpredictable maternal emergencies.

Overcoming the present fragmentation of care for newborns is no easy task. What is done before and at childbirth should be linked with what will happen afterwards in the home and within the services that assume responsibility for providing health care for the newborn and, later, the child. The first challenge, though, is to roll out skilled maternal and newborn care fast enough to put an end to the exclusion of nearly half of the world's newborns from the life-saving care to which they are entitled.

PLANNING FOR UNIVERSAL ACCESS

Benchmarks for supply-side needs

It would be ill-advised to separate the plan for scaling up access to newborn care from that of care during pregnancy, childbirth and the postpartum. Planning requires benchmarks. The current recommendations suggest that maternal and newborn health facilities should be organized with at least one "comprehensive" and four "basic" essential obstetric care facilities per 500 000 population, that is, one facility for 3000 births per year. These recommendations do not fit the reality of health districts, which are often considerably smaller. In sub-Saharan Africa, where most of the stagnation occurs, the average district has around 120 000 inhabitants; in South-East Asia they are often much smaller units.

Estimating the need for first-level care for mothers and babies is straightforward: eventually all should have access. The problem is to decide on the optimal level of decentralization – the compromise between access and efficiency.

The requirement for back-up care is more difficult to assess, since only some expectant mothers and their babies will eventually need such interventions – but they cannot be identified beforehand. The percentage of mothers and their babies who need such care is the subject of debate. Estimates vary considerably, without a strong empirical basis *(37)*. According to current guidelines from the United Nations Children's Fund, the United Nations Population Fund and WHO, the percentage of mothers who develop serious complications is 15% – but this does not mean that all need back-up care: many of these complications can be resolved within the first-level package. On the basis of more recent evidence and ongoing research, this percentage can probably be revised downwards, to a low-end estimate of 7%, including 2–3% who are surgical cases. The proportion of newborns requiring back-up care is often very much underestimated – while the need for sophisticated equipment to save their lives is overestimated. The percentage of newborns for whom back-up care would make the difference between survival and a high risk of dying is probably between 9% and 15%, but the evidence is scarce.

In a district of 120 000 inhabitants, and assuming a birth rate of 30 per 1000 inhabitants, there would be a workload of 3600 mothers and newborns requiring first-level care, of whom some 600–650 would also require back-up. Midwives working in a team can easily assist at least 175 births per year *(38)*. Such a district would require some 20 midwives, or equivalent skilled attendants, to provide first-level care to all mothers and their newborns in the district, in hospital and in decentralized midwifery-led birthing facilities of 60–80 beds.

A practical and cost-effective arrangement would be for one team of 9–10 midwives (or equivalent staff) to be stationed in the hospital *(38)*. The others would be stationed in other birthing facilities in the district. In a more dispersed population, smaller birthing facilities, with perhaps five midwives each, would be an option that would still provide round-the-clock service, but with higher quality control and emergency evacuation costs. In large, sparsely populated districts, the only solution may be to station individual midwives in villages – as has been the policy in Indonesia. This greatly improves access, but poses problems of quality assurance, 24-hour availability and the effectiveness and cost of emergency referral links.

A district like this would require the services of one full-time equivalent doctor and his or her supporting team to provide back-up care for the 600 or more mothers and babies with problems that go beyond the competence of the first-level staff. Given the imperative of 24-hour availability and the range of skills required for back-up care, a single gynaecologist-obstetrician per district is not a viable option. Alternatives, such as improving the skills of all-round medical staff or specialized technicians, have successfully been tried out in a large number of resource-poor countries, with considerable success. Such upgrading of skills has to cover both obstetric and neonatal care, a consideration that has received too little attention so far.

Room for optimism, reasons for caution

Where credible services are offered, uptake can increase dramatically. For example in Dakar, Senegal, the opening of a surgical theatre in an urban maternity unit immediately led to an 80% increase in the number of births in the unit. There is obviously a huge demand waiting to be tapped.

Globally the availability of nationally representative data for skilled attendants at birth is high and data are available for 93.5% of all live births. From this we know that 61.1% of births worldwide are attended by a professional who, at least in principle, has the skills to do so. Extrapolating from data available on 58 countries representing 76% of births in the developing world, the use of a skilled attendant at delivery – the key feature of first-level care – increased significantly, from 41% in 1990 to 57% in 2003, a 38% increase between 1990 and 2003. The greatest improvements occurred in South-East Asia (from 34% in 1990 to 64% in 2003) and northern Africa (from 41% in 1990 to 76% in 2003). These trends represent an increase of more than 85% in both regions. Hardly any change was observed, however, in sub-Saharan Africa, where rates remained at around 40% – among the lowest in the world. Within these regional averages there are significant differences between countries and between urban and rural areas. Almost all of the increases in births with a skilled attendant are driven by increases in the presence of medical doctors at birth. In fact, most regions, with the exception of sub-Saharan Africa, show decreasing use of other types of professional assistance. There is a marked increase in the proportion of deliveries that take place in health facilities, both in rural and urban areas (see Figure 5.6).

This tendency towards increased use of professional maternal and newborn care services should not give rise to excessive optimism. There are many places where hospitals with trained professional staff exist, and yet mortality remains staggeringly high. In 1996, for example, Brazzaville, Congo, had a maternal mortality ratio of

Figure 5.6 **The proportion of births in health facilities and those attended by medical doctors is increasing**

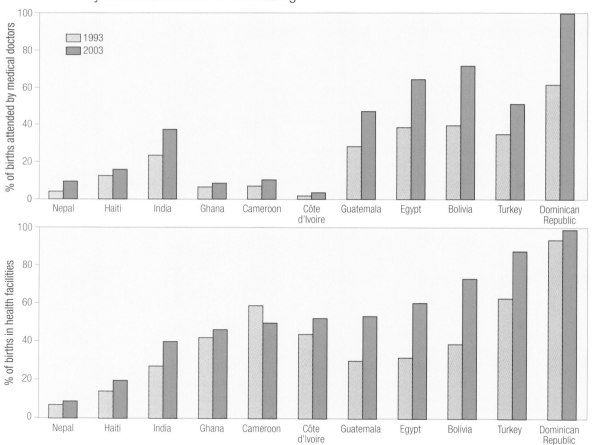

Source: Extrapolated from consecutive Demographic and Health Surveys.

645 per 100 000, university hospital and health care facilities notwithstanding *(39)*. Delivery care is not merely a matter having a hospital with trained clinicians, it is also a question of how professional staff perform and behave *(40)*.

Two tendencies are particularly worrying. First, there is the difference between what the qualification of midwife, nurse-midwife or doctor guarantees and the actual level of skills and competence. In a seminal study of their capacities in four countries, there was little correspondence between knowledge and skills, and all types of providers showed large differences between their actual skill levels and international reference standards. This was also the case for crucial life-saving skills, for newborns, and also for their mothers *(41)*.

Second, maternal and newborn care is an area where commercialization of health care delivery – overt or covert – finds a readily exploitable public. Payments for a spontaneous vaginal delivery amount to at least 2% of annual household cash expenditure in Benin and Ghana; in cases of interventions for complications, costs reached a high of 34% of annual household cash expenditure *(42)*. With an ample potential clientele, supply-induced overuse of medical technology is rife, with consequent risk of iatrogenesis and financial exploitation of clients. The worldwide epidemic of caesarean section is a typical example, but not the only one (see Box 5.3).

Closing the human resource and infrastructure gap

Information is now becoming available on the infrastructure and personnel available to provide this kind of care, but it is still very fragmentary. In Bangladesh, Benin, Bhutan, Chad, Morocco, Nicaragua, Niger, Senegal and Sri Lanka, for example, five years of monitoring the adequacy of emergency care shows a mixed picture, but with a consistent lack of first-level care in most settings and an inappropriate spread of facilities *(54–56)*. The situation is very different from country to country, but appears to be worse in the countries whose outcomes were stagnating or in reversal between 1990 and 2002.

The number of beds available in the maternity wards of health facilities of many countries is well below their needs and unevenly distributed. The main constraint, however, is the shortage of skilled professionals. Examples of the extent of the shortage in human resources can be seen in Figure 5.7, which compares the benchmarks set out above with an exhaustive on-the-spot inventory of staff in both public and private facilities. The gaps are most pronounced, in all countries, for the personnel typically entrusted with first-level maternal and newborn care.

It will take time and money to make up for these shortages: midwives are in short supply, especially outside the capital cities, and in many countries the scarcity is becoming more pronounced. It will also take time and money to establish the health care network infrastructure, both for first-level and back-up care. This is particularly true for countries in sub-Saharan Africa and others in stagnation or reversal.

Scenarios for scaling up

WHO has established scenarios to make up for these shortages in 75 countries, and move towards universal access to both first-level and back-up maternal and newborn care (details on the scenarios and associated costs are available at: http/www.who.int/whr). Together, these countries account for more than 75% of the world's population, almost 90% of all births worldwide, and approximately 95% of all maternal and neonatal deaths. At present, some 43% of births in these countries take place in health facilities, with skilled attendants, though the level of skills is highly

Box 5.3 Overmedicalization

Childbirth is an event that easily lends itself to overmedicalization. Women and their families readily follow medical advice that promotes interventions portrayed as important for the life of mother and baby. Irrational demand, commercial exploitation or defensive medicine are not uncommon. Many medical procedures are indeed life-saving and necessary. But unnecessary interventions can cause unnecessary harm and expenditure and can have serious consequences. Supply-induced demand is one of the main reasons to question the supposed better quality of the private sector, especially in the case of "for profit" providers. Four interventions are particularly subject to overuse.

Throughout the world caesarean section rates are increasing. A life-saving intervention in cases of obstructed labour or other indications, it carries risks and can lead to morbidity of its own. It also leads to what are often major and at times catastrophic expenditures for clients. Yet in some countries the number of women delivering by caesarean section is increasing beyond all reason. In the early 1990s very high caesarean section rates were essentially a Latin American phenomenon. It appears that the epidemic is now expanding throughout the world. With the exception of the African Region, caesarean section rates in the urban areas of most countries are now well above 10%; they are on the increase in rural areas as well. This means that in many countries, most of these interventions are carried out for non-medical reasons, without clear health benefits. The causes are complex, but doctors creating demand for their own financial gain certainly contribute to the epidemic. These are countries where consumer protection is becoming the priority. In contrast, caesarean section rates remain low in sub-Saharan Africa, with rates below 5% in urban areas, and below 2% in rural areas (43). These are countries where the first problem to tackle is the supply gap.

In many rich countries such unnecessary interventions carry very little risk, but elsewhere the potential for unintended adverse consequences for both infant and woman are very real. Furthermore, unnecessary caesarean sections may divert scarce resources in situations where many people cannot get the caesarean section they need for a life-threatening condition. Strategies to reduce unnecessarily high caesarean section rates have been proposed but few have been properly evaluated, or where they have been evaluated, have shown only limited success (44, 45).

Caesarean sections are not the only interventions that are becoming more frequent without medical indication and have little benefit, and which can have harmful effects and often lead to greater expenditures for patients. Episiotomy is routinely practiced without strong evidence that it protects the perineum (40, 46), and is associated with increased risk of HIV transmission, trauma and perineal tears, and dyspareunia. There is also no evidence that routine early amniotomy is useful in women whose labour is progressing normally; it does, however, increase the risk of fetal distress (47) and HIV transmission.

Another case is the abuse of oxytocin. This drug is useful during the third stage of labour to reduce postpartum haemorrhage (48). It can also be used to induce or augment labour, with beneficial effects in well-defined indications, that are guided by monitoring of labour with a partograph. The use of oxytocin is becoming increasingly common in settings where medical supervision during deliveries is minimal and partographs are not used or not even known (49, 50). In some parts of India, Mali, Nepal and Senegal, one third of women have received oxytocin during childbirth (51,52). Inappropriate use of oxytocin, especially in settings without medical supervision, can lead to fetal distress, stillbirth, uterine rupture and maternal death (52, 53).

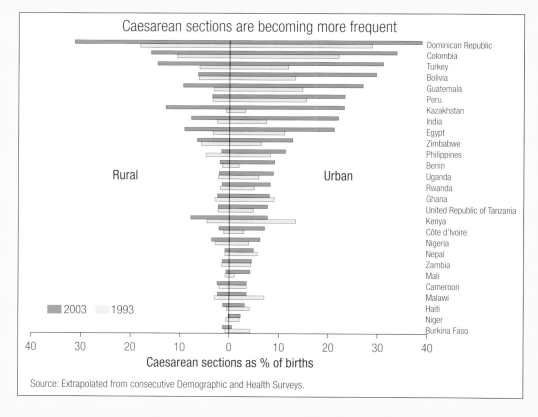

Source: Extrapolated from consecutive Demographic and Health Surveys.

variable, and only a fraction of these mothers and their babies have access to the full range of maternal and newborn health interventions. There is thus a double agenda of reaching all mothers and newborns, and of improving the quality and range of interventions made available.

The pace of scaling up depends on the specific circumstances and difficulties each country is facing. It is likely to be slowest in the countries that currently face the greatest challenges: the lowest levels of coverage, poorly developed and fragile health systems, and unfavourable circumstances. Taking into account the specific situation of the 75 countries, it seems realistic, in 12 countries, to provide access to the full set of first-level and back-up care for 95% of mothers and newborns by 2010, and to do the same in 18 other countries by 2015. For 25 countries, however, it is unlikely that coverage could be scaled up beyond 65% by 2015, and to universal access before 2025; in a fourth group of 20 countries, where current coverage is lowest, the supply gap most pronounced, health systems weakest and the environment most unfavourable, it seems possible to reach 50% by 2015, but full coverage may well require a further 15 years.

According to these scenarios, coverage with maternal and newborn care in the 75 countries taken together would grow from its present 43% (with a limited package of care) to around 73% (with a full package of care) in 2015. Table 5.1 shows some of the implications this has for the stock of health professionals and for the infrastructure for first-level and back-up maternal and newborn care. A first estimate of the potential impact of this scaling up suggests a reduction of maternal mortality, in these 75 countries, from a 2000 aggregate level of 485 to 242 per 100 000 births by 2015, and of neonatal mortality from 35 per thousand live births to 29 by the same date.

(text continues on page 98)

Figure 5.7   The human resource gap in Benin, Burkina Faso, Mali and Niger, 2001

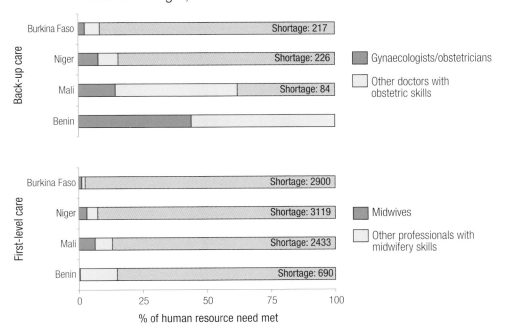

Source: Adapted from The Unmet Obstetric Need Network (http://www.itg.be/uonn/).

Table 5.1 Filling the supply gap to scale up first-level and back-up maternal and newborn care in 75 countries (from the current 43% to 73% coverage by 2015 and full coverage in 2030)

Benchmarks	Supply gap
First-level maternal and newborn care for all mothers and newborns:	Upgrading and redeployment of 140 000 of the estimated 265 000 professionals currently attending to 43% of births
1 birthing centre per 1750 births, 1 midwife or other professional with midwifery skills per 175 births	Production of midwives or professionals with midwifery skills: 700 000 by 2030 (330 000 to increase the stock and 370 000 to make up for attrition), 334 000 being produced within the first 10 years
	Upgrading and creation of 37 000 birthing units, 24 000 within the first 10 years
Back-up maternal and newborn care for at least 7% of mothers and 9–15% of newborns:	Upgrading of 47 000 doctors and technicians providing back-up services, 27 000 within the first 10 years
1 hospital per 120 000 inhabitants	Upgrading of 18 000 maternity units in hospitals, 11 000 within the first 10 years

Figure 5.8 Cost of scaling up maternal and newborn care, additional to current expenditure

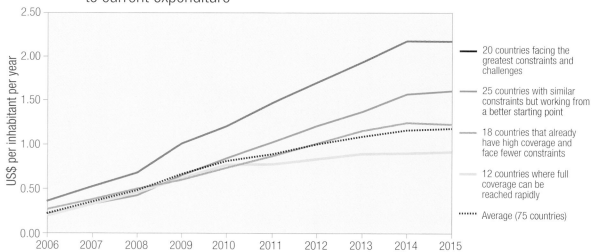

Box 5.4 A breakdown of the projected costs of extending the coverage of maternal and newborn care

The scenarios for moving towards universal coverage with maternal and newborn care in 75 countries were built around the scaling up of first-level and back-up skilled attendance at birth, and include a full range interventions aimed at reducing mortality and improving health: a package of 67 different interventions during pregnancy, birth and the postpartum and postnatal periods. The cost of implementing these scenarios, additional to current levels of expenditure in the 75 countries, increases from US$ 1 billion in 2006 to US$ 6.1 billion in 2015. Over the whole 10-year period covered by the costing exercise, 4% of the additional costs are for programme development and support. Investment in health systems (training, transport and communication, and health care network infrastructure) accounts for 22%; according to the scenarios, the yearly health system investment costs double between 2006 and 2015, but their share of the total drops from 46% to 12%.

The vast majority of the additional costs are for expanded service delivery: US$ 460 million out of the US$ 1 billion in 2006, rising to US$ 5.2 billion of the US$ 6.1 billion in 2015 (56% for first-level care and 44% for back-up care). The costs for service delivery will continue to grow, both in absolute and relative terms, after 2015, as coverage continues to expand. During the 2006–2015 period, 48% of all additional costs are accounted for by drugs, commodities and supplies, and 25% by the salaries and remuneration of the extra workforce. The latter, however, is an estimate based on current levels of remuneration, which are unlikely to be sufficient to recruit, retain and deploy health workers to the areas where they are most needed.

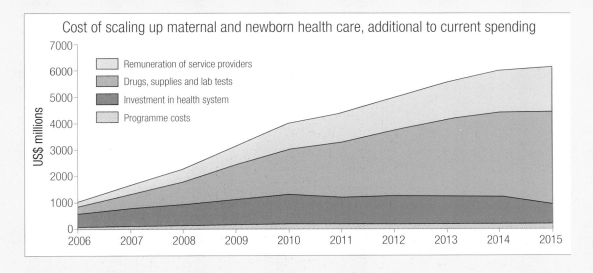

Cost of scaling up maternal and newborn health care, additional to current spending

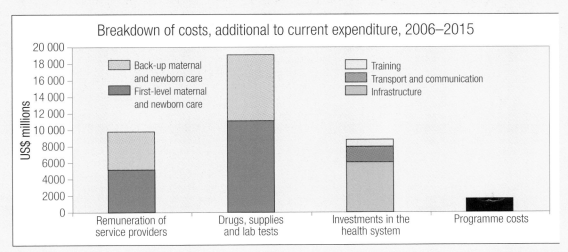

Breakdown of costs, additional to current expenditure, 2006–2015

Costing the scale up

The cost of implementing these scenarios up to 2015 is estimated at US$ 39 billion (US$ 1 billion in 2006 increasing, as coverage expands, to US$ 6 billion in 2015), additional to current expenditure on maternal and newborn health. This corresponds to around US$ 0.22 per inhabitant per year initially, expanding to US$ 1.18 in 2015 (see Figure 5.8; a breakdown of the estimated costs is given in Box 5.4).

Of this investment, 18% would be to scale up access to 50% in the 20 countries facing the greatest challenge (the equivalent of US$ 1.25 per inhabitant per year); 17% for the 25 countries that would reach 65% coverage (US$ 0.87 per inhabitant per year); 9% for the 18 countries that can reach 95% coverage by 2015 (US$ 0.74 per inhabitant per year); and 56% for the 12 countries that can reach full coverage as of 2010 (US$ 0.61 per inhabitant per year). This outlay corresponds to a growth in the level of public expenditure on health, compared with current levels, of respectively 30%, 5%, 7% and 3% per year.

The largest effort is needed in the poorest and most aid-dependent countries, despite the fact that cost estimates in these countries may be biased downwards because they reflect the current prices of labour and commodities, which are much lower than elsewhere. National authorities and the international community have to be aware that, if the scenarios are implemented, the results obtained will be slowest in the countries where the largest effort is made. In a superficial analysis this may appear an inefficient way of allocating the world's resources to maternal and newborn health – but it is necessary in order to reduce the growing gaps between countries and to move towards the MDGs in all countries of the world.

References

1. *Best practices: detecting and treating newborn asphyxia*. Baltimore, MD, JHPIEGO, 2004 (http://www.mnh.jhpiego.org/best/detasphyxia.pdf, accessed 16 February 2005).
2. Verhoeff FH, Le Cessie S, Kalanda BF, Kazembe PN, Broadhead RL, Brabin BJ. Post-neonatal infant mortality in Malawi: the importance of maternal health. *Annals of Tropical Paediatrics*, 2004, 24:161–169.
3. Grantham-McGregor SM, Lira PI, Ashworth A, Morris SS, Assuncao AM. The development of low birth weight term infants and the effects of the environment in northeast Brazil. *Journal of Pediatrics*, 1998, 132: 661–666.
4. Godfrey KM, Barker DL. Fetal nutrition and adult disease. *American Journal of Clinical Nutrition*, 2000, 71(Suppl.):1344S–1352S.
5. UNICEF/WHO. *Low birthweight: country, regional and global estimates*. New York, NY, United Nations Children's Fund, 2004.
6. Caulfield L. Nutritional interventions in reducing perinatal and neonatal mortality. In: *Reducing perinatal and neonatal mortality. Report of a meeting, Baltimore, MD, 10–12 May 1999*. Baltimore, MD, Johns Hopkins School of Public Health, 1999 (Child Health Research Project Special Report, Vol. 3, No. 1).
7. Tinker A. *Safe motherhood is a vital social and economic investment*. Paper presented at: Technical Consultation on Safe Motherhood, Safe Motherhood Inter-Agency Group, Colombo, Sri Lanka, 18–23 October, 1997 (http://safemotherhood.org/resources/pdf/aa-06_invest.pdf, accessed 15 February 2004).
8. Lawn J, Zupan J, Knippenberg R. *Newborn survival*. In: Jamison D, Measham AR, Alleyne G, Breman J, Claeson M, Evans DB et al, eds. *Disease control priorities in developing countries*, 2nd ed. Bethesda, MD, National Institutes of Health, 2005.

9. Masuy-Stroobant G. Infant health and child mortality in Europe: lessons from the past and challenges for the future. In: Corsini C, Viazzo PP, eds. *The decline of infant and child mortality: the European experience 1750–1990*. The Hague, Kluwer Law International/Martinus Nijhoff, 1997.

10. Hall S. *Neonatal mortality in developing countries: what can we learn from DHS data?* Southampton, Southampton Statistical Sciences Research Institute, 2005 (Applications & Policy Working Paper, A05/02; http://eprints.soton.ac.uk/14214, accessed 15 February 2005).

11. Hill K, Pande R. *The recent evolution of child mortality in the developing world*. Arlington, VA, BASICS (Basic Support for Institutionalizing Child Survival), 1997 (Current Issues in Child Survival Series).

12. Curtis S. *An assessment of the quality of data used for direct estimation of infant and child mortality in DHS II surveys*. Calverton, MD, Macro International Inc., 1995 (Demographic and Health Surveys Occasional Paper, No. 3).

13. Reher D, Perez-Moreda V. Assessing change in historical context: childhood mortality patterns in Spain during demographic transition. In: Corsini C, Viazzo PP, eds. *The decline of infant and child mortality: the European experience 1750–1990*. The Hague, Kluwer Law International/Martinus Nijhoff, 1997.

14. Hanmer L, White H. *Infant and child mortality in sub-Sarahan Africa. Report to Sida*. The Hague, Institute of Social Studies, 1999.

15. Simms C, Milimo JT, Bloom G. *The reasons for the rise in childhood mortality during the 1980s in Zambia*. Brighton, University of Sussex, Institute of Development Studies, 1998 (Working Paper 76).

16. Costello A, White H. Reducing global inequalities in child health. *Archives of Disease in Childhood*, 2001, 84:98–102.

17. Ticconi C, Mapfumo M, Dorrucci M, Naha N, Tarira E, Pietropolli A et al. Effect of maternal HIV and malaria infection on pregnancy and perinatal outcome in Zimbabwe. *Journal of Acquired Immune Deficiency Syndromes*, 2003, 34:289–294.

18. Brocklehurst P, French R. The association between maternal HIV infection and perinatal outcome: a systematic review of the literature and meta-analysis. *British Journal of Obstetricts and Gynaecology*, 1998, 105:836–848.

19. Rutstein SO. Factors associated with trends in infant and child mortality in developing countries during the 1990s. *Bulletin of the World Health Organization*, 2000, 78:1256–1270.

20. Cornia A, Mwabu G. *Health status and health policy in sub-Saharan Africa: a long-term perspective*. Helsinki, United Nations University/World Institute for Development Economics Research, 1997.

21. Anand S, Bärnighausen T. Human resources and health outcomes: cross country econometric study. *Lancet*, 2004, 364:1603–1609.

22. Bulatao RA, Ross JA. Which health services reduce maternal mortality? Evidence for ratings of maternal health services. *Tropical Medicine & International Health*, 2003, 8:710–721.

23. Shiffman J. Can poor countries surmount high maternal mortality? *Studies in Family Planning*, 2000, 31:274–289.

24. Filmer D, Pritchett L. The impact of public spending on health: does money matter? *Social Science and Medicine*, 1999, 49:1309–1323.

25. Matthews Z, Ensor T, Amoako-Johnson F, Van Lerberghe W. socioeconomic and health system determinants of maternal, newborn and child mortality (unpublished IMMPACT/WHO background paper for *The World Health Report*).

26. Werner D, Sanders D. *Questioning the solution: the politics of health care and child survival*. Palo Alto, CA, Heathwrights, 1987.

27. Loudon I. *Death in childbirth: an international study of maternal care and maternal mortality, 1800–1950*. Oxford, Clarendon Press, 1992.

28. MacFarlane A. *Birth counts: statistics of pregnancy and child birth* [CD-Rom]. London, The Stationery Office, 2000.

29. Mahy M. *Childhood mortality in the developing world: a review of evidence from the Demographic and Health Surveys*. Calverton, MD, Macro International Inc., 2003 (DHS Comparative Reports, No.4).

30. Inter-Agency Group on Safe Motherhood. *The safe motherhood action agenda: priorities for the next decade. Report of the Safe Motherhood Technical Consultation, 18–23 October 1997, Colombo, Sri Lanka* (http://www.safemotherhood.org/resources/pdf/e_action_agenda.PDF, accessed 16 February 2005).

31. MacDonagh S. *Creating synergies in maternal and neonatal health services.* London, Department for International Development, 2003 (unpublished Options working paper undertaken on behalf of DFID).

32. Harvey SA, Ayabaca P, Bucagu M, Djibrina S, Edson WN, Gbangbade S et al. Skilled birth attendant competence: an initial assessment in four countries, and implications for the Safe Motherhood movement. *International Journal of Gynecology and Obstetrics*, 2004, 87:203–210.

33. Bautista LE. Duration of maternal breast-feeding in the Dominican Republic. *Revista Panamericana de Salud Pública/Pan American Journal of Public Health*, 1997, 1:104–111.

34. *Working with individuals, families and communities to improve maternal and newborn health.* Geneva, World Health Organization, 2003 (WHO/FCH/RHR/03.11).

35. O'Rourke K, Howard-Grabman L, Seoane G. Impact of community organization of women on perinatal outcomes in rural Bolivia. *Revista Panamericana de Salud Pública/Pan American Journal of Public Health*, 1998, 3:9–14.

36. Manandhar DS, Osrin D, Shrestha BP, Mesko N, Morrison J, Tumbahangphe KM et al. and MIRA. Effect of a participatory intervention with women's groups on birth outcomes in Nepal: cluster randomised controlled trial. *Lancet*, 2004, 364:970–979.

37. Maine D, McCarthy J, Ward V. *Guidelines for monitoring progress in reduction of maternal mortality.* New York, NY, United Nations Children's Fund, 1992.

38. Van Lerberghe W, Lafort Y. The role of the hospital in the district; delivering or supporting primary health care? *Current Concerns SHS Papers*, 1990:1–36.

39. Le Coeur S, Pictet G, M'Pelé P, Lallemant M. Direct estimation of maternal mortality in Africa. Lancet, 1998, 352:1525–1526.

40. Buekens P. Over-medicalisation of maternal care in developing countries. *Studies in Health Services Organisation and Policy*, 2001, 17, 195–206.

41. Harvey SA, Ayabaca P, Bucagu M, Djibrina S, Edson WN, Gbangbade S et al. Skilled birth attendant competence: an initial assessment in four countries, and implications for the Safe Motherhood movement. *International Journal of Gynaecolology and Obstetrics*, 2004, 87:203–210.

42. Borghi J, Hanson K, Acquah CA, Ekanmian G, Filippi V, Ronsmans C et al. Costs of near-miss obstetric complications for women and their families in Benin and Ghana. *Health Policy and Planning*, 2003, 18:383–390.

43. Buekens P, Curtis S, Alayon S. Demographic and Health Surveys: caesarean section rates in sub-Saharan Africa. *BMJ*, 2003, 326:136.

44. Kristensen MO, Hedegaard M, Secher NJ. Can the use of cesarean section be regulated? A review of methods and results. *Acta Obstetricia Gynecologica Scandinavica*, 1998, 77:951–960.

45. Walker R, Turnbull D, Wilkinson C. Strategies to address global cesarean section rates: a review of the evidence. *Birth*, 2002, 29:28–39.

46. Carroli G, Belizan J. Episiotomy for vaginal birth (Cochrane Review). Cochrane Database of Systematic Reviews, 1999, 3:CD000081.

47. Fraser WD, Turcot L, Krauss I, Brisson-Carrol G. Amniotomy for shortening spontaneous labour (Cochrane Review). *Cochrane Database of Systematic Reviews*, 1999, 4:CD000015.

48. Elbourne DR, Prendiville WJ, Carroli G, Wood J, McDonald S. Prophylactic use of oxytocin in the third stage of labour. *Cochrane Database of Systematic Reviews*, 2001, 4:CD001808.

49. Jeffery P, Jeffery R, Lyon A. Labour pains and labour power, London, Zed Books, 1989.

50. Van Hollen C. Invoking vali: painful technologies of modern birth in south India. *Medical Anthropology Quarterly*, 2003, 17:49–77.

51. Bouvier-Colle MH, Prual A, de Bernis L et le groupe MOMA. *Morbidité maternelle en Afrique de l'Ouest. Resultats d'une enquete en population a Abidjan, Bamako, Niamey, Nouakchott, Ougadougou, Saint-louis et Kaolack [Maternal mortality in West Africa. Results from a population-based survey in Abidjan, Bamako, Niamey, Nouakchott, Ougadougou, Saint-louis et Kaolack].* Paris, Ministère des Affaires Etrangères – Cooperation et Francophonie, 1998.

52. Ellis M, Manandhar N, Manandhar DS, Costello AM. Risk factors for neonatal encephalopathy in Kathmandu, Nepal, a developing country: unmatched case-control study. *BMJ*, 2000, 320:1229–1236.

53. Dujardin B, Boutsen M, De S, I, Kulker R, Manshande JP, Bailey J et al. Oxytocics in developing countries. *International Journal of Gynecology and Obstetrics*, 1995, 50:243–251.

54. AMDD Working Group on Indicators. Program note. Using UN process indicators to assess needs in emergency obstetric services in Morocco, Nicaragua and Sri Lanka. *International Journal of Gynecology and Obstetrics*, 2003, 80:222–230.

55. AMDD Working Group on Indicators. Program note. Using UN process indicators to assess needs in emergency obstetric services: Bhutan, Cameroon and Rajasthan, India. *International Journal of Gynecology and Obstetrics*, 2002, 77: 277–284.

56. Goodburn EA, Hussein J, Lema V, Damisoni H, Graham W. Monitoring obstetric services: putting the UN guidelines into practice in Malawi. I: developing the system. *International Journal of Gynecology and Obstetrics*, 2001, 74:105–117.

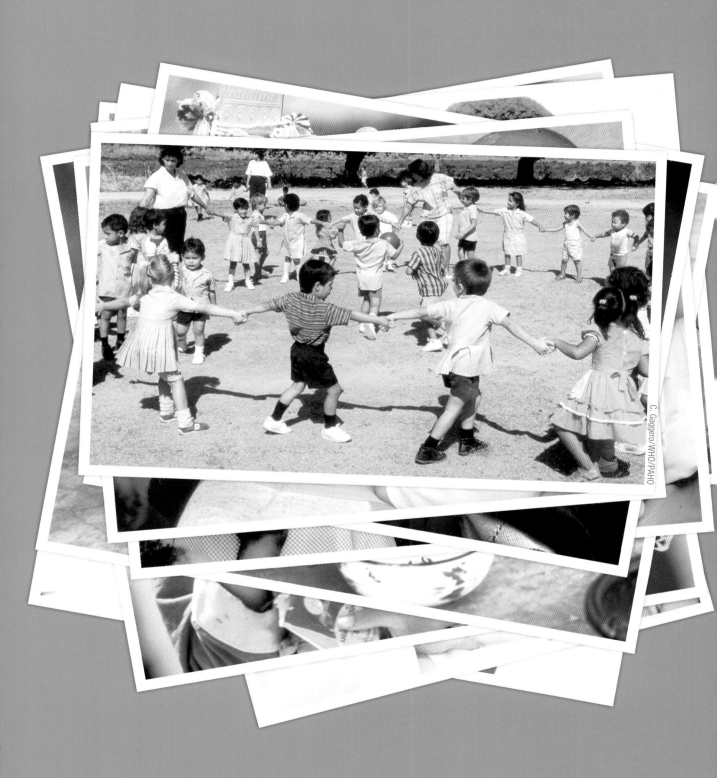

chapter six
redesigning child care:
survival, growth and development

The knowledge and effective interventions for reducing child mortality are available and technically appropriate to the countries and areas that need them most. This chapter says that what is now needed is to implement them to scale. Over the last half-century there has been a shift in focus from diseases to children, and from health centres alone to a continuum of care that implicates families and communities, health centres, and referral-level hospitals. Our understanding of the underlying skills that mothers need to care adequately for their children has grown and changed. As child health programmes continue to move towards integration, we need to move from small-scale projects to universal implementation that will also reach those children we are currently not reaching. Finally, the chapter provides the additional costs of scaling up that will be needed to reach all children with the appropriate interventions and meet the challenge of the Millennium Development Goal.

IMPROVING THE CHANCES OF SURVIVAL

The ambitions of the primary health care movement

During the 1970s, socioeconomic development and improved basic living conditions – clean water, sanitation and nutrition – were seen as the keys to improving child health. The primary health care movement, with its commitment to tackle the underlying social, economic and political causes of poor health, integrated this notion but outlined a strategy which would also respond more equitably, appropriately and effectively to basic health care needs. Along with intersectoral action for health, community involvement and self-reliance, primary health care stood for universal access to care and coverage on the basis of need. Much of the primary health care strategy was designed with the health of children as the priority of priorities.

The ambitions of the primary health care movement were vast. To implement its strategy, resources would have had to be redistributed, health personnel reoriented and the whole design, planning and management of the health system overhauled. This was clearly a long-term endeavour that would have required a major increase in funds being made available to the sector.

The successes of vertical programmes

The economic situation at the end of the 1970s, however, did not allow for such a development. Setting up primary health care systems in a context of shrinking resources was a daunting task. While countries struggled with the complexities of long-term socioeconomic development, child health – and particularly child survival – was such an obvious emergency that pressure for immediate action mounted. Therefore, by the early 1980s, many countries shifted their focus from primary health care systems to vertical, "single-issue", programmes that promised cheaper and faster results.

The most visible illustration of this shift was the Child Survival Revolution of the 1980s, spearheaded by the United Nations Children's Fund (UNICEF), and built around a package of interventions grouped under the acronym GOBI (growth monitoring, oral rehydration therapy for diarrhoea, breastfeeding, and immunization). Donors and ministries of health responded enthusiastically, particularly to initiatives prioritizing immunization and oral rehydration therapy. Many countries set up programmes for this purpose. Like the malaria and smallpox programmes of the 1950s and 1960s, each one had its own administration and budget and a large amount of autonomy from the conventional health care delivery system.

These programmes benefited from the support of dedicated programmes within WHO: the Expanded Programme on Immunization of the mid-1970s, and, later, those created to reinforce national programmes for Control of Diarrhoeal Disease and Acute Respiratory Infections. At country level these vertical programmes successfully tackled a number of priority diseases.

The Expanded Programme on Immunization started in 1974 and widened the range of vaccines routinely provided, from smallpox, BCG and DTP to include polio and measles. It set out to increase coverage in line with the international commitment to achieve the universal child immunization goal of 80% coverage in every country. The 1980s did indeed see a huge increase in coverage (see Figure 2.2 in Chapter 2). In 1988, when the World Health Assembly resolved to eradicate polio, there were some 350 000 cases worldwide; by January 2005 there were only 1185 cases reported. Thanks to sustained efforts to promote immunization, deaths from measles decreased by 39% between 1999 and 2003 *(1)*; compared to levels in 1980, measles mortality has declined by 80%. Efforts continue to increase coverage and widen the range of vaccines provided. The vaccination schedule is under constant revision as new vaccines become available, for example those against Hepatitis B and *Haemophilus influenzae* type b, and, in the near future, rotavirus (diarrhoea) and pneumococcus (pneumonia).

These vertical programmes used a combination of state-of-the-art management and simple technologies based on solid research. The prototype for this was oral rehydration therapy, the "medical discovery of the century" *(2, 3)* – a cheap and effective way to tackle mortality from diarrhoea. Widespread introduction of oral rehydration therapy largely contributed to reducing the number of deaths due to diarrhoea from 4.6 million per year in the 1970s to 3.3 million per year in the 1980s and 1.8 million in 2000.

As mortality from diarrhoea and vaccine-preventable diseases decreased, pneumonia came to the foreground as a cause of death, and in the early 1980s programmes were developed around simplified diagnostic and treatment techniques. In the meantime promotion of breastfeeding continued, backed up by international initiatives such as the International Code of Marketing of Breast-milk Substitutes (adopted by the World Health Assembly in 1981) and the Global Strategy for Infant and Young Child Feeding (endorsed by the World Health Assembly and by the UNICEF Executive Board in 2002). Advances were made possible by new insights into the optimal duration of exclusive breastfeeding and feeding for babies born to HIV-infected women. Countries widely implemented the Baby-Friendly Hospitals initiative to support promotion of breastfeeding in maternities. In 1990, less than one fifth of mothers gave exclusive breastfeeding for four months; by 2002 that figure had doubled to 38%.

Some countries had impressive successes with such programmatic approaches, and went beyond the small number of priority programmes that had international attention. Tunisia, for example, used the managerial experience gained in its first successful programmes to expand the range of health problems addressed, organizing delivery of these programmes through its network of health centres and hospitals. The country reduced the under-five mortality rate by 50% between 1970 and 1980, 48% between 1980 and 1990 and 46% between 1990 and 2000.

TIME FOR A CHANGE OF STRATEGY

Combining a wider range of interventions

For all their impressive results, the inherent limitations of these vertical approaches soon became apparent. In their daily practice health workers have to deal with a large range of situations and health problems. A feverish and irritable child that has difficulty eating can be suffering from a single illness, such as dysentery, or from a combination of diseases, such as malaria and pneumonia *(3–8)*. Single-issue programmes were not designed to provide guidance on how to deal with such situations. There was

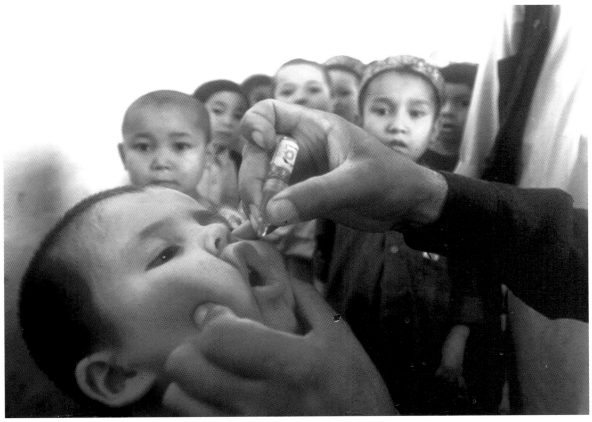

J.M. Giboux/WHO

In 1988 when the World Health Assembly resolved to eradicate polio, there were some 350 000 cases worldwide; by January 2005 there were only 1185 cases reported.

Box 6.1 What do children die of today?

Despite the substantial reductions in the number of deaths observed in recent decades, around 10.6 million children still die every year before reaching their fifth birthday. Almost all of these deaths occur in low-income and middle-income countries. A global picture of what these children die from has emerged during the past few years in a collaborative effort between WHO, UNICEF, and a group of independent technical experts, the Child Health Epidemiology Reference Group (CHERG).

Most deaths among children under five years are still attributable to just a handful of conditions and are avoidable through existing interventions. Six conditions account for 70% to over 90% of all these deaths. These are: acute lower respiratory infections, mostly pneumonia (19%), diarrhoea (18%), malaria (8%), measles (4%), HIV/AIDS (3%), and neonatal conditions, mainly preterm birth, birth asphyxia, and infections (37%).

Malnutrition increases the risk of dying from these diseases. Over half of all child deaths occur in children who are underweight. The relative importance of the various causes of death has changed with the decline in mortality from diarrhoea and many of the vaccine-preventable diseases. The relative contribution of HIV/AIDS to the total mortality of children under five years of age, especially in sub-Saharan Africa, has been increasing steadily: in 1990 it accounted for around 2% of under-five mortality in the African Region, but in 2003 the figure had reached about 6.5%.

Summarizing data across regions and countries masks substantial differences in the distribution of causes of death. Approximately 90% of all malaria and HIV/AIDS deaths in children, more than 50% of measles deaths and about 40% of pneumonia and diarrhoea deaths are in the African Region. On the other hand, deaths from injuries and noncommunicable diseases other than congenital anomalies account for 20–30% of under-five deaths in the Region of the Americas and in the European and Western Pacific Regions.

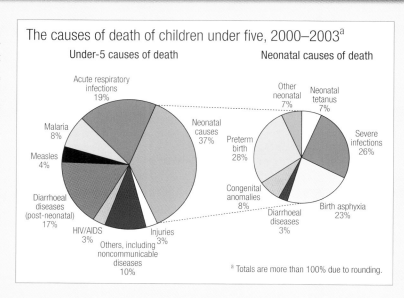

The causes of death of children under five, 2000–2003[a]

Under-5 causes of death

Neonatal causes of death

[a] Totals are more than 100% due to rounding.

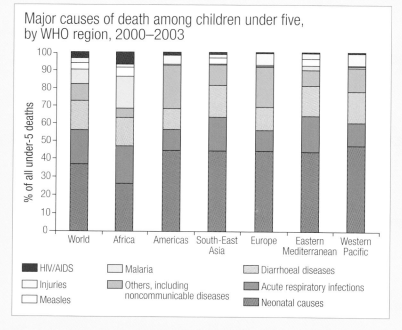

Major causes of death among children under five, by WHO region, 2000–2003

clearly a need for a more comprehensive view of the needs of the child, one that would correspond to problems as they were encountered in the field *(4)* and would offer a wider range of responses than the existing programmes. These had been designed to target the most important causes of death and, partly as a result of their success, the profile of mortality was changing. Diarrhoea, for example, now causes 18% of childhood deaths, as opposed to 25% in the 1970s (see Box 6.1).

The response to this new situation was to package a set of simple, affordable and effective interventions for the combined management of the major childhood illnesses and malnutrition, under the label of "Integrated Management of Childhood Illness" (IMCI). IMCI combines effective interventions for preventing death and for improving healthy growth and development: oral rehydration therapy for diarrhoea; antibiotics for sepsis, pneumonia, and ear infection; antimalarials and insecticide-treated bednets; vitamin A, treatment of anaemia, promotion of breastfeeding and complementary feeding for healthy nutrition and for recovery from illness, and immunization. Some countries have included guidelines to treat children with HIV/AIDS, others for dengue fever, wheezing, or sore throat, or for the follow-up of healthy children.

Dealing with children, not just with diseases

The second justification for a more comprehensive approach was the recognition that the health of children is not merely a question of targeting a limited number of diseases that are immediate causes of mortality.

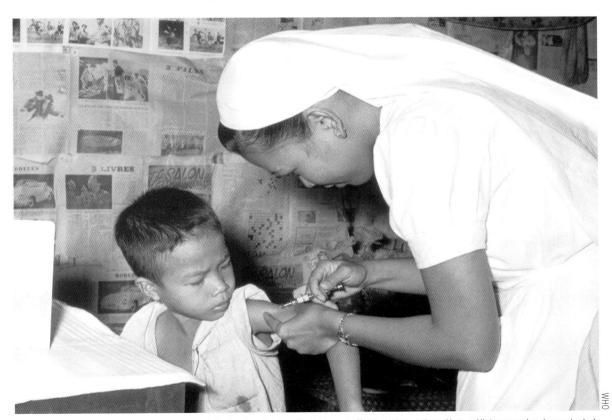

WHO

Packaging simple, affordable and effective interventions. Here, a Vietnamese boy is vaccinated.

As appropriate technologies became more widely available, a gradual evolution also took place in the content and methods of communication between health workers and parents. Previously, a family who brought a child for curative care had generally received basic treatment with minimal instruction and explanation for use of prescribed treatments at home. The introduction of oral rehydration therapy, however, added a new element to the relationship between the family and the clinic. During the clinic visit, families now learnt how to prepare and give oral rehydration salts solution *(9–11)*, to recognize signs of illness, and to treat their children without delay at home; they also learnt to make use of fluids available in the home, to make treatment more accessible. This led to the development of a systematic process of advising and counselling, and to new partnerships between health workers and households.

Child health programmes see many malnourished children. Some of these children may be malnourished as a result of lack of access to food, but more often it is because of infection and poor feeding practices, or a combination of the two *(4, 12)*. Counselling on feeding practices naturally became an element of IMCI. As with oral rehydration therapy, this forced health workers to enter into a different kind of partnership with mothers. It was no longer a matter of asking a few simple questions and prescribing a treatment: feeding problems had to be identified and acceptable solutions negotiated with the mother. Counselling carried out in this way requires specific training for the health worker, and the right kind of environment, but it is more effective *(13, 14)*.

The next logical step was to pay more attention to the physical and psychosocial development of children. A child's health and development is strongly influenced by the relationship between child, parents and other caregivers. The key is for the caregiver to be receptive to the child's state and needs, to interpret them correctly and be quick to react appropriately *(15)*. This is a critical factor in healthy growth *(16–19)*; the absence of sensitive, responsive care is associated with malnutrition and failure to thrive *(20–22)*. The influence of such care on healthy cognitive and social development as well as on survival has been well documented *(18, 23)*.

New evidence accumulated during the 1990s shows that mothers can be helped to communicate better with and to stimulate their young children *(24)*. The skills needed for appropriate feeding, psychosocial care and care-seeking are closely linked *(24)*, and improving one of these positively influences the others. Sensitivity and responsiveness can be effectively promoted and taught to caregivers, even in difficult social and economic conditions, or when a mother's ability to care for her child is compromised by depression *(24)*. Specific efforts are required to work with foster-parents, or with children who are heads of households. The challenge is to integrate these new findings into public health programming.

Parents are naturally concerned about the growth and psychosocial development of their children; however, health workers who operate in resource-constrained environments have long considered this more of a luxury or something that they could not influence. IMCI changed that: in doing so it created new challenges for what was no longer just a technical programme but became a partnership between parents and health workers.

ORGANIZING INTEGRATED CHILD CARE

The notion of integration has a long history. Integration is supposed to tackle the need for complementarity of different interdependent services and administrative structures, so as to better achieve common goals. In the 1950s these goals were defined in terms of outcome, in the 1960s of process and in the 1990s of economic impact

(25–27). Integration has different meanings at different levels *(28)*. At the patient level it means case management. At the point of delivery it means that multiple interventions are provided through one delivery channel – for example where vaccination is used as an opportunity to provide vitamin A and insecticide-treated bednets during "EPI-plus" activities, boosting efficiency and coverage *(29, 30)*. At the system level integration means bringing together the management and support functions of different sub-programmes, and ensuring complementarity between different levels of care. IMCI is now the only child health strategy that aims for improved integration at these three levels simultaneously.

IMCI has successfully integrated case management and tasks in first-level facilities by providing health workers with guidelines, tools and training. Progress towards integration between different levels is facilitated by the complementary guidelines for case management at first-level and referral facilities. Health workers at first-level facilities have guidelines for referring severely ill newborns and children, as well as those with complex problems. Health workers at the district hospital in turn get the guidelines and training to manage these referred children.

IMCI has gone a step further. More than just adding more programmes to a single delivery channel, it has sought to transform the way the health system looks at child care. IMCI retained its original name, but with the ambition of going beyond the management of illness *(3, 5, 31, 32)*. Based on experience from single-issue programmes, IMCI designed an approach with three components: improving the skills of health workers, strengthening the support of health systems, and helping families and communities to bring up their children healthily and deal with ill-health when it occurs. In doing so, IMCI had to move beyond the traditional notion of a health centre's staff providing a set of technical interventions to their target population.

Households and health workers

As they increasingly entered into dialogue with households, health workers in child programmes realized how crucial what happens in the household is for the health of a child. Food, medicine and a stimulating environment are all necessarily mediated by what households and communities do or do not do. When a child is ill, for example, someone in the household must recognize that there is a problem, provide appropriate care, identify signs indicating that the child needs medical care, take the child to a health worker, work out a proper course of action with the health worker (which may be to obtain medication and comply with the instructions on how to use it, or to take the child to hospital), provide support during convalescence, and return to the health worker if necessary. Households and communities thus determine whether the health system's intervention can make a difference. Without all this, even the best health centre will get poor results. To look at child health from this perspective may seem obvious today, but for the vertical programmes of the 1980s this was a radical change. It stimulated a flurry of interest in how households can contribute to the improvement of the health of their children: the so-called "key family practices" summarized in Box 6.2.

These family practices tackle behaviour that promotes physical growth and mental development, and prevents illness. The importance of this is obvious and has long been recognized. What is new is that seeking care from health services is also considered to be one of the ways households contribute to the health of their children. Poor or delayed care-seeking contributes to up to 70% of child deaths *(33)*. Most children die at home, and many without prior contact with competent medical care.

Promoting appropriate care-seeking and ensuring that health facilities are accessible are therefore crucial. The potential of appropriate home care, whether by the caregiver or by a lay community worker, is also increasingly recognized. For example, home management of malaria can reduce the incidence of severe malaria and malaria mortality, as experience in Burkina Faso and Ethiopia has shown *(34, 35)*. Prompt antibiotic treatment of pneumonia by well-trained and supervised community health workers can substantially reduce pneumonia-related mortality *(36)*.

Recognizing the importance of what households do is one thing, identifying how they can be helped to do so is another *(37)*. One approach is to improve the communication skills of health workers. Experiences in Brazil and the United Republic of Tanzania show that this results in improved care by families in the home *(13)*. Another approach is to work through community development programmes. In Bangladesh, for example, training of health workers in combination with community activities tripled the uptake of services from 0.6 to 1.8 visits per child per year *(38)*. While households carry the primary responsibility for what they do or do not do at home, the health system needs to enable households to meet these responsibilities. This is not a simple question of health education, but a more complex process of empowerment, for which the health worker also needs to change his or her way of working *(38)*.

With the support of a responsive health system, much can be done. In Makwanpur, Nepal, for example, women's groups supported by a facilitator discussed what factors contributed to perinatal mortality in their own living environment and formulated strategies to deal with them. This improved the way newborns were cared for at home and the appropriate use of health services, leading to a reduction of neonatal mortality *(39)*.

Box 6.2 How households can make a difference

Households can promote **physical growth and mental and social development** by ensuring exclusive breastfeeding for six months, by starting complementary feeding at six months of age and continuing breastfeeding until the child is aged two years or more. They can ensure that children receive adequate amounts of micronutrients either in their diet or through supplementation. They can also respond to a child's needs for care through talking, playing and providing a stimulating environment. The entire household, including men, has a role to play.

Households and communities can help **prevent child abuse and neglect**, and can take appropriate action when it has occurred.

Households can improve adequate **uptake of health care services** by recognizing when sick children need treatment outside the home and seeking timely care from appropriate providers. It is important for households to take children as scheduled to complete a full course of immunizations before their first birthday, and to follow health workers' advice about treatment, follow-up and referral.

Households can improve **care for sick children at home** by continuing to feed and offer more fluids (including breast milk) to children when they are sick, by giving them appropriate home treatment for infections, and by taking appropriate action in case of injury or accidents.

Households can **prevent illness** by disposing of faeces safely, and by washing hands after defecation, before preparing meals and before feeding children. They can bring their children for vaccination. In malaria-endemic areas they can ensure that children sleep under insecticide-treated bednets. Households and communities can take measures to prevent injuries and accidents.

Much depends, though, on the environment in which members of poor households live. An example is indoor air pollution. Half of the world's population rely on dung, wood, crop waste or coal to meet their most basic energy needs. In the highlands of western Guatemala, for example, most households use an open fire, fuelled by wood, for cooking and heating. Cooking with these so-called solid fuels leads

to levels of particulate matter that are 100 times higher than typical outdoor air concentrations in European cities. With little ventilation, the smoke makes breathing difficult, burns the eyes and covers the dwelling in black soot. Young children, often carried on their mothers' backs during cooking, are most exposed. Moreover, women and children often spend many hours collecting fuel – time that could be spent on education, child care or income generation. Lack of a good source of lighting limits educational activities beyond daylight hours.

In the short term, well-designed stoves with chimneys can significantly reduce emissions and help protect children. But to reduce indoor air pollution drastically, it is necessary to switch to cleaner and more efficient fuels: liquid petroleum gas, electricity or solar power. Poor households often do not have the resources to do so, and this situation will continue until the roots of poverty are tackled.

In Haryana, India, health workers provided counselling during immunization sessions and curative care consultations, while community health workers did the same during weighing sessions and home visits. This increased exclusive breastfeeding at three months, reduced rates of diarrhoea *(40)*, improved complementary feeding practices at nine months of age *(41)*, and increased uptake of curative and preventive health care services *(42)*.

IMCI has focused much of its training and capacity-building efforts on the first contact level: the health centre, and the nurse or doctor who first sees the sick child. For IMCI to work optimally, it has to build the continuum of care in two directions: towards facilitating referral, and towards bringing care closer to households, and thus to children (see Figure 6.1).

Referring sick children

The focus on primary health care and, more recently, on the role of households themselves, has often meant that child health programmes have overlooked how important it is to be able to refer a sick child to a well-functioning hospital. This is important for the child and the child's family, but also for the front-line health workers; it can have a substantial impact on child mortality *(43)*. Facilitating referral is straightforward, at least in principle, if a district system has been put in place. It does, however, depend on removing delays and obstacles that are not always considered to be part of the health worker's responsibilities.

Deaths in hospital often occur within 24 hours of admission. Many of these deaths could be prevented if good-quality care were provided in good time. To achieve this, dangerous delays must be avoided: first, by helping mothers or other caregivers identify early the signs which show that children need medical attention; second, by ensuring that public health services are open when they are needed, such as when parents are home from the fields or from work, and when children feel ill (often in the evening); third, by making sure that health workers refer promptly when there is an indication to do so. Implementation of IMCI guidelines should result in referral of 10% of children aged between two months and five years *(44, 45)*. In many of the countries that have made little or

Figure 6.1 An integrated approach to child health

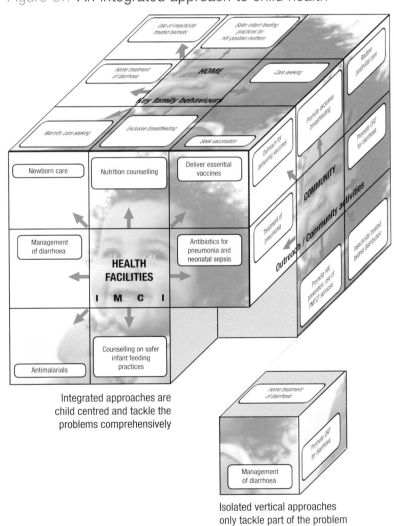

Integrated approaches are child centred and tackle the problems comprehensively

Isolated vertical approaches only tackle part of the problem

no progress in terms of child health, there is a substantial amount of under-referral, particularly in rural areas, and the referral rates one would expect from the IMCI guidelines are rarely reached.

A further source of delay is the journey to hospital, a problem for which many health workers do not feel they are responsible. Yet problems can be avoided in many cases if they are anticipated. Health workers can help to organize transport and to find arrangements for the other children and domestic duties while parents take a child to the hospital.

Finally, much can de done to reduce delays in starting appropriate treatment within hospitals *(46, 47)*. In Malawi, for example, the number of deaths before admission was reduced from 10 per month to five as a result of rapid triage as soon as the child arrived. Inpatient mortality was brought down from 11–18% to 6–9%, with improved staff morale as an added bonus. Management of severe malnutrition *(48–50)* and of pneumonia *(51)*, as well as neonatal care *(52)* can be substantially improved with better ward organization, clinical guidelines and standards, active staff participation, and (often limited) additional resources *(53)*.

Bringing care closer to children

More difficult, and perhaps more important, is to bring care closer to the children. The familiar answer is outreach. For health workers to visit households and communities in their catchment area is probably the fastest way to scale up coverage with interventions that can be planned, such as vaccination. The drawback, though, is that it cannot provide the full range of services needed to improve child health and survival. The potential of this mode of delivery to scale up coverage is very variable from place to place, but probably big on a global scale, particularly for population groups that are currently excluded.

The less familiar way is to empower households, and help them take better care of their children. Health workers tend to be less comfortable with this kind of approach. They are understandably reluctant to relinquish parts of their professional prerogatives, and they do not know how to do so. Classic health education to obtain changes in behaviour has only a limited potential, and many health workers have experienced this. Empowerment is much more challenging than health education: it requires time, and an attitude that is new and has to be learnt.

Community health workers can function as a bridge between health centre and households where the health centre network is not readily accessible. In Ethiopia, for example, community health workers diagnose and treat fever. This has increased the coverage of malaria treatment services well beyond the reach of many health facilities. From 1991 to 1998, the number of febrile patients receiving antimalarials steadily increased from 76 000 to 949 000 *(54)*. In Pakistan, Lady Health Workers are a pivotal component of the national health system. They are selected and supported by the government, and provide basic primary health care services, including home visits, to the community in which they live. The programme covers approximately one fifth of the population *(55)*. Such programmes can boost coverage; by themselves, however, they are no substitute for extending the health care network and helping the households themselves to take care of their children better.

ROLLING OUT CHILD HEALTH INTERVENTIONS

IMCI has now been adopted by more than 100 countries. The guidelines are designed for adaptation at national and sub-national levels. The establishment of task forces at national level to adapt the guidelines to national contexts has created ownership and helped overcome problems with, for example, the availability of essential drugs. Where IMCI has been evaluated, results are on the whole positive. Training has led to improved health worker performance and quality of care, without increasing costs. For example, IMCI-trained health workers in Uganda and the United Republic of Tanzania gave correct treatment with antibiotics or antimalarials to much larger proportions of children than their colleagues, and prescribed fewer antibiotics to children not needing them *(56)*. The impact is impressive: in the United Republic of Tanzania, in a setting where utilization of health services was high, IMCI implementation reduced mortality by 13% over a two-year period, compared with control districts, and indications are that results may further improve over a longer period.

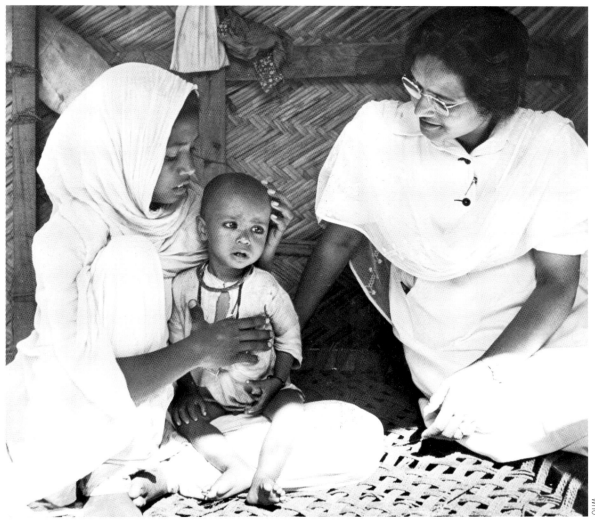

For the Integrated Management of Childhood Illness (IMCI) to work optimally, it has to build a continuum of care that extends through families and communities, first-level facilities and hospitals.

However, the expansion of IMCI has proceeded more slowly than expected. Only 16 out of 100 countries had started implementation in more than 50% of their districts in 2003; moreover, most have focused on improving health worker skills, and little has usually been done to strengthen health systems or empower households *(57, 58)*. This can be explained in part by the slow development of district health care systems, particularly in the countries most in need of scaling up IMCI (see Chapter 3). IMCI fits perfectly with the district concept, giving the same central place to the health centre, considering the continuum of care in the same terms, and with the same balance between responding to epidemiology and responding to demand. The downside is that it is subject to the same constraints: infrequent or inadequate supervision, rapid turnover and low morale of staff, a culture of non-responsiveness, and underfunding *(59)*.

A second reason for the slow expansion of IMCI results from its emphasis on integration and horizontality. In its insistence on full integration at the point of delivery, IMCI has dismantled or weakened pre-existing organizational structures of vertical programmes *(60)*, and has in the process lost the programmatic visibility that allowed these to thrive and attract funding. The absence of full-time coordinators, operational plans or specific budget lines hampered sustained implementation *(60)*. The lesson learnt is that a careful trade-off is required between integrating at point of delivery and maintaining the programmatic structures that define the technical norms and standards, drive expansion of coverage and provide a logistic platform. It requires considerable capacity and skills to integrate immunization services, for example, within the local political, social and health infrastructure, while at the same time protecting strategic elements within existing national and regional strategic plans and

Figure 6.2 Proportion of districts where training and system strengthening for IMCI had been started by 2003[a]

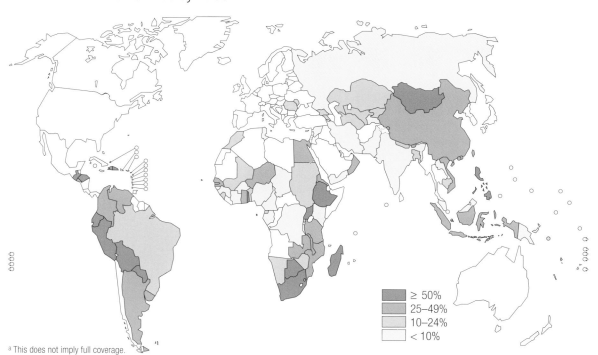

≥ 50%
25–49%
10–24%
< 10%

[a] This does not imply full coverage.

workplans. One of the strategies to facilitate this is to plan coverage on a district-by-district basis, as some countries do in the Reaching Every District initiative launched in 2002. It combines the re-establishment of outreach services, supportive supervision, community links with service delivery, monitoring and use of data for action, and planning and management of resources. To date more than 30 countries in four WHO regions have adopted this strategy, and plan and monitor vaccination coverage on a district-by-district basis.

The reality is that today many children do not yet benefit from comprehensive and integrated care. They are even excluded from the care necessary to ensure survival – that is, the core interventions around which IMCI is built.

Scaling up a set of essential interventions to full coverage (see Table 6.1) would lower sufficiently the incidence and case-fatality of the conditions causing children under five years of age to die, to allow progress towards and beyond the Millennium Development Goals.

Table 6.1   Core interventions to improve child survival

- **Nurturing newborns and their mothers:** skilled attendance during pregnancy, childbirth and the immediate postpartum period (not costed in this chapter).

- **Infant feeding:** exclusive breastfeeding during the first six months of a child's life, with appropriate complementary feeding from six months and continued breast-feeding for two years or beyond, with supplementation with vitamin A and other micronutrients as needed.

- **Vital vaccines:** increased coverage of measles and tetanus vaccines, as well as immunization against common vaccine-preventable diseases.

- **Combating diarrhoea:** case management of diarrhoea, including therapeutic zinc supplementation and antibiotics for dysentery.

- **Combating pneumonia and sepsis:** case management of childhood pneumonia and neonatal sepsis with antibiotics.

- **Combating malaria:** use of insecticide-treated bednets, intermittent preventive malaria treatment in pregnancy, and prompt treatment of malaria.

- **Prevention and care for HIV:** treatment, care, infant feeding counselling and support for HIV-infected women and their infants.

THE COST OF SCALING UP COVERAGE

One of the major challenges the world faces is to scale up these interventions to full coverage as soon as possible. Theoretically it is possible to fill the gap between present levels and near-universal coverage within the next 10 years. In some countries the coverage gap is relatively small and the health system strong enough to bridge it quickly. In others the challenge is much greater, all the more so as health systems there are less developed and more fragile. Even in these cases, however, it is possible to reach full coverage through a combination of extension of the health care network, stepped-up outreach and, in some situations and for some interventions, by relying on lay community health workers.

Scaling up interventions to full coverage will not, however, be possible without massively increasing expenditure on child health. From the perspective of planning and resource mobilization it is crucial to be aware of the additional costs that will be entailed (over and above current levels of expenditure).

For the 75 countries that together account for almost 95% of child deaths in the world, it is possible to formulate scenarios for scaling up each of the interventions to 95% coverage between 2006 and 2015. Such countries include those with the highest numbers of child deaths and those with the highest under-five mortality rates; they comprise all the countries in which the mortality rates of children under five years of age have been stagnating or reversing during the 1990s, as well as many of those making slow progress or which are already well on track. Together they have a population of around 4.6 billion (in 2005), including 496 million children under five years of age. These countries have been classified in four groups using a set of criteria that include the level of mortality, the strengths and weaknesses of the health system, and the challenges imposed by the environment in which they operate. For each country a group-specific scenario for scaling up coverage was applied to current levels of coverage with each intervention.

The sum of the additional costs for implementing these scaling-up scenarios is estimated to be at least US$ 52.4 billion: US$ 2.2 billion in 2006 increasing, as coverage expands, to US$ 7.8 billion in 2015. This corresponds to US$ 1.05 per inhabitant per year (US$ 0.47 initially, increasing to US$ 1.48 in year 10, when 95% of the child population would be covered with the full range of interventions in every country). This in turn corresponds to an average increase of 12% per year of current median public health expenditure in the 75 countries, which is currently around US$ 8.4 per inhabitant (see Figure 6.3 and Box 6.3). Assumptions and methods for the costing exercise are summarized on the *World Health Report* web site (http://www.who.int/whr). Countries in the two groups in which the starting situation is relatively

Figure 6.3 Cost of scaling up child health interventions, additional to current expenditure

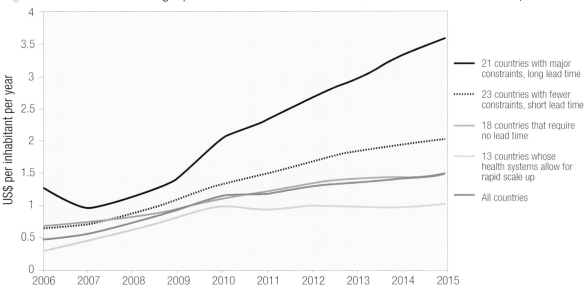

favourable, but where labour, drugs and supplies are more expensive, account for 60% of the global price tag of US$ 52.4 billion. Approximately US$ 21 billion would be required in the countries in the two groups where conditions are currently most challenging. These are low-income countries with high mortality levels, low coverage and relatively weak health systems – but where the current prices of labour and supplies are lower.

In the 13 middle-income countries that belong to the group currently in the most favourable situation, expenditure on child health would have to increase by US$ 0.79 per inhabitant per year on average (US$ 0.29 at the beginning, rising over time to US$ 1.01). This corresponds to an increase of 3% per year (1% at the beginning, rising to 4% in 2015) of current median public expenditure on health in these countries, which is around US$ 23 per inhabitant.

Low-income countries in the group where the situation is currently most difficult, such as Angola, Chad, Côte d'Ivoire, the Democratic Republic of the Congo, Ethiopia, Mali, Niger, Nigeria and Somalia, would have to spend US$ 2.16 per inhabitant per year on top of current expenditure: US$ 1.27 in the early years and, as they move towards full coverage, US$ 3.58 per inhabitant per year 10 years later. This corresponds to a 46% growth (27% to start with, rising to 76% in 2015) of current median public expenditure on health in these countries, which is around US$ 4.7 per inhabitant (the median private expenditure in these countries is US$ 5.5 per inhabitant per year).

These estimates are only as good as the assumptions and projections underlying them. In some countries scaling up can go faster than projected, in others it will be slower: much depends on political will and commitment, and on the social, political and economic contexts. Population dynamics may change, as well as cost structures. Technical innovations and changes in patterns of health care provision and human resource availability may influence coverage expansion as well as cost estimates. Furthermore, the cost projections currently do not take account of the effects of scaled-up intervention sets on changes in disease epidemiology and do not include gains in efficiency that would derive from integration of the different interventions at the point of delivery.

Nevertheless, these projections provide a benchmark for the additional cost, on top of current expenditure, of a massive scale up. It is a low-end benchmark, because it assumes that current coverage levels can be sustained without additional investments, and that there are no constraints to the capacity to produce supplementary staff and infrastructure. Furthermore, it does not account for the cost of training new multipurpose health professionals involved in child care, nor for the increases in salaries and other benefits that in many countries are necessary to redeploy and motivate staff.

FROM COST PROJECTIONS TO SCALING UP

Every country faces unique challenges in increasing access to care and coverage, but all will need a sustained political commitment to mobilize the considerable resources that are required. While such a financing effort seems to be within reasonable reach in some countries, in many it will go beyond what can be borne by governments alone. Relying on increased out-of-pocket expenditure for mobilizing such resources seems unrealistic in many countries; to do this through increased public spending is more realistic in others, but in many cases the additional cost is such that external assistance will be necessary.

Box 6.3 A breakdown of the projected cost of scaling up

Increasing coverage means that more children and households have to be reached. The result is that the cost of scaling up coverage, additional to current levels of expenditure, will grow over time. This is particularly the case for personnel and commodities, less so for programme costs.

Of these additional costs, 13% are for programme development and support, 87% for service delivery (roughly three quarters for service delivery through health facilities and one quarter for community level interventions).

Of the extra service delivery costs, 38% are for salaries and honorariums for the professional staff, 10% for community health worker programmes to complement the services provided by the professional health care workers, and 39% for drugs, lab tests and other supplies.

The distribution of these additional costs over different interventions changes over time. In absolute terms, the projections assume roughly a tenfold increase between 2006 and 2015 in resource requirements for counselling

for breastfeeding and complementary feeding, as well as for case management of neonatal infections, diarrhoea and acute respiratory infections. The additional resources required to scale up immunization and target malaria will double over the same period, but their share of the total would be reduced by two thirds to 9% and 12%, respectively. Only treatment of complications of measles would require less funding in 2015 than in 2006: prevention pays off in the long run.

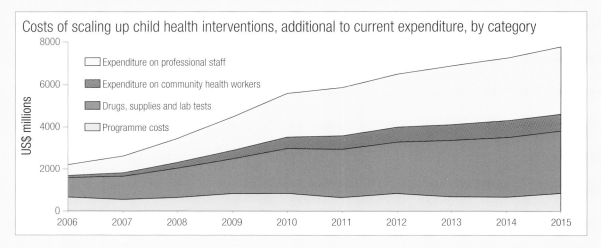

Costs of scaling up child health interventions, additional to current expenditure, by category

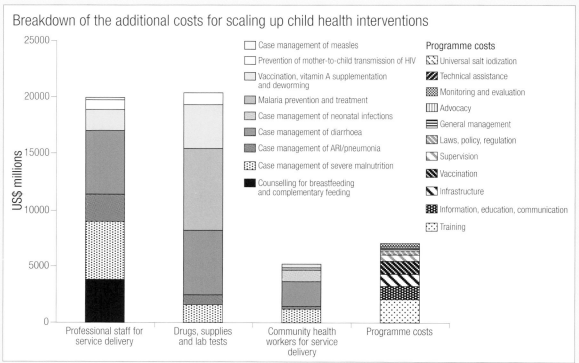

Breakdown of the additional costs for scaling up child health interventions

In any event, the institutional capacity will have to be created not only to mobilize such funds, but also to plan and implement the integration of the various interventions, and to complete the reorientation of child health services from solely survival to survival, growth and development. This cannot be done in isolation from the development and strengthening of health systems. First, health services need to be able to provide care that addresses multiple risks and conditions, and for this they have to rely on well functioning health systems that ensure a continuum of care between the home, first-level facilities and district hospitals. Second, it cannot be done without establishing a better continuity with the interventions aimed at improving maternal and newborn health. Third, it requires a cultural revolution among health workers to start working with households and communities as partners, and to look at children as children, and not merely as a collection of diseases.

The evolution within child health programmes – from the comprehensive view of early primary health care, over the interim strategies of selective interventions targeting priority disease, to today's more comprehensive integrated management of childhood illness – reflects the awareness that successful strategies to improve child survival are likely to involve a combination of approaches that move towards greater integration. Without it, too many children will not reach services or, when they do, too many opportunities to protect their health will be missed. Many countries have already started to reorient their services to build or strengthen this continuum of care. It is now up to governments and the global community to support these efforts, and to mobilize resources accordingly.

References

1. Progress in reducing global measles deaths: 1999–2002. *Weekly Epidemiological Record*, 2004, 79:20–21.
2. Water with sugar and salt [editorial]. *Lancet*, 1978, 2:300–301.
3. Wolfheim C. From disease control to child health and development, *World Health Forum*, 1998, 19:174–181
4. *The evolution of diarrhoeal and acute respiratory disease control at WHO – achievements 1980–1995 in research, development and implementation*. Geneva, World Health Organization, 1999 (WHO/CHS/CAH/99.12).
5. Tulloch J. Integrated approach to child health in developing countries. *Lancet*, 1999, 354(Suppl. 2):SII16–20.
6. Hahn S, Kim Y, Garner P. Reduced osmolarity oral rehydration solution for treating dehydration due to diarrhoea in children: systematic review. *British Medical Journal*, 2001, 323:81–85.
7. Fontaine O. Effect of zinc supplementation on clinical course of acute diarrhoea. *Journal of Health Population and Nutrition*, 2001, 19:339–346.
8. Pakistan Multicentre Amoxicillin Short Course Therapy (MASCOT) pneumonia study group. Clinical efficacy of 3 days versus 5 days of oral amoxicillin for treatment of childhood pneumonia: a multicentre double-blind trial. *Lancet*, 2002, 360:835–841.
9. Victora CG, Bryce J, Fontaine O, Monasch R. Reducing deaths from diarrhoea through oral rehydration therapy. *Bulletin of the World Health Organization*, 2000, 78:1246–1255.
10. Touchette P, Douglass E, Graeff J, Monoang I, Mathe M, Duke LW. An analysis of home-based oral rehydration therapy in the Kingdom of Lesotho. *Social Science & Medicine*, 1994, 39:425–432.
11. Bronfman M, Castro R, Castro V, Guiscafre H, Munoz O, Gutierrez G. Prescripción médica y adherencia al tratamiento en diarrea infecciosa aguda: impacto indirecto de una intervención educativa [Medical prescription and treatment compliance in acute infectious diarrhoea: indirect impact of an educational intervention]. *Salud Pública de México*, 1991, 33:568–575.

12. World Health Organization, Department of Child and Adolescent Health and Development web site (http://www.who.int/child-adolescent-health, accessed 28 January 2005).

13. Pelto GH, Santos I, Goncalves H, Victora C, Martines J, Habicht JP. Nutrition counseling training changes physician behavior and improves caregiver knowledge acquisition. *Journal of Nutrition*, 2004, 134:357–362.

14. Santos I, Victora CG, Martines J, Goncalves H, Gigante DP, Valle NJ et al. Nutrition counseling increases weight gain among Brazilian children. *Journal of Nutrition*, 2001, 131:2866–2873.

15. Richter L. *The importance of caregiver-child interactions for the survival and healthy development of young children: a review*. Geneva, World Health Organization, 2004.

16. Begin F, Frongillo EA Jr, Delisle H. Caregiver behaviors and resources influence child height-for-age in rural Chad. *Journal of Nutrition*, 1999, 129:680–686.

17. Lamontagne JF, Engle PL, Zeitlin MF. Maternal employment, child care, and nutritional status of 12–18-month-old children in Managua, Nicaragua. *Social Science and Medicine*, 1998, 46:403–414.

18. Zeitlin M, Ghassemi H, Mansour M. *Positive deviance in child nutrition – with emphasis on psychosocial and behavioural aspects and implications for development*. Tokyo, United Nations University Press, 1990.

19. Black M, Dubowitz H. Failure-to-thrive: lessons from animal models and developing countries. *Journal of Developmental and Behavioral Pediatrics*, 1991, 2:259–267.

20. Chase HP, Martin HP. Undernutrition and child development. *New England Journal of Medicine*, 1970, 282:933–939.

21. Richter L, Griesel D. Malnutrition, low birthweight and related influences on psychological development. In: Dawes A, Donald D, eds. *Childhood and adversity: psychological perspectives from South African research*. Cape Town, David Philip, 1994:66–91.

22. Pollitt E, Eichler AW, Chan CK. Psychosocial development and behaviour of mothers of failure-to-thrive children. *American Journal of Orthopsychiatry*, 1975, 45:525–537.

23. NICHD Early Child Care Research Network. Nonmaternal care and family factors in early development: An overview of the NICHD Study of Early Child Care. *Journal of Applied Developmental Psychology*, 2001, 22:457–492.

24. Pelto G, Dickin K, Engle P. *A critical link: interventions for physical growth and psychological developmen: a review*. Geneva, World Health Organization, 1999 (WHO/CHS/CAH/99.3).

25. *Methodology of planning an integrated health programme for rural areas. Second report of the Expert Committee on Public Health Administration*. Geneva, World Health Organization, 1954 (WHO Technical Report Series, No. 83).

26. *Integration of mass campaigns against specific diseases into general health services. Report of a WHO Study Group*. Geneva, World Health Organization, 1965 (WHO Technical Report Series, No. 294).

27. *Integration of health care delivery. Report of a WHO Study Group*. Geneva, World Health Organization, 1996 (WHO Technical Report Series, No. 861).

28. Scherpbier RW, Ottmani SE, Pio A, Raviglione MR. *Practical approach to lung health (PAL). A primary health care strategy for integrated management of priority respiratory illnesses*. Geneva, World Health Organization, 2003.

29. Gorstein J, Shreshtra RK, Pandey S, Adhikari RK, Pradhan A. Current status of vitamin A deficiency and the National Vitamin A Control Program in Nepal: results of the 1998 National Micronutrient Status Survey. *Asia Pacific Journal of Clinical Nutrition*, 2003, 12:96–103.

30. Swami HM, Thakur JS, Bhatia SP. Mass supplementation of vitamin A linked to National Immunization Day. *Indian Journal of Pediatrics*, 2002, 69:675–678.

31. Gove S. Integrated management of childhood illness by outpatient health workers. technical basis and overview. The WHO Working Group on Guidelines for Integrated Management of the Sick Child. *Bulletin of the World Health Organization*, 1997, 75 (Suppl. 1):7–24.

32. Lambrechts T, Bryce J, Orinda V. Integrated management of childhood illness: a summary of first experiences. *Bulletin of the World Health Organization*, 1999, 77:582–594.

33. Terra de Souza AC, Peterson KE, Andrade FM, Gardner J, Ascherio A. Circumstances of post-neonatal deaths in Ceara, Northeast Brazil: mothers' health care-seeking behaviors during their infants' fatal illness. *Social Science & Medicine*, 2000, 51:1675–1693.

34. Sirima SB, Konate A, Tiono AB, Convelbo N, Cousens S, Pagnoni F. Early treatment of childhood fevers with pre-packaged antimalarial drugs in the home reduces severe malaria morbidity in Burkina Faso. *Tropical Medicine and International Health*, 2003, 8:133–139.

35. Kidane G, Morrow RH. Teaching mothers to provide home treatment of malaria in Tigray, Ethiopia: a randomised trial. *Lancet*, 2000, 356:550–555.

36. *WHO-UNICEF joint statement: management of pneumonia in community settings*. New York, NY, United Nations Children's Fund; Geneva, World Health Organization (UNICEF/PD/Pneumonia/01; WHO/FCH/CAH/04.06).

37. Hill Z, Kirkwood B, Edmond K. *Family and community practices that promote child survival, growth and development: a review of the evidence*. Geneva, World Health Organization, 2004.

38. El Arifeen S, Blum LS, Hoque DM, Chowdhury EK, Khan R, Black RE et al. Integrated Management of Childhood Illness (IMCI) in Bangladesh: early findings from a cluster-randomised study. *Lancet*, 2004, 364:1595–1602.

39. Manandhar DS, Osrin D, Shrestha BP, Mesko N, Morrison J, Tumbahangphe KM et al. Effect of a participatory intervention with women's groups on birth outcomes in Nepal: cluster-randomised controlled trial. *Lancet*, 2004, 364:970–979.

40. Bhandari N, Bahl R, Mazumdar S, Martines J, Black RE, Bhan MK et al. Effect of community-based promotion of exclusive breastfeeding on diarrhoeal illnesses and growth: a cluster randomised controlled trial. *Lancet*, 2003, 361:1418–1423.

41. Bhandari N, Mazumder S, Bahl R, Martines J, Black RE, Bhan MK et al. An educational intervention to promote appropriate complementary feeding practices and physical growth in infants and young children in rural Haryana, *Indian Journal of Nutrition*, 2004,134:2342–2348.

42. Bhandari N, Mazumder S, Bahl R, Martines J, Black RE, Bhan MK et al. Use of multiple opportunities for improving feeding practices in undertows within child health programs is feasible, effective and beneficial to the health system. *Health Policy and Planning* (submitted).

43. Nolan T, Angos P, Cunha AJ, Muhe L, Qazi S, Simoes EA et al. Quality of hospital care for seriously ill children in less-developed countries. *Lancet*, 2001, 357:106–110.

44. Simoes EA, Peterson S, Gamatie Y, Kisanga FS, Mukasa G, Nsungwa-Sabiiti J et al. Management of severely ill children at first-level health facilities in sub-Saharan Africa when referral is difficult. *Bulletin of the World Health Organization*, 2003, 81:522–531.

45. Peterson S, Nsungwa-Sabiiti J, Were W, Nsabagasani X, Magumba G, Nambooze J et al. Coping with paediatric referral – Ugandan parents' experience. *Lancet*, 2004, 363: 1955–1956.

46. Tamburlini G, Di Mario S, Maggi RS, Vilarim JN, Gove S. Evaluation of guidelines for emergency triage assessment and treatment in developing countries. *Archives of Disease in Childhood*, 1999, 81:478–482.

47. Robertson MA, Molyneux EM. Triage in the developing world – can it be done? *Archives of Disease in Childhood*, 2001, 85:208–213.

48. Ahmed T, Ali M, Ullah MM, Choudhury IA, Haque ME, Salam MA et al. Mortality in severely malnourished children with diarrhoea and use of a standardised management protocol. *Lancet*, 1999, 353:1919–1922.

49. Wilkinson D, Scrace M, Boyd N. Reduction in in-hospital mortality of children with malnutrition. *Journal of Tropical Pediatrics*, 1996, 42:114–115.

50. Puoane T, Sanders D, Chopra M, Ashworth A, Strasser S, McCoy D et al. Evaluating the clinical management of severely malnourished children – a study of two rural district hospitals. *South African Medical Journal*, 2001, 91:137–141.

51. Duke T, Mgone J, Frank D. Hypoxaemia in children with severe pneumonia in Papua New Guinea. *International Journal of Tuberculosis and Lung Disease*, 2001, 5:511–519.

52. Duke T, Willie L, Mgone JM. The effect of introduction of minimal standards of neonatal care on in-hospital mortality. *Papua and New Guinea Medical Journal*, 2000, 43:127–136.

53. *Management of the child with a serious infection or severe malnutrition: guidelines for care at the first-referral level in developing countries*. Geneva, World Health Organization, 2001 (WHO/FCH/CAH/00.1).

54. Ghebreyesus TA, Witten KH, Getachew A, O'Neill K, Bosman A, Teklehaimanot A. Community-based malaria control programme in Tigray, northern Ethiopia. *Parassitologia*, 1999, 41:367–371.

55. Pakistan: evaluation of the Prime Minister's programme for family planning and primary health care. Interim report. Oxford, *Oxford Policy Management*, 2000.
56. Tanzania IMCI Multi-Country Evaluation Health Facility survey Study Group. The effect of Integrated Management of Childhood Illness on observed quality of care of under-fives in rural Tanzania. *Health Policy and Planning*, 2004, 19:1–10.
57. Armstrong Schellenberg JR, Adam T, Mshinda H, Masanja H, Kabadi G, Mukasa O et al. Effectiveness and cost of facility-based Integrated Management of Childhood Illness (IMCI) in Tanzania. *Lancet*, 2004, 364:1583–1594.
58. Claeson M, Waldman R. The evolution of child health programmes in developing countries: from targeting diseases to targeting people. *Bulletin of the World Health Organization*, 2000, 78:1234–1245.
59. *Multi-country evaluation of IMCI effectiveness, cost and impact (MCE). Progress report May 2002–April 2003*. Geneva, World Health Organization, 2003 (WHO/FCH/CAH/03.5).
60. Victora CG, Hanson K, Bryce J, Vaughan JP. Achieving universal coverage with health interventions. *Lancet*, 2004, 364:1541–1548.

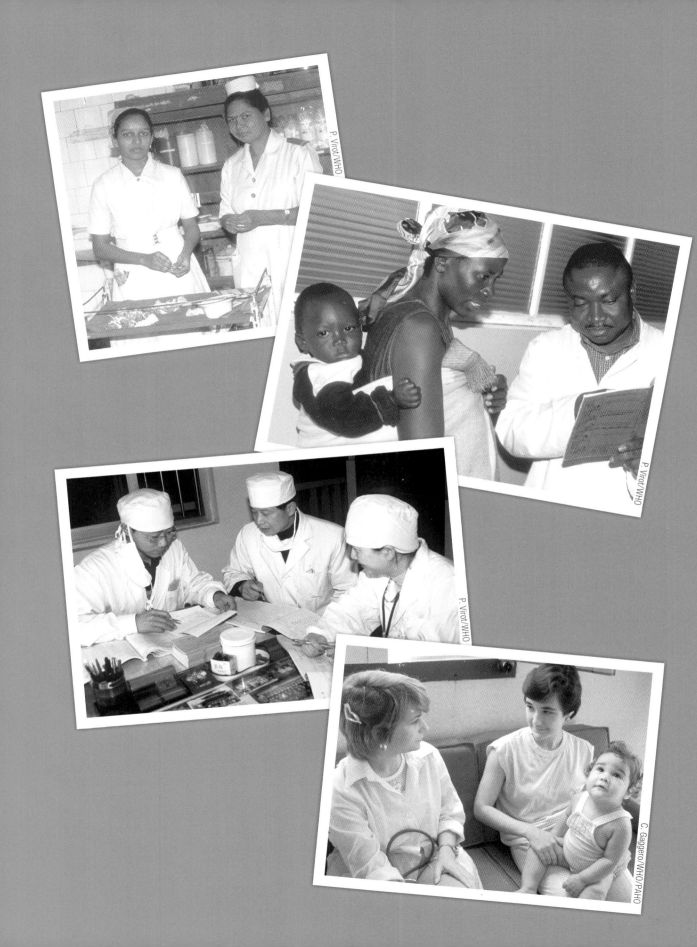

chapter seven

reconciling maternal, newborn and child health with health system development

This last chapter looks at the place of maternal, newborn and child health within a wider context of health system development. Today, maternal, newborn and child health are no longer discussed in purely technical terms, but as part of a broader agenda of universal access. This frames it within a straightforward political project: responding to society's demand for the protection of the health of citizens and access to care, a demand that is increasingly seen as legitimate.

REPOSITIONING MNCH

Maternal and child health programmes have long lacked a clear strategic focus and a consistent policy articulation (1). Tensions between programmes that concentrate on the health needs of mothers and those developed for their children have proved counterproductive for both: sets of distinct, legitimate needs had often turned into competing demands for care and attention (2). Programmes for women and children have now been repositioned. First, the specific needs of newborns are now recognized: this has led to the introduction of an N for newborn into the well-worn acronym of MCH so that it becomes MNCH. Second, it is now generally acknowledged that the interests of mother and child are closely intertwined, and that the MNCH agenda cannot be separated from the right of access to reproductive health care for all which was promoted by the Cairo International Conference on Population and Development (ICPD). Third, there is now a general consensus that MNCH programmes will be effective only if a continuum of care is established within strengthened health systems.

This forces programmes with different histories, strategies and constituencies to work together and to tackle the dilemma of competition for the attention of decision-makers and donors. Funding for maternal, newborn and child health is difficult to track: it tends to be diluted within the overall health system and fragmented in a juxtaposition of programmes and initiatives. For all the rhetoric about integration, donors and agencies have shown little interest in smoothing out the evident distortions within the funding envelopes, and in particular the

Box 7.1 International funds for maternal, newborn and child health

External Official Flows (EOF)[1] on health from grants and loans increased from US$ 3.2 to US$ 6.3 billion between 1990 and 2002 (in constant 2002 US$), which equates to a rise from US$ 0.62 to US$ 0.88 per capita. These amounts do not include spending on sectors such as water and sanitation, or spending on health in the context of budget support programmes. Although globally this is a small fraction of global health expenditure (0.4–0.6%, excluding the 22 richest OECD countries' total health expenditures), in many countries it is of strategic importance, for two reasons. First, because the average masks a huge variation: in some countries external resources represent a very large percentage (38% in Niger in 2002, for example). Second, because within the health sector some areas depend almost exclusively on donors. This is the case for child health in most poor African countries (5).

Allocation of resources by sector changed significantly between 1990–1992 and 2000–2002. The share of EOF going to population and reproductive health, which includes support to maternal health, increased from 30% to 39%. This corresponds to a doubling of funding, from US$ 1 billion to US$ 2 billion per year (in constant 2002 US$) between 1990–1992 and 2000–2002. This is mainly a result of increases for programmes targeting sexually transmitted infections, including HIV/AIDS. Some 4% of EOF for health were directed to such programmes in 1990-1992, compared with 19% (nearly US$ 1.4 billion per year) in 2000–2002. Funds allocated to family planning and other reproductive health care areas, which include maternal health, decreased both in relative and absolute terms.

The proportion allocated to basic health care has increased from 23% to 37% (US$ 0.14 to US$ 0.32 per capita) between 1990–1992 and 2000–2002. Most of the increase was committed to basic and primary health care programmes and infectious disease control. It is not possible to disaggregate these funds so as to ascertain the evolution of funding intended for child health, but it is likely that funding actually increased, albeit in a less visible and traceable way. Private international funding for child health through nongovernmental organizations and large foundations, such as the Bill & Melinda Gates Foundation, has also increased (6). Spending by smaller private foundations on child health decreased, but their global impact on child health is relatively small. For national programme managers the dilution of child health funds in system or sectoral support, channelling through vertical sub-programmes such as the polio eradication efforts, and increased channelling of external aid through international nongovernmental organizations, have led to a perception that their access to and control over resources needed for the development of integrated child health programmes have actually diminished (5).

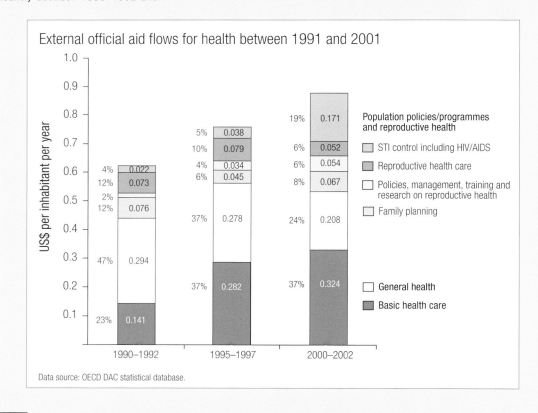

External official aid flows for health between 1991 and 2001

Data source: OECD DAC statistical database.

---

[1] Made up mostly of Official Development Assistance, but also including Other Official Flows (loans) as described in the OECD DAC statistical database (www.oecd.org/dac/stats).

disappointing contributions for maternal health and family planning within reproductive health funding *(3, 4)* (see Box 7.1).

In contrast to the route chosen by the advocates of a number of other major public health priorities, such as malaria, tuberculosis or HIV/AIDS, champions of maternal, newborn and child health – including the various global partnerships (see Box 7.2) – prefer to tap into the greater funds available for overall health sector development rather than to create new, parallel funding mechanisms. Whether this is for tactical reasons or for more fundamental considerations, it fits well with the growing importance of the health sector reform movement *(13)*. The emphasis on health sector development as the platform for maternal, newborn and child health coincides with the recognition among key multilateral and bilateral donors that poverty reduction is the primary goal of development assistance *(14)*. It comes at a moment when the wave of health care reforms in the aftermath of primary health care, rooted in a neo-liberal ideology of rolling back the presence of the state, is well under way. These reforms were promoted in contexts of transition from socialist to market economies – in countries such as Mongolia or Tajikistan – and of rebuilding services in post-conflict areas such as Cambodia, or as part of the structural adjustment programmes of many African and Asian countries that were facing severe resource crunches. MNCH consequently evolves in a context dominated by discussions on the role and responsibility of the state in tackling underfunding of the health sector, accessibility of services, inequities and exclusion, inefficiencies, and lack of accountability.

The result is that maternal, newborn and child health can no longer be framed in purely technical terms. The appearance of a shared commitment to solving health sector problems that are obviously relevant to maternal, newborn and child health contributes to the assumption that MNCH policy interests are synonymous with those

Box 7.2 Building pressure: the partnerships for maternal, newborn and child health

Against the backdrop of slow progress towards the Millennium Development Goals concerning maternal and child health, the need for an urgent, global coordinated response has prompted several agencies and international organizations to join forces and create partnerships for maternal, newborn and child health. Over the past few decades, it has become clear that the support required for the development of a resource-constrained country is so multifaceted and complex, that it cannot be successfully taken on by one agency alone *(7)*. Within the field of maternal, newborn, and child health, three partnerships are currently active: the Partnership for Safe Motherhood and Newborn Health, the Healthy Newborn Partnership, and the Child Survival Partnership. The recently established Partnership for Safe Motherhood and Newborn Health aims to strengthen and expand maternal and newborn health efforts. The Healthy Newborn Partnership has been established to promote awareness and attention to newborn health, exchange information, and improve communi-

cation and collaboration among organizations beginning to work in newborn health. The new Child Survival Partnership intends to galvanize global and national commitment and action for accelerated reduction of child mortality worldwide. All three put their work in a context of poverty reduction, equity, and human rights. They collaborate closely to ensure a coordinated approach to the continuum of care and universal coverage with cost-effective interventions at the country level.

The first function of these partnerships is to stimulate and sustain the political will to keep the maternal, newborn and child health agenda as a central priority. They do so through dialogue at the highest level of government. As many countries have to step up their efforts in combating exclusion, monitoring inequities in maternal, newborn and child health and uptake of services, as well as tracking resources flows have become matters of prime concern *(8, 9)*. By keeping track of progress made, the partnerships can help to hold countries and their partners accountable *(10)*.

The partnerships can also assist in bridging the gap between knowledge and action *(11)* by facilitating the interaction between policy-makers, researchers, funders and other stakeholders who can influence the uptake of research findings – and reorient research towards solving the operational and systemic constraints that hold back the scaling up of effective interventions.

Finally, the partnerships can help bring together the various parties involved in maternal, newborn and child health (ministries of health, finance and planning, national non-governmental organizations, health professional groups, donor agencies, United Nations agencies, faith-based groups and others), or provide technical support to existing coordination mechanisms. This creates national partnerships through which funding, planning and implementation of national and subnational maternal, newborn and child health plans can be accelerated *(12)*.

of reforms. In countries where external assistance plays an important role, it also gives the impression that the policy interests of maternal, newborn and child health are those of the poverty reduction strategies (PRSPs) and sector-wide approaches (SWAps) through which reforms are steered *(13)* (see Boxes 7.3 and 7.4). The reality, however, is not so clear-cut.

Different constituencies, different languages

The constituencies from which champions of reform and those of maternal, newborn and child health draw support are quite different. Safe motherhood and child health programmes have been rather conservatively technical in emphasis *(4, 31)*, with solutions presented consistently in terms of technical strategies and cost-effectiveness *(32–36)*. For all the logical imperatives driving it, integration of the sub-programmes in the areas of maternal, newborn and child health and reproductive health has long been problematic *(37–40)*. Well-established vertical health programmes are frequently resistant to change, and there is apprehension (often with good cause) that the transition to integrated management and information systems carries the risk of losing corporate and technical skills that previously sustained their activities *(28, 40)*. Where integrated programmes have been established, they frequently bring with them parallel human resources, finance, logistics and monitoring systems *(28)*. To be fair, this has often helped to consolidate health systems. There remains, however, a persistent perception of selectivity and verticality in these programmes that inhibits their easy accommodation into comprehensive sectoral approaches.

The convergence of the maternal, newborn and child health agenda with that of the Cairo ICPD has added a second dimension. Policy discussions have become more inclusive, politicized and rights-driven in orientation. Firmly rooted in a vision where

Box 7.3 MNCH, poverty and the need for strategic information

The requirement for countries to formulate Poverty Reduction Strategy Papers (PRSPs) as a precursor to debt relief and the shared commitment to the Millennium Development Goals have cemented the links between pro-poor policy and maternal, newborn and child health (MNCH) priorities.

PRSPs systematically include maternal and child health (often not including a focus on newborn health) among their priorities, but the strategies to access the poor and the excluded are often a mere continuance of current (and not demonstrably successful) practice *(15)*. The significant shift, though, is that the PRSP process relocates MNCH priorities, poverty and exclusion securely on the national agenda, giving the health sector a seat at the table when the government discusses budget allocation to pro-poor policies *(16)*. No longer are MNCH programmes developed in isolation on the basis of vertical interventions: they are now being considered in the broader context of pro-poor health policy, and, more importantly, their significance for the overall governmental

poverty reduction policies is being recognized. Little gain has as yet been drawn from this new strategic advantage. Ministries of health often find it difficult to conceive that poverty reduction is their core business; they are often late in their participation in the PRSP drafting process, at a relatively low level of representation. But the potential exists, because by their very nature MNCH programmes fit naturally within a poverty reduction framework: they share similar values of entitlement and elimination of exclusion.

The first cycle of PRSPs has been criticized for their "striking sameness" and superficiality, with global strategies dominating over locally developed and more productive options *(15, 17)*. In decentralized Uganda, for example, the introduction of PRSPs brought with it generic, rather than specific, solutions, eroding advances achieved through the local initiatives that had been taken under the decentralized District Development Programme.

The analysis required for PRSPs has exposed the scarcity of relevant strategic information

in many developing countries. While in some cases – such as Gambia's – it has been possible to disaggregate key health information by age, gender, economic quintile and geographical division, few health information systems have that flexibility or specificity *(18–20)*. Information on MNCH, and particularly on maternal health, remains problematic, as is shown by the difficulties in documenting maternal mortality and establishing effective vital registration systems *(21)*. An even bigger obstacle, from a planning perspective, is the sketchiness of crucial information on resource availability within health care systems: estimates of the total number of skilled attendants for Burkina Faso, for example, range between 78 and 476, according to the data source. Information on the public network is often sketchy, while that on the private, not-for-profit and commercial sectors is often non-existent. WHO is now helping countries to fill these gaps, for example through Service Availability Mapping exercises or, more broadly, by helping establish health metrics networks.

public or quasi-public services would play a major role, they make increasingly explicit reference to entitlements to access care and health systems. As a result, the language used by champions of maternal, newborn and child health has become a combination of technical arguments and advocacy. The specificity and focus of maternal, newborn and child health thus reinforce an appearance of vertical special interest programmes, despite attempts to locate them more broadly within health systems. This generates resistance in the comprehensive ethos of sectoral approaches.

In contrast to the technical focus of maternal, newborn and child health programmes, health care reforms are driven by cross-cutting economic and managerial imperatives. The focus of operations for reform is the entire health sector, and its primary advo-cates are used to working at the systems level, both within national health systems and from outside. They naturally concentrate on a number of the systemic problems that constrain the health systems on which maternal, newborn and child health care relies, but the technical and service delivery considerations that are at the centre of the MNCH agenda are a secondary preoccupation *(13)*. Most importantly, the opera-tional articulation between community-level intervention, primary care and hospital referral services – the essence of district health systems and the organization of a continuum of care – is often inadequately dealt with.

The gap between the system-level focus and managerial language of reform, the on-the-ground service delivery preoccupations of district-level managers and the

Box 7.4 Sector-wide approaches

Poverty Reduction Strategy Papers (PRSPs) appeared when "sector-wide approach" (SWAp) mechanisms were emerging as the coordination and financing mechanisms to harmonize and align development assistance around a coherent sectoral reform *(20, 22, 23)*.

SWAp partners in a country – government, civil society and donor agencies – commit their resources to a collaborative programme of work. This includes policy development, capacity building and institutional reform: usually a mix of decentralization, restructuring of the civil service and ministries of health, broadening of health financing options, and the recognition that health systems are pluralistic *(24)*. SWAps are underpinned by the preparation of mid-term expenditure plans and corresponding financial, procurement, disbursal and accounting mechanisms. Implicit in the collaboration is the development of processes to negotiate strategic and management issues, and monitoring and evaluation of progress against agreed criteria *(23, 25)*.

The shared recognition by both donors and recipient governments of the need for coordination of resources was a critical factor in the early acceptance of SWAps *(26)*. Donors were – in theory – prepared to sacrifice profile by investing in pooled (or otherwise

coordinated) development assistance, in return for greater policy leverage and the opportunity to influence sectoral reform. Local ministries of health gained at least nominal leadership of the collaboration and access to an expanded resource pool, though they have lost the tactical advantage that previously accrued through negotiations with individual agencies *(26, 27)*. This simultaneous recognition of local "ownership" of sectoral reforms and the commitment of both donors and government to finance necessary reforms is significant: it marks a shift in development practice, moving from the coordination of resources to their active management by a government-led coalition of stakeholders *(28)*.

Even if results are by no means always satisfactory, indications are that the trend to use such cooperation mechanisms and shift to budget support is going to continue in the countries that make up the bulk of those in which progress is stagnating or in reverse *(29)*. The PRSPs have the potential to give SWAps a unifying policy focus against which the outcomes of reform might be measured *(18)*, while the processes required for the achievement of the Millennium Development Goal targets are sufficiently complex to reflect the overall outcomes of the health systems reforms coordinated under the SWAps.

SWAps came into being partly as a result of broad discontent with the efficiencies of project-based development assistance, and with the fragmentation and lack of coordination among donors, which was tackled in the coordination offered by their sectoral approach *(23)*. The second element in their development, however, was the World Bank's experience with its structural adjustment and macroeconomic processes *(19, 22)*. The combination of these strategies gave SWAps the potential to steer reform across the whole sector, with sufficient collective influence and financial leverage to drive long-term policy change with ministries of health.

The SWAp structure also does not always fit comfortably with the development assistance profile of other bilateral or nongovernmental agencies committed to maternal, new-born and child health and supportive of the values that underlie SWAps. They may find themselves limited by domestic legislation or administrative regulation in the extent to which they are able to commit to pooled funding mechanisms or shared monitoring and evaluation processes *(30)*. Crucially, in many countries nongovernmental organizations actively engage in maternal and child health, but usually have only limited access to SWAp governance mechanisms.

advocacy language in maternal, newborn and child health, puts champions of MNCH in an uncomfortable position *(31, 41)*. The strategic discussions take place in a highly politicized arena, where ministries of health compete with other ministries that have an interest in health, planning or financing; programmes are in tension with integrated services, hospitals with community-based services; central planning and budgeting contrasts with peripheral autonomy; and governments and nongovernmental organizations compete for the same donor funds *(42)*. Real pooling of resources through government financial systems is exceptional, even in countries where SWAp mechanisms attempt to apply this principle *(43)*. Despite the rhetoric of collaboration and consensus in shared priority setting, maternal, newborn and child health programmes often try to safeguard support through continued vertical donor funding *(44)*. Institutional agendas being what they are, this is probably inevitable to some degree *(45)*. The net effect, however, is often that maternal, newborn and child health programmes remain sceptical about their capacity to draw on sectoral resources, while sector managers may be tempted to locate such activities outside their core preoccupations. To keep maternal, newborn and child health at the centre of a policy agenda of health system development is particularly difficult for governments that have gone through decades of working on shoestring budgets and whose health systems are carved up in a patchwork of projects. These are precisely the countries that now face the biggest problems and the slowest progress, and are the most dependent on donors and their shifting agendas.

SUSTAINING POLITICAL MOMENTUM

Long-term sustained improvements in maternal, newborn and child health require long-term commitments that go well beyond the political lifespan of many decision-makers. Countries such as Cuba, Malaysia and Sri Lanka have rooted their impressive results in a stepwise extension of health systems coverage, over many years. They went through different phases – laying a foundation by building up a cadre of professional health workers, developing an accessible network of primary and referral-level services, and consolidating advances by improving the quality of care *(46)* – all in conjunction with improvements in living conditions and the status of women *(47)*. They prioritized broad social safety nets that ensured equitable access to health and education, making health services widely available, reducing barriers to key services, and providing primary and secondary schooling to all children *(48)*. Even in some of the poorest countries in Latin America, where monetary crises, weak institutions, social inequalities and poverty continue to hinder progress, there have been notable successes in countries that move towards generalized access to care.

These countries share a long-term commitment to build up health systems over many years, with sustained "political will" and "ownership" *(49–56)*. Most analysts would agree that a reasonable degree of macroeconomic and political stability and budget predictability is a precondition for mobilizing the institutional, human and financial resources that strengthening the health system requires. In many of the countries that experience problems in accelerating progress towards the MDGs, this precondition does not exist. Without sustained political momentum, however, effective leadership is unlikely to be present, be it at the centre where the broad sectoral decisions are made, or at the operational level, in the districts where the interaction with the population takes place.

What does it take to encourage national leaders to act to ensure the health rights of mothers and children – rights to which they are committed? There is extensive

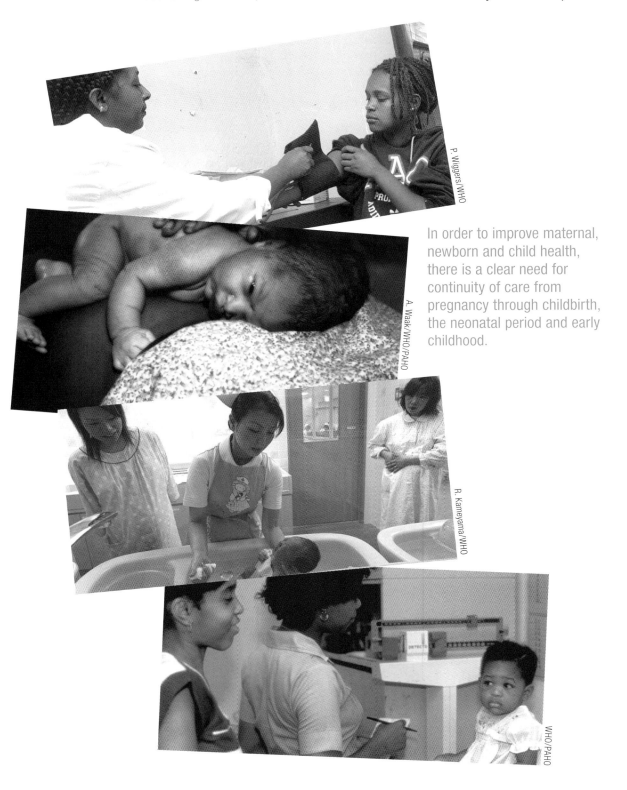

P. Wiggers/WHO

A. Waak/WHO/PAHO

In order to improve maternal, newborn and child health, there is a clear need for continuity of care from pregnancy through childbirth, the neonatal period and early childhood.

R. Kameyama/WHO

WHO/PAHO

knowledge of the technical and contextual interventions required to improve maternal, newborn and child health. In contrast, little is known about what can be done to make national political leaders give it their sustained support. The international community knows how to put things on the global policy agenda – the MDGs are proof of that – but there is a lot more to learn about how to bridge the gap between global attention and national action, and on how to maintain attention spans long enough to make a difference.

Political will first requires information on the magnitude, distribution and root causes of the problems that mothers and children face, and on the consequences, in terms of human capital and economic development, of failing to confront them effectively. Maternal, newborn and child health can boast a large network of advocates at the international level that has done much to produce and disseminate such information. Considerable progress has also been made in developing a battery of interventions, to demonstrate their cost-effectiveness, and to share that knowledge *(10, 36)*. Finally, much has been done to emphasize the need for a wide range of interventions to be implemented simultaneously at household level, in communities, and through health centres and hospitals.

This work is important and must continue. Framing discussions on maternal, newborn and child health in terms of a wide range of technical interventions, however, has given the impression of a complex and expensive undertaking. To attract the sustained attention of policy-makers, it needs to be articulated in a different language. The programmes have to be perceived by national decision-makers as effective and affordable ways of tackling well-recognized problems, but also as an agenda that commands a wide constituency and provides political mileage.

The common project that can bring together the interests and preoccupations of the MNCH programmes, as well as those of sector managers and health care providers, is that of universal access to care for mothers and children, embedded within an overall strategy of universal access for the whole population. Presenting MNCH in terms of progress towards universal access to care is not only a question of language. It frames the health of mothers, newborn babies and children within a broader, straightforward political project that is increasingly seen as a legitimate concern and is the subject of a wide social debate: responding to society's demand for the protection of the health of all its citizens.

REHABILITATING THE WORKFORCE

Not just a question of numbers

Providing universal access requires a viable and effective health workforce. Yet, as demand has increased and as more ways of delivering effective treatment and prevention have become available to respond to increasing needs and demand, the size, skills and infrastructure of the workforce have not kept pace. Indeed, in many countries economic and financial crises have destabilized and undermined the workforce during the past two decades. The resulting human resources crisis affects the whole spectrum of health care activities and MNCH programmes in particular. It has long been a major concern for health workers in the field, as well as for officials in ministries of health, but the problem has proved so intractable that the international community started to recognize it explicitly only in the late 1990s.

The most visible features are the staggering shortages and imbalances in the distribution of health workers. With insufficient production, downsizing and caps on recruitment under structural adjustment and fiscal stabilization policies, and with frozen salaries and losses to the private sector, migration and HIV/AIDS, filling the supply gap will remain a major challenge for years to come *(57–61)*. The scaling up of projected requirements for maternal, newborn and child health described in Chapters 5 and 6, for example, assumes the production, in the next 10 years, of at least 334 000 additional midwives (or professionals with midwifery skills), and the upgrading of 140 000 others. Some 27 000 doctors and technicians have to learn the skills to provide back-up maternal and newborn care, and the 100 000 full-time equivalent multipurpose professionals (many more under scenarios that rely less on community health workers), have to learn to follow up maternal and newborn care with integrated child care.

Along with the shortages, it appears that many countries have also witnessed a deterioration in the effectiveness of their workforce. The public expects skills, knowledge and competencies in maternal, newborn and child health care that health workers often lack, putting lives at risk. Upgrading can improve the effectiveness of the present workforce, but the current levels of skills are so poor and the mix so inappropriate that the potential of upgrading is limited. In-service training and supervision are generally considered key elements in improving outcomes, but there is a dire lack of evidence on cost-effec-

Box 7.5 Rebuilding health systems in post-crisis situations

Building the district health systems required for maternal, newborn and child health, let alone their equivalent in more pluralistic settings, supposes a reasonable degree of macroeconomic and political stability and a reasonable degree of budget predictability. In many of the countries where progress is stagnating, various forms of instability rule out systematic long-term approaches to rolling out health systems coverage and coordinating efforts through sector-wide approaches. Complex emergencies require the initial focus to be on repair, on getting things working, not on reform.

Even in countries in crisis, many professionals work tirelessly at field level, often without salaries. To achieve progress, the first requirement is for cash to get institutions working, to enable those who work in them to feed themselves and to avoid their having to resort to levying user charges or pilfering supplies. Paying decent wages to staff in place is then better than bringing in volunteers: sustainability is less an issue in these situations than preventing the disappearance of the basic public health system.

The first priority often is to establish institutional islands of dependable critical services: medical supply depots and hospitals, even if this sometimes conflicts with the urge to launch population-wide immunization programmes. Efforts should not be diluted but concentrated where the threshold for basic functioning can

be maintained or reinstated. All this works better with short-term planning horizons such as the 90-day cycle used in Liberia or Darfur, Sudan, involving nongovernmental organizations and humanitarian agencies, and engaging directly with peripheral service networks.

In the phase of post-crisis recovery the situation changes and a difficult transition has to be made from relief to development, in a context of competing priorities and scarce resources. Offering minimum health services in rural areas requires immediate strengthening of the health care network and, crucially, of the workforce.

Mozambique's recovery from years of war shows that support of recurrent expenditure, decentralized planning and strengthening of the information base, even at the peak of a crisis, can pay off. These measures can be the starting point for rationalizing aid flows, and can pave the way for integrated planning and incremental sector-wide approaches. Disbursement of aid for post-conflict reconstruction is often slow, and disproportionate to what the public health sector in these countries can mobilize by itself. Aid flows are particularly important for sustaining primary health care and maternal, newborn and child health care services. International actors have disproportionate power in these circumstances. But the transition from relief to development aid is particularly difficult: public administrative structures are very weak, so it takes time to re-establish the relations

that make it possible to channel funds into the health sector.

Cambodia, recovering after the decimation of its health workforce as a consequence of the actions of the Khmer Rouge, introduced accelerated training to build capacity in the early 1980s. By the time sectoral reforms were introduced, its health workforce was bloated, poorly trained and maldistributed. The upgrading of nurses to doctors eroded competent leadership in nursing. Donor-supported changes in the nursing curriculum resulted in the closure of one-year primary midwife training, and the introduction of a postgraduate midwifery diploma that will serve to reinforce the current concentration of midwives in urban areas, where private practice provides welcome additional income *(62, 63)*. While aware of the critical dilemma it faces, the Cambodian Ministry of Health has been unable to mount a strategic response that will effectively redress this shortage.

The responsibility for quickly restoring acceptable standards of health services falls on under-resourced ministries of health. In such circumstances the expansion of the network to cover remote areas is far slower and more expensive than would usually be expected. If recurrent costs are underestimated when investment decisions are made, this undermines the sector's long-term sustainability.

tive approaches to improving competency, particularly in conditions where pre-service training is poor and working conditions inadequate. The situation may be less critical for child care, but in many places large parts of the workforce do not reach the competency threshold required for effective and safe maternal and newborn care. Clearly, it is vital that the new professionals who will fill the numbers gap do reach that threshold.

Planning is an essential prerequisite to correct the shortages and to improve the skills mix and the working environment; so is building the institutional capacity to manage human resources for health. But to plan is not sufficient: today's problems require solutions for today. Developing countries and countries in transition frequently have disruptive histories that have challenged cohesive workforce development. After years of neglect, the resulting problems require immediate attention, at the same time as planning and reform prepare the future (see Box 7.5). These immediate and thorny problems include working and employment conditions in the public sector, and the resulting distortions in the behaviour and productivity of the health workforce.

Recovering from the legacy of past neglect

In many countries the public sector health workforce is often labelled "unproductive", "poorly motivated", "inefficient", "client unfriendly", or even "corrupt". "Unfair" salaries are presented as the justification of "inevitable" predatory behaviour and public-to-private brain-drain *(64)*. This has eroded the implicit psychological and social contracts that underlie the public service values of well-functioning public organizations *(65)*. Most observers would agree that often public sector salaries are definitely unfair and insufficient for daily living expenses, let alone for living up to the expectations of health professionals; in many countries they have been falling, in real terms, over recent decades. For example, nurses in Mozambique have seen the purchasing power of their salaries eroded by 85–90% over 15 years. In such a context, demotivation, overall lack of commitment and low productivity are to be expected.

It should come as no surprise that in order to compensate for unrealistically low salaries, health workers increasingly rely on individual coping strategies to boost their income, for example by competing for access to seminars or training courses with attractive per diems or by engaging in dual practice *(64, 66, 67)*. Many combine salaried public sector work with a fee-for-service private clientele. Others stay away from work to earn a living in other ways, or resort to predatory behaviour such as extracting under-the-counter payments or misappropriating drugs or other supplies. The problems such behaviour creates are increasingly recognized, although the subject remains taboo for many ministries of health and development agencies *(68)*.

When health workers set up in dual practice to improve their living conditions – or merely to make ends meet – this does not necessarily interfere with their duties; it may even help to retain valuable elements in public service. Most often, however, it entails at least competition for time and a loss of resources for the public sector, while reinforcing a rural-urban and public-private brain-drain of the best-trained and most competent workers. This in turn reinforces the attraction of a job "on the side", which quickly becomes not only more rewarding financially, but also professionally and in terms of social prestige.

There are even more serious consequences when health workers resort to predatory behaviour: financial exploitation of patients builds a barrier to access to care, and may have catastrophic effects for patients if they have to pay for care that is not needed or effective but is always expensive. In the long run, this affects the legitimacy and credibility of the public sector and harms the essential relation of trust between users and providers.

Pretending that the problem does not exist, or that it is merely a question of individual ethics, does not do justice to the nature and extent of the problem and will not make it go away. Prohibition of dual practice is equally unlikely to meet with success, certainly where salaries are patently insufficient. As an isolated measure, the use of restrictive regulations – when not blatantly ignored – only drives dual practice underground and makes it difficult to correct its negative effects. Despite this, many governments still resort to prohibition as their main means of controlling dual practice. Another disappointing approach is to downsize the workforce (in the hope that dividing the salary mass among a smaller number will leave a better individual income for those who remain). Such initiatives often generate so much resistance that they do not reach a stage of implementation. Where retrenchment becomes a reality it is rarely followed by substantial salary increases, so that the problem remains and the public health system is even less capable than before of assuming its mission.

On the other hand, it is remarkable that many people do remain in public service, given the gap between current salary levels and what they could earn in alternative employment. There obviously are other sources of motivation: social responsibility, self-fulfilment, professional satisfaction, working conditions and prestige *(69)*. In fact, most health workers implicitly or explicitly condemn dual practice and predatory behaviour, though they may attempt to explain and justify them in various ways. There is often a disconnection between health workers' self-image as honest public servants wanting to do a decent job and the brutal facts of life that force them to betray that image. The manifest unease that this provokes offers important prospects. It suggests that, even in difficult circumstances, behaviours that depart from traditional public servant deontology have not been interiorized as a norm. This ambiguity suggests that interventions to mitigate the erosion of proper conduct would be welcomed *(70)*.

A piecemeal approach using a combination of measures – career possibilities, prospects for training, and others – can go a long way towards rehabilitating the working environment. A prerequisite to dealing with these situations is to confront the problem openly. That is the only way to create the possibility of containing and discouraging income-generating activities that present conflicts of interest, in favour of ad hoc solutions that have less negative impact on the functioning of the health services. Besides minimizing conflicts of interest, open discussion can diminish the feeling of unfairness among colleagues. It can help to build a social environment that reinforces professional behaviour free from the clientelism and the arbitrariness that is prevalent in the public sector of many countries. Peer influence, for example through professional societies, can be effective in improving professional accountability, particularly if it is seen as building up public reputation and status *(71)*. It then becomes possible to manage human resources in a more transparent and predictable way. There are indications that the newer generations of professionals have more modest expectations and are realistic enough to see that the market for dual practice is finite and to a large extent occupied by their elders. This gives scope for the introduction of systems of incentives that are consistent with the health system's social goals *(72)*.

Where, for example, financial compensation for work in deprived areas is introduced in a context that provides a clear sense of purpose and the necessary recognition, this may help to reinstate lost public service values. The same goes for the introduction of performance-linked financial incentives. These can, in principle, overcome the problem of competition for working time, one of the major drawbacks of dual practice. However, such approaches require well functioning and transparent bureaucracies, so they are, a priori, most difficult to implement on a large scale in the countries most in need of them.

Destabilization with the best of intentions

The individual strategies of health personnel to cope with their financial predicament – dual practice, predatory behaviour or other coping strategies – are compounded by donor interventions in the labour markets of developing countries. Often, such interventions have fractured existing workforces by promoting structural reforms or establishing programmes that bypass existing employer-employee relationships. The result has been a workforce that is not available to take on its basic tasks and lacks the solidarity, resilience and resources to accept new challenges *(61)*.

International development agencies have become more sensitized to the problem over recent years. They are also changing their recruitment practices to help minimize the brain drain consequent on their poaching the most competent and productive ministry of health staff. Many development organizations implement, at least in principle, recruitment policies that divert government staff from their basic duties only for short-term tasks, leaving them to return before the civil service functions suffer negative consequences *(73)*. Donors are also essential partners in the search for solutions: policy dialogue between donors and government is particularly important to support good governance and capacity-building. As well as providing an opportunity to document and analyse best practices, such dialogue can make both reformers and champions of MNCH aware of the consequences of programme development on the specific circumstances in which the health workforce operates.

The situation of profound crisis that characterizes the workforce in many countries requires long-term planning and structural reform as well as immediate short-term management. Countries need to find solutions to human resources challenges that are appropriate to their own circumstances, their political culture and their economic ability. Building up a global knowledge base on best practices, however, may assist donors and governments by informing their analysis and problem-solving and assessment of the potential consequences – intended and unintended – on the workforce of initiatives to tackle health problems and develop health systems. This may help them face up to the problems caused by dual practice and fragmentation of the health care system before these become part of the organizational culture of the public sector *(74)*.

Tackling the salary problem

If nothing is done, disinvestment in the workforce is more likely to increase than to diminish *(75)*, and thus to jeopardize hopes of improving maternal, newborn and child health. There is no getting around the fact that low salaries and poor working conditions remain a major disincentive to the public sector workforce. Sustainable ways will have to be devised of offering competitive remuneration and incentive packages that can attract, motivate and retain competent and effective health workers.

The challenge is considerable. At present levels of remuneration, the increase in salary mass required for the extension of coverage projected in Chapters 5 and 6 amounts to a total of US$ 35 billion over the next decade. Particularly important in countries that are losing human resources for health, the gap between these salaries and expectations, as well as the gap between these salaries and what health workers can earn in the private sector, in alternative employment or by migrating to richer countries, is often huge. Medical doctors and health system managers in middle-income countries can easily earn three times their salary by running a small private practice; in low-income countries they can earn six or seven times their salary by doing so *(69)*. In Thailand a complex system of incentives did not close the gap between public salaries for doctors and income from private practice, but proved enough to retain doctors in rural practice. It did, however, require a multiplication of the basic salary by a factor of four to five, while nurses' salaries were boosted by 70% *(76, 77)*. In Brazil, multiplying salaries by a factor of two to three has had some effect in retaining staff, but was still considered insufficient *(78)*. In Cambodia, salaries plus allowances would have to be multiplied by between eight and ten in order to make up for the cost of living *(79)*. In Georgia it has been suggested that salaries and allowances should be multiplied by five within the next few years. There is no general rule of thumb to say how much salaries of health personnel in poor countries have to be increased to become fair and competitive: it varies very much from country to country. But it is safe to say that in many of the countries where progress towards the MDGs is disappointing, very substantial increases are urgently needed.

This means that out of the projected additional costs for scaling up MNCH (US$ 91 billion) the part that is earmarked for salaries and other staff benefits, i.e. US$ 35 billion, is well below what is required to recruit, retain and redeploy staff in the 75 countries for which the scale-up scenarios were developed. Even an attempt to close the remuneration gap by doubling or even tripling the total workforce's salary mass and benefits might still be insufficient to attract, retain and redeploy quality staff. But it would correspond to an increase of 2%, rising over 10 years to 17%, of current public expenditure on health, merely for raising payment of the MNCH workforce to a fairer level. This is obviously a challenge of a magnitude that most poor countries cannot face alone.

The collaborative engagement provided by SWAps does have the potential to move towards consistency between the salary and conditions offered by ministries of health, donors and nongovernmental organizations, but that is only a partial solution. A salary increase by itself would not automatically reinstate the sense of purpose that is required to make public services function *(75)*. Health workers have to be confident that improvements will not be a one-off, short-term stop-gap solution. There has to be a clear, predictable and sustainable assurance that work in the health sector will become rewarding – in terms of living conditions, but also socially and professionally. This will require a refinancing of the whole health sector, in a way that guarantees long-term stability.

FINANCIAL PROTECTION TO ENSURE UNIVERSAL ACCESS

Funding is the killer assumption underlying the planning of maternal, newborn and child health care and of a solution to the human resource crisis, a fact that donors and governments are often reluctant to acknowledge *(80–82)*. Ensuring universal access to maternal, newborn and child health care, however, is not merely a question of increasing the supply of services and paying health care providers. For services to be taken up, financial barriers to access have to be reduced or eliminated and users given predictable financial protection against the costs of seeking care: universal access has to go with financial protection *(83)*. Only then can health services be made universally available on the basis of need rather than on the basis of people's ability to pay, and households and individuals protected from financial hardship or impoverishment.

There are essentially two broad options to organize this: through a general tax-based system or through a social health insurance system. Both provide financial risk protection and promote equity through prepayment of health care costs and pooling of health risks. The clearest difference between the two systems lies in the way revenues are collected. In tax-based systems, the main source of funds is general tax revenue, with tax funds allocated by the government for purchasing or providing health services. In social health insurance, pre-payments for health care come directly from workers, the self-employed, enterprises and governments, on a compulsory basis. Both can be called insurance systems because they pool contributions across a large number of people: the difference is that in tax-based systems the insurance is implicit, whereas in social health insurance it is explicit. There are also mixed systems: the organization of financial protection for part of the population is covered via a tax-based system, while other groups are covered by various types of health insurance or other forms of social protection.

Whichever organization of the health financing system is adopted, two things are important: first, that ultimately no population groups are excluded; second, that maternal, newborn and child health services are part of the set of services to which citizens are entitled and that are financed in a coherent way through the selected system. If these conditions are met, whether services are provided by public-sector employees or purchased from nongovernmental providers in the non-profit sector, or from other private providers becomes a secondary issue. The reality is that in most countries health care delivery systems are pluralistic. The choice of what is, at a given moment, the optimal balance, depends on its specific circumstances, experience and history. Provided the organization of the health financing system guarantees the whole population its health entitlements in an equitable way, the organization of health care delivery in pluralistic systems is not a matter of principle, but of carefully monitoring positive and negative effects and of negotiation and regulation.

With time, most countries tend to widen prepayment and pooling schemes and move towards universal financial protection, in parallel with the extension of their health care supply networks. It can take many years, however, to move from a situation of a limited supply of services, high out-of-pocket payments and exclusion of the poor to a situation of universal access and financial protection. Countries at varying stages of economic development and in different social and political contexts have different problems and may resort to other schemes to shore up supply of, and access to, services. They may levy user fees or implement a variety of prepayment and pooling schemes for selected population groups.

Replacing user fees by prepayment, pooling and a refinancing of the sector

In the poorest countries, where large numbers of people are excluded from access to health care, financial protection is often absent. The limited supply of "free" services is usually tax-based and underfunded. Current estimates show that out-of-pocket expenditure in these countries is between two and three times the total expenditure by government and donors, a substantial proportion of these out-of-pocket expenses being captured by commercial providers or through the payment of informal fees. The latter have become a major obstacle which has prevented the poor from accessing scarce public services, with the unpredictability of the cost compounding their reluctance to seek care.

The out-of-pocket expenditures that are channelled into the provision of public services rarely amount to a substantial increase in their funding. In some cases, the introduction of user fees has been accompanied by an improvement in the quality of services, the elimination of informal fees, and a transparent fee structure; the revenue has then permitted the revitalization of moribund services. Even in these cases, however, the drawbacks overshadow the benefits: in most countries, for example in Kenya, Papua New Guinea, the United Republic of Tanzania and other countries, the introduction of user fees has resulted in increased exclusion, including a diminished uptake of maternal, newborn and child health services by the poorest population groups.

Efforts to mitigate the exclusion that goes with the introduction of user fees have been disappointing. Exemption schemes for the poor rarely work, partly because of the dilemmas that staff face when they realize that the exemptions they approve directly reduce the income of the health service or their own. The main beneficiaries of exemption schemes are frequently capable of paying – including staff of health facilities and their relatives *(84)*. To mitigate conflicts of interest, countries such as Cambodia experiment with funds cosponsored by key donors and held in trust by local nongovernmental organizations, distinct from the health services, who decide on exemptions *(85)*. With eligible clients often comprising more than 30% of attendances, however, this solution raises major concerns of sustainability. An alternative to exemption schemes are loans. Loan schemes to assist with the costs associated with childbirth have been piloted in Sierra Leone *(86)*. The loans enable repayment of costs incurred over a longer time frame, with incremental repayments and without interest. There have been some initial successes, but implementation depends on strong community leadership and mobilization, and scaling up on a significant scale has not been reported.

By and large, the introduction of user fees is not a viable answer to the underfunding of the health sector: it institutionalizes exclusion of the poor and does not accelerate progress towards universal access and financial coverage. Nevertheless, abolishing user fees where they already exist is not a panacea: it needs to be accompanied, from the very day they are brought to an end, by structural changes and a refinancing of the health services. The South African government, for example, has eliminated user fees for maternal and child health care in a targeted approach to reduce health inequalities. This has led to increased use of antenatal and child health services but also to resistance by health care providers, whose workload has increased with no corresponding increase in benefits or support. Health workers expressed concerns about over-servicing, on-selling of free medications and in-migration from neighbouring states. Without other necessary structural reforms – increased 24-hour availability of services, improved resourcing and referral, enhanced technical capacity, and changed attitudes to patients – gains made by removing financial barriers alone may not be adequate *(87)*. Without a refinancing of health services and the introduction of financial protection systems, abolishing existing systems of user fees only makes a bad situation worse.

Making the most of transitory financial protection mechanisms

As countries expand their health care networks, they often also supplement the limited coverage of public or quasi-public health insurance (social health insurance based on taxation, or mixed systems) through a multitude of voluntary insurance schemes: community, cooperative, employer-based and other private schemes. These usually provide limited financial protection from catastrophic expenditure, support equity in the distribution of spending, and facilitate the provision of affordable quality care to the enrolled population. They emerge in countries that are usually no longer at a stage of massive deprivation – their supply of health care is better – but present the transitional queuing pattern of exclusion with the large inequalities described in Chapter 2.

The introduction of social insurance schemes for poor people in Viet Nam, for example, has ensured access to maternal and newborn health services. But the near-poor, who are not covered by these social insurance schemes, remain ill-equipped to cope with catastrophic health costs; furthermore, there has been a perceived decline in quality in peripheral health services, and there have been reports that patients seeking care under insurance provisions are discriminated against in terms of waiting times *(88)*. Another initiative is the National Maternal and Child Health Insurance Programme in Bolivia, which covers antenatal care, labour and delivery (including caesarean sections and emergency care), postnatal care and newborn care *(89)*. Funded by pooled prepayments and central tax revenues through municipality funds, facilities are reimbursed on an annual basis for services provided. The poorest quintiles of the population almost doubled their uptake of skilled care for birthing, from 11% to 20%. The major beneficiaries of the insurance scheme, however, at least in the initial phase, were people in the upper income quintiles.

Schemes such as these offer protection to only a limited section of the population or only for a limited package of benefits. Yet by introducing prepayment and pooling in a context of a growing supply of services, they may help to accelerate the transition to universal access with financial protection.

Generalizing financial protection

In countries where the health care network is well developed, and exclusion from access to care is limited to a relatively marginal group, the need to generalize financial protection persists, also for the non-excluded. Even households that can afford to access services may be forced to reduce other basic expenditure, on education for example, or may incur catastrophic expenses.

Catastrophic payments for health care – which push about 100 million people in the world into poverty every year – occur wherever health services require out-of-pocket payments, there are no mechanisms for financial risk-pooling, and households have a limited capacity to pay *(90)*. Several middle-income countries and countries in transition with a well-developed supply of services fulfil these conditions. In Brazil and Colombia, for example, as many as 10% and 6% of households, respectively, face catastrophic payments *(91)*. As the supply of health services expands, the frequency of catastrophic expenditure actually rises unless social protection mechanisms are developed at the same time. Complications of childbirth, trauma and accidents or chronic diseases in children, in particular, easily lead to catastrophic expenditure. While the poorest people are most in need and are most often excluded, all income groups may be affected by the financial consequences of ill-health, if copayments are high or if financial protection coverage is limited. Financial protection should not therefore be limited to the poorest. Universal access requires financial protection mechanisms that are designed in ways that protect all households from catastrophic spending.

CHANNELLING FUNDS EFFECTIVELY

The key to moving towards universal access and financial protection is the organization of financing. Current government expenditure and international flows cannot guarantee universal access and financial protection, because they are insufficient and because they are too unpredictable. At the same time, historical patterns of financial management – incremental adjustments of the recurrent programme budgets, supplemented by donor-funded projects – have often been slow to adapt to initiatives aimed at scaling up universal access to health care *(92)*. Funding flows have not only to increase, they have to be channelled in a different way.

Some countries, such as Thailand, have made a quantum leap in extending financial coverage, by merging various partial schemes and extending entitlements to the whole population. This obviously requires the fiscal space to increase public funding sufficiently so as to ensure an adequate supply of services, with a benefit package that covers a wide range of services, including those required to improve maternal, newborn and child health. The challenge is to capture the different sources of funding so as to scale up both access and financial protection in a stable and predictable way. In most countries, financial sustainability will only be achieved in the short and middle term by looking at all sources of funding: external and domestic, public and private.

Channelling resources through discrete programmes or projects has shown its limitations, not least because it fails to take account of the cross-cutting structural workforce issues. Pooling funds into financial protection mechanisms that are developed alongside increased access makes the situation more predictable and allows the problem of workforce financing to be given due consideration. It leaves room for flexible approaches, such as resorting to direct recruitment of staff or purchasing of services outside the public sector, according to the specific circumstances of the country. Pooling can improve the absorptive capacity of countries and the management of the impact of funding flows on inflation, exchange rates and economic growth. But it is no panacea. In many countries, the institutional capacity to create, expand and manage coherent schemes for moving towards universal access and financial protection needs to be built.

If governments are to live up to their responsibilities as the ultimate stewards of their countries' health systems and to complete universal coverage, merging financial protection schemes is a task that becomes unavoidable at some point. Few countries have found it easy to merge fragmented channels of financial protection if they are already well developed: vested interests often prevail over managerial considerations. To minimize the difficulties it is important to create the institutional capacity to run financial protection schemes at a very early stage, with governments firmly in the lead but also with inbuilt systems of checks and balances.

To frame maternal, newborn and child health services in terms of universal access and financial protection may command the wide constituency and promise the political visibility that mobilization of decision-makers requires. The drawback is that the central position of maternal, newborn and child health is not automatically guaranteed. Pooling of funds through insurance schemes that support the drive towards universal access and financial protection has to go together with a clear specification of the population's entitlements to maternal, newborn and child health care. The international community can contribute to this, but ultimately pressure will have to come from civil society within countries. This depends on political entrepreneurship and institutional capacity; it also requires a place at the negotiating table for civil society organizations. As the donor community moves from project funding towards poverty reduction strategies, general budget support, and sector reform, these civil society organizations run the risk of being sidelined. Civil society organizations can and should, however, do more than provide services *(93)*: they are essential to maintaining a sustained political commitment to improving maternal, newborn and child health.

It is important that stakeholders from civil society are represented in steering financial protection mechanisms, and particularly in the priority-setting processes. This is to ensure that many less popular, politically sensitive aspects of maternal, newborn and child health (including issues such as unsafe abortion, adolescent pregnancy, sexual coercion and violence, child abuse and neglect, etc.) are not forgotten. It is also a way to improve the chances that health sector policies are linked to strategies that tackle the social determinants of gender inequality, poverty and exclusion.

Furthermore, it is important that stakeholders from civil society contribute to a system of checks and balances on the functioning of health services – both public and in private. They have an important role to play in helping mothers and children take up their entitlements and in protecting consumers against financial exploitation and overmedicalization. This watchdog function requires involvement not only in planning, but also in assessment and monitoring of projects, programmes and services.

In many countries, civil society organizations have little institutional capacity to support priority setting, monitoring, and assisting mothers and children to claim their entitlements. In these cases, then, there is a need for investment in national civil society organizations, partly by earmarking donor funds to do so (see Box 7.6). Some

Box 7.6 Civil society involvement requires support

In May, 2004, the 57th World Health Assembly endorsed WHO's first strategy to accelerate progress in reproductive health *(94)*. It recommends action in key areas, including the mobilization of political will as a prerequisite for success in strengthening health system capacity; setting the right priorities; creating supportive legislative and regulatory frameworks; and strengthening monitoring, evaluation, and accountability.

Experience from Bangladesh in the mid-1990s shows that time and money invested in mobilizing constituencies is well worth it; failing to do so can have serious negative consequences.

Bangladesh formulated its first Health and Population Sector Strategy (HPSS) in 1996 *(95)*, and a five-year Health and Population Sector Programme (HPSP) in 1998 *(96)*. The country established "improving the health of women, children, and the poor" as the main goal and earmarked about 60% of the national health budget for an essential services package to be delivered through the primary health care system. The centrepiece was reproductive health care: safe motherhood, including expansion of emergency obstetric care; family planning; prevention and control of reproductive-tract infections and sexually transmitted diseases, including HIV/AIDS; maternal nutrition; menstrual regulation and management of the complications of unsafe abortions; adolescent care; and infertility and newborn care.

The HPSP introduced major structural changes: unification of health and family planning cadres under a single management to deliver integrated essential services; sector-wide planning, management, and financing; community and stakeholder participation in policy and programme formulation, implementation, and monitoring; decentralization of health services and autonomy in hospital

management; partnerships with nongovernmental organizations and mainstreaming gender issues.

Government and international donors agreed that civil society had to be involved in the design stage, to build the consensus needed for structural change. They therefore allocated time, funds and personnel in order to work with civil society for nearly two years. The task force on community and stakeholder participation organized nationwide consultations with 34 stakeholder groups, including service users and providers, women, adolescents, and indigenous populations, professional and nongovernmental organizations, and the media *(97)*.

The strong civil society voice in programme formulation helped secure backing by top political leaders under a new government: Bangladesh shifted its health policy priorities and investment from a narrow focus on family planning to comprehensive services for sexual and reproductive health. Sector-wide programming and unification of lower levels of health and family planning cadres made notable progress, as did various programme initiatives. Outcome indicators improved: the maternal mortality ratio (from 4.1 to 3.2 per 1000 live births); the fertility rate (from 3.3 to 2.9 per woman aged 15–49 years); severe malnutrition (from 20.6% to 12.9%); the under-five mortality rate (from 96 to 83 per 1000 live births); antenatal care coverage (from 26.4% to 47.5%); and met need for essential obstetric care (from 5.1% to 26.5%) *(98)*.

To plan and steer continuing consultation during implementation of the plan, the government had established a national committee, which created 25 community-based primary stakeholder committees in different regions of the country as "health watch groups". However, contrary to what happened during the design phase, the consultative process was

not prioritized, funded or officially recognized. The first two annual programme reviews did not organize the previously agreed stakeholder dialogues.

This left the programme vulnerable when a new government came to power. Opponents of reform, particularly the family planning lobby, persuaded the new government to oppose the pivotal ingredient: integrated service delivery for sexual and reproductive health through unification of health and family planning cadres. As a result, implementation stalled and, in 2003, the government reversed the unification decision *(99)*. Donors protested, temporarily suspending aid, but with little effect. Excluded from systematic consultation since 1999, civil society alliances had nearly disappeared. Constituency building now needs to be restarted, almost from scratch.

Several lessons can be drawn from the Bangladesh experience *(50)*. First, changing agendas requires a popular base. In Bangladesh, nongovernmental and women's organizations composed the mass base of support and forged broader alliances for political weight. Second, constituency and alliance building requires sustained funding not only for advocacy but also for capacity building. Third, for credibility and staying power, mobilization is best delegated to be led by civil society organizations. Fourth, the primary gatekeepers – governments and donors – must give the relevant civil society organizations access to decision-making processes, and also involve them in policy-making, programme implementation, and monitoring. Only in this way is it possible to sustain political will long enough to survive changes in governments and donor interests, and make a significant contribution to achieving universal access.

Source: *(50)*.

countries have done this through social funds and similar mechanisms, others have institutionalized collaboration and contracting with non-profit organizations in the field of service delivery, expanding that collaboration naturally into policy dialogue. In most countries, however, much needs to be done, and there is an urgent need for better documentation of what works and what does not.

Universal access for mothers and children requires health systems to be able to respond to the needs and demands of the population, and to offer protection against the financial hardship that results from ill-health. To make this possible, investments in health systems and in human resources for health need to be stepped up. Maternal, newborn and child health should constitute the core of the health entitlements protected and funded through universal coverage systems. In many countries this will require a mix of external and domestic funding and will not succeed without greatly increased global support and solidarity. But it will build the basis for an end to the widespread exclusion of many mothers and children throughout the world from access to a continuum of care that extends from pregnancy through childbirth, the neonatal period and childhood. People want and societies need mothers and children to be healthy. That is why every mother and every child counts so much in our ambitions for a better tomorrow.

References

1. Maine D, Rosenfield A. The Safe Motherhood Initiative: why has it stalled? *American Journal of Public Health*, 1999, 89:480–482.

2. Berer M, Sundari Ravindran TK. Preventing maternal mortality: evidence, resources, leadership, action. In: Berer M, Sundari Ravindran TK, eds. *Safe motherhood initiatives: critical issues*. London, Blackwell Science, 1999 (Reproductive Health Matters: 3–9).

3. McDonagh M, Goodburn E. Maternal health and health sector reform: opportunities and challenges. In: De Brouwere V, Van Lerberghe W, eds. *Safe motherhood strategies: a review of the evidence*. Antwerp, ITG Press, 2001 (Studies in Health Services Organisation and Policy, 17:371–385.

4. AbouZahr C. Cautious champions: international agency efforts to get safe motherhood onto the agenda. In: Van Lerberghe W, De Brouwere V, eds. *Safe motherhood strategies: a review of the evidence*. Antwerp, ITG Press, 2001 (Studies in Health Services Organisation and Policy, 17:387–414).

5. Picazzo O. Child health financing and cost-effectiveness: supplement to the report on the Analytic Review of IMCI (unpublished).

6. *The analytic review of the Integrated Management of Childhood Illness strategy. Final report, November 2003*. Geneva, World Health Organization, 2003 (http://www.who.int/child-adolescent-health/New_Publications/IMCI/ISBN_92_4_159173_0.pdf, accessed 4 February 2005).

7. McKinsey & Company. *Developing successful global health alliances*. Seattle, Bill & Melinda Gates Foundation, 2002 (http://www.gatesfoundation.org/nr/downloads/globalhealth/GlobalHealthAlliances.pdf, accessed 4 February 2005).

8. Wagstaff A, Bustreo F, Bryce J, Claeson M; WHO-World Bank Child Health and Poverty Working Group. Child health: reaching the poor. *American Journal of Public Health*, 2004, 94:726–736.

9. Gwatkin DR, Bhuiya A, Victora CG. Making health systems more equitable. *Lancet*, 2004, 364:1273–1280.

10. The Bellagio Study Group on Child Survival. Knowledge into action for child survival. *Lancet*, 2003, 362:323–327.

11. Haines A, Kuruvilla S, Borchert M. Bridging the implementation gap between knowledge and action for health. *Bulletin of the World Health Organization*, 2004, 82:724–732.

12. Lawn JE, Cousens S, Bhutta ZA, Darmstadt GL, Martines J, Paul V et al. Why are 4 million newborn babies dying each year? *Lancet*, 2004, 364:1121.

13. Goodburn E, Campbell O. Reducing maternal mortality in the developing world: sector-wide approaches may be the key. *BMJ*, 2001, 322:917–920.

14. OECD/DAC Working Party on Aid Evaluation. *Review of the DAC principles for the evaluation of development assistance, conclusions and recommendations*. Paris, Organisation for Economic Co-operation and Development, 1998.

15. Laterveer L, Niessen LW, Yazbeck AS. Pro-poor health policies in poverty reduction strategies. *Health Policy and Planning*, 2003, 18:138–145.

16. Walford V. Health in Poverty Reduction Strategy Papers (PRSPs): an introduction and early experience. London, DFID Health Systems Resource Centre, 2002.

17. Craig D, Porter D. Poverty Reduction Strategy Papers: a new convergence. *World Development*, 2003, 31:53–69.

18. *Poverty Reduction Strategy Papers: their significance for health: second synthesis report*. World Health Organization, Geneva, 2004 (WHO/HDP/PRSP/04.1).

19. Peters D, Chao S. The sector-wide approach in health: what is it? Where is it leading? *International Journal of Health Planning and Management*, 1998, 13:177–190.

20. Cassels A, Janovsky K. Sectoral investment in health: prescription or principles? *Social Science and Medicine*, 1997, 44:1073–1076.

21. Graham W, Hussein J. The right to count. *Lancet*, 2004, 363:989.

22. Harrold P and Associates. *The broad sector approach to investment lending*. World Bank, New York, NY, 1995 (World Bank Discussion Papers, Africa Technical Department Series, No. 302).

23. Cassels A. *A guide to sector-wide approaches for health development: concepts, issues and working arrangements*. World Health Organization, Geneva, 1997.

24. Cassels A. Health sector reform: key issues in less developed countries. *Journal of International Development*, 1995, 7: 329–347.

25. Foster M, Brown A, Conway T. *Sector-wide approaches for health development: a review of experience*. World Health Organization, Geneva, 2000 (WHO/GPE/00.1).

26. Hill PS. The rhetoric of sector-wide approaches to health development. *Social Science and Medicine*, 2002, 54:1725–1737.

27. Buse K, Gwin C. The World Bank and global cooperation in health: the case of Bangladesh. *Lancet*, 1998, 351:665–669.

28. Lush L, Cleland J, Walt G, Mayhew S. Integrating reproductive health: myth and ideology. *Bulletin of the World Health Organization*, 1999, 77:771–777.

29. Abrantes AV. Strategic options for World Bank support to Africa in health, nutrition and population. Paper presented at: Forum Barcelona, Barcelona, 8 June 2004 (http://www.barcelona2004.org/eng/eventos/dialogos/docs/ponencias/154p_aabranteseng.pdf, accessed 2 October 2004).

30. Brown A, Foster M, Norton A, Naschold F. *The status of sector wide approaches*. Overseas Development Institute, London, 2001 (Working Paper 142).

31. Standing H. An overview of changing agendas in health sector reforms. *Reproductive Health Matters*, 2002, 10:19–28.

32. Rosenfield A, Maine D. Maternal mortality – a neglected tragedy. Where is the M in MCH? *Lancet*, 1985, 2:83–85.

33. *Reduction of maternal mortality: a joint WHO/UNFPA/UNICEF/World Bank statement*. Geneva, World Health Organization, 1999.

34. Koblinsky MA, Campbell O, Heichelheim J. Organizing delivery care: what works for safe motherhood? *Bulletin of the World Health Organization*, 1999, 77:399–406.

35. De Brouwere V, Van Lerberghe W, eds. *Safe motherhood strategies: a review of the evidence*. Antwerp, ITG Press, 2001 (Studies in Health Services Organisation and Policy, 17).

36. Jones G, Steketee RW, Black RE, Bhutta ZA, Morris SS, and the Bellagio Child Survival Study Group. How many child deaths can we prevent this year? *Lancet*, 2003, 362:65–71.

37. Mayhew SH, Lush L, Cleland J, Walt G. Implementing the integration of component services for reproductive health. *Studies in Family Planning*, 2000, 31:151–162.

38. Mayhew S. Integrating MCH/FP and STD/HIV services: current debates and future directions. *Health Policy and Planning*, 1996, 11:339–353.

39. Berer M. Integration of sexual and reproductive health services: a health sector priority. *Reproductive Health Matters*, 2003, 11:6–15.

40. Huque ZA, Leppard M, Mavalankar D, Akhter HH, Chowdhury TA. Safe motherhood programmes in Bangladesh. In: Berer M, Sundari Ravindran TK, eds. *Safe motherhood initiatives: critical issues*. London, Blackwell Science, 1999 (Reproductive Health Matters: 53–61).

41. Cook RJ, and Bevilacqua MBG. Invoking human rights to reduce maternal deaths. *Lancet*, 2004, 363:73.

42. Jeppsson A. SWAp dynamics in a decentralized context: experiences from Uganda. *Social Science and Medicine*, 2002, 55:2053–2060.

43. Peters D, Chao S. The sector-wide approach in health. What is it? Where is it leading? *International Journal of Health Planning and Management*, 1998, 13:177–190.

44. Walt G, Pavignani E, Gilson L. Buse K. Managing external resources in the health sector: are there lessons for SWAps? *Health Policy and Planning*, 1999, 14:273–284.

45. Penrose P. *Sector development programmes: definitions and issues*. Oxford, Oxford Policy Management, 1997.

46. Pathmanathan I, Liljestrand J, Martins JM, Rajapaksa LC, Lissner C, de Silva A et al. *Investing in maternal health: learning from Malaysia and Sri Lanka*. Washington, DC, The World Bank, 2003 (Human Development Network, Health, Nutrition and Population Series).

47. Miller S, Sloan NL, Winikoff B, Langer A, Fikree FF. Where is the 'E' in MCH? The need for an evidence-based approach in safe motherhood. *Journal of Midwifery and Women's Health*, 2003, 48:10–18.

48. Campbell OMR. What are maternal health policies in developing countries and who drives them? A review of the last half-century. In: De Brouwere V, Van Lerberghe W, eds. *Safe motherhood strategies: a review of the evidence*. Antwerp, ITG Press, 2001 (Studies in Health Services Organisation and Policy, 17:415–448).

49. AbouZahr C. Safe motherhood: a brief history of the global movement 1947–2002. *British Medical Bulletin*, 2003, 67:13–25.

50. Jahan R, Germain A. Mobilising support to sustain political will is the key to progress in reproductive health. *Lancet*, 2004, 364:742–744

51. *The Millennium Development Goals for health: rising to the challenges*. Washington, DC, World Bank, 2004.

52. *Reducing maternal deaths – evidence and action. A strategy for DFID*. London, United Kingdom Department for International Development, 2004 (Draft, 26 May 2004).

53. *Shaping policy for maternal and newborn health: a compendium of case studies*. Baltimore, MD, JHPIEGO, 2003.

54. *Skilled care during childbirth policy brief: saving women's lives, improving newborn health*. New York, NY, Safe Motherhood Inter-Agency Group, 2002.

55. Van Lerberghe W, De Brouwere V. Of blind alleys and things that have worked: history's lessons on reducing maternal mortality. In: De Brouwere V, Van Lerberghe W, eds. *Safe motherhood strategies: a review of the evidence*. Antwerp, ITG Press, 2001 (Studies in Health Services Organisation and Policy, 17:7–33).

56. Hardee K, Agarwal K, Luke N, Wilson E, Pendzich M, Farrell M. *Post-Cairo reproductive health policies and programs: a comparative study of eight countries*. Washington, DC, The POLICY Project, 1998.

57. Lowell G, Findlay A. *Migration of highly skilled persons from developing countries: impact and policy responses*. Geneva, International Labour Office, 2001.

58. *The health sector human resources crisis in Africa: an issue paper*. Washington, DC, United States Agency for International Development, Bureau of Africa, Office of Sustainable Development, 2003.

59. Zurn P, Dal Poz MR, Stilwell B, Adams O. Imbalance in the health workforce. *Human Resources for Health*, 2004, 2:13.

60. Tawfik L, Kinoti SN. *The impact of HIV/AIDS on the health sector in sub-Saharan Africa: the issue of human resources*. Washington, DC, United States Agency for International Development, Bureau for Africa, Office of Sustainable Development, 2001.

61. The Joint Learning initiative. *Human resources for health: overcoming the crisis* (http://www.globalhealthtrust.org/Report.html, accessed 7 February 2005).

62. *First biennial review of the health workforce development plan 1996–2005*. Phnom Penh, Ministry of Health, 1999.

63. Van Lerberghe W. *Safer motherhood component of the health sector support programme, Cambodia*. London, DFID Centre for Sexual and Reproductive Health, 2001.

64. Ferrinho P, Van Lerberghe W. *Providing health care under adverse conditions: health personnel performance & individual coping strategies*. Antwerp, ITG Press, 2000 (Studies in Health Services Organisation and Policy, 16).

65. Webber T. Strategies for surviving and thriving in organizations. *Career Development International*, 1997, 2:90–92.

66. Tracy J, Antonenko M. In Russian health care, you get what you pay for, even when it is free. In: Hodess R, Banfield J, Wolfe T, eds. *Global corruption report 2001*. Berlin, Transparency International, 2001:115.

67. Alcázar L, Andrade R. Induced demand and absenteeism in Peruvian hospitals. In: Di Tella R, Savedoff WD, eds. *Diagnosis corruption. Fraud in Latin America's public hospitals*. Washington, DC, Inter-American Development Bank, 2001:123–162.

68. Van Lerberghe W, Conceição C, Van Damme W, Ferrinho P. When staff is underpaid: dealing with the individual coping strategies of health personnel. *Bulletin of the World Health Organization*, 2002, 80:581–584.

69. Macq J, Ferrinho P, De Brouwere V, Van Lerberghe W. Managing health services in developing countries: between the ethics of the civil servant and the need for moonlighting. *Human Resources for Health Development Journal*, 2001, 5:1–3;17–24.

70. Ferrinho P, Omar, MC, de Jesus Fernandes M, Blaise P, Bugalho AM, Van Lerberghe W. Pilfering for survival: how health workers use access to drugs as a coping strategy. *Human Resources for Health*, 2004, 2:4.

71. Brugha R, Zwi A. Improving the quality of private sector delivery of public health services: challenges and strategies. *Health Policy and Planning*, 1998, 13:107–120.

72. Adams O, Hicks V. *Pay and non-pay incentives, performance and motivation*. Paper prepared for: Global Health Workforce Strategy Group, World Health Organization, Geneva, December 2001 (http://www.who.int/hrh/documents/en/pay_non_pay.pdf, accessed 7 February 2005).

73. Adams O. Internal brain-drain and income topping-up: policies and practices of the World Health Organization. In: Ferrinho P, Van Lerberghe W, eds. *Providing health care under adverse conditions: health personnel performance & individual coping strategies*. Antwerp, ITG Press, 2000 (Studies in Health Services Organisation and Policy, 16:203–206).

74. Van Lerberghe W, Adams O, Ferrinho P. Human resource impact assessment. *Bulletin of the World Health Organization*, 2002, 80:525.

75. Segall M. From cooperation to competition in national health systems – and back? Impact on professional ethics and quality of care. *International Journal of Health Planning and Management*, 2000, 15:61–79.

76. Nitayarumphong S, Srivanichakom S, Pongsupap Y. Strategies to respond to health manpower needs in rural Thailand. In: Ferrinho P, Van Lerberghe W, eds. *Providing health care under adverse conditions: health personnel performance & individual coping strategies*. Antwerp, ITG Press, 2000 (Studies in Health Services Organisation and Policy, 16:55–72).

77. Kittimunkong S. Coping strategies in Hua Thalay urban health centre, Korat, Thailand. In: Ferrinho P, Van Lerberghe W, eds. *Providing health care under adverse conditions: health personnel performance & individual coping strategies*. Antwerp, ITG Press, 2000 (Studies in Health Services Organisation and Policy, 16:231–238).

78. Dal Poz MR. Cambios en la contraction de recursos humanos: el caso del programa de salud de la familia en Brasil [Changes in the hiring of health personnel: the family health programme in Brazil]. *Gaceta Sanitaria*, 2002, 16:82–88.

79. Hardeman W, Van Damme W, Van Pelt M, Por I, Kimvan H, Meessen B. access to health care for all? User fees plus a Health Equity Fund in Sotnikum, Cambodia. *Health Policy and Planning*, 2004, 19:22–32.

80. Brown A. *Current issues in sector-wide approaches for health development: Tanzania case study*. Geneva, World Health Organization, 2000 (WHO/GPE/00.6).

81. Brown A. *Current issues in sector-wide approaches for health development: Mozambique case study*. Geneva, World Health Organization, 2000 (WHO/GPE/00.4).

82. Brown A. *Current issues in sector-wide approaches for health development: Uganda case study*. Geneva, World Health Organization, 2000 (WHO/GPE/00.3).

83. *Universal coverage: options for the organization of health financing systems*. Geneva, World Health Organization, 2004 (Health System Financing, Expenditure and Resource Allocation, Technical Brief for Policy, No. 1, Draft, November 2004).

84. Briasco C, Floate H, Tate A. Feeding the System. Brisbane, University of Queensland, 2004 (unpublished MPH dissertation).

85. Meesen B, Van Damme W, Por I, Van Leemput L, Hardeman W. *The new deal in Cambodia: the second year. Confirmed results, confirmed challenges*. Phnom Penh, Médecins sans Frontières, 2002.

86. Fofana P, Samai O, Kebbie A, Sengeh P. Promoting the use of obstetric services through community loan funds, Bo, Sierra Leone. *International Journal of Gynecology and Obstetrics*, 1997, 59(Suppl. 2): S225–S230.

87. Schneider H, Gilson L. The impact of free maternal health care in South Africa. In: Berer M, Sundari Ravindran TK, eds. *Safe motherhood initiatives: critical issues*. London, Blackwell Science, 1999 (Reproductive Health Matters: 93–101).

88. Conway T. *Current issues in sector-wide approaches for health development: Viet Nam case study*. Geneva, World Health Organization, 2000 (WHO/GPE/00.5).

89. Seoane G, Equiluz R, Ugalde M, Arraya JC. Bolivia, 1996–2000. In: Koblinsky MA, ed. *Reducing maternal mortality*. Washington, DC, World Bank, 2003:83–92.

90. *Reducing catastrophic health expenditure in the design of health financing systems*. Geneva, World Health Organization, 2004 (Health System Financing, Expenditure and Resource Allocation, Technical Brief for Policy, No. 2, Draft, November 2004).

91. Xu K, Evans DB, Kawabata K, Zeramdini R, Klavus J, Murray CJ. Household catastrophic health expenditure: a multicountry analysis. *Lancet*, 2003, 362:111–117.

92. Brown A, Foster M, Norton A, Naschold F. *The status of sector-wide approaches*. London, Overseas Development Institute, 2001 (Working Paper 142).

93. *Thailand's health care reform project, 1996–2001. Final report, July 2001*. Bangkok, Ministry of Public Health, 2001.

94. *Reproductive health: report by the Secretariat*. Geneva, World Health Organization, 2004 (http://www.who.int/reproductive-health/A57_13_en.pdf, accessed 9 February 2005).

95. *Bangladesh: health and population sector strategy 1996*. Dhaka, Government of Bangladesh, 1997.

96. Health and population sector programme 1998–2003: programme implementation plan. Dhaka, Government of Bangladesh, 1998.

97. Ahmed N. Voices of stakeholders in Bangladesh health sector reform. In: Yazbeck A, Peters D, Wagstaff A, eds. *Health policy research in South Asia: guiding reforms and building capacity*. Baltimore, MD Johns Hopkins University Press, 2003, 14:369–400.

98. Streatfield PK, Mercer A, Siddique AB, Khan ZUA, Ashraf A. *Health and Population Sector Programme 1998–2003. Bangladesh: status of performance indicators 2002; a report for the Health Programme Support Office for the annual programme review 2002*. Dhaka, ICDDR,B-Centre for Health and Population Research, 2003 (ICDDR,B special publication, no. 116).

99. Jahan R. Restructuring the health system: experiences of advocates for gender equity in Bangladesh. *Reproductive Health Matters*, 2003, 11:183–191.

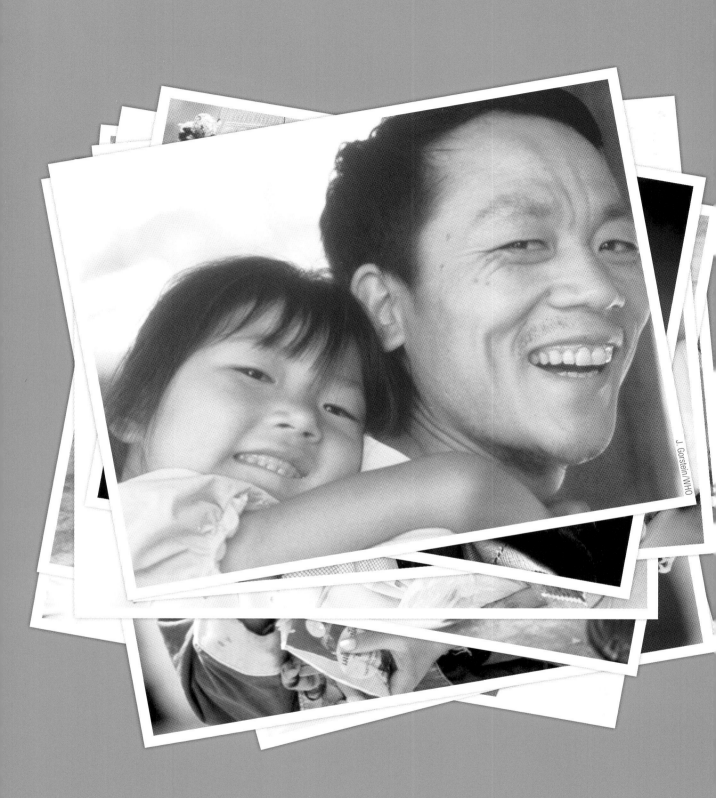

statistical annex
explanatory notes

The tables in this statistical annex present information on population health in WHO Member States and regions for the year 2003 (Annex Tables 1, 2a and 2b), under-five and neonatal causes of deaths for 2000–2003 (Annex Tables 3 and 4), selected national health accounts aggregates for 1998–2002 (Annex Tables 5 and 6), and selected indicators related to reproductive, maternal and newborn health (Annex Tables 7 and 8). These notes provide an overview of concepts, methods and data sources, together with references to more detailed documentation. It is hoped that careful scrutiny and use of the results will lead to progressively better measurement of core indicators of population health and health system financing.

The theme of *The World Health Report 2005* is maternal and child health. The latest estimates of under-five mortality and causes of death are now available, so special consideration is given both to estimates and to the empirical basis of under-five mortality and causes of death. Annex Table 3 on the estimated number and distribution of deaths by cause focuses on the deaths of children under the age of five years. For the first time, the estimated numbers of deaths for neonates by cause are being published (as Annex Table 4). Consequently, the table on estimated deaths by cause, sex and mortality stratum that appeared in earlier *World Health Reports* is not being published here.

Of the eight major goals set at the United Nations Millennium Summit in 2000, six relate directly to the health and well-being of women and children. These Millennium Development Goals (MDGs) reflect a thorough recognition by governments that improving the well-being of individuals is a prerequisite to economic development. In order to monitor progress in achieving the MDGs as well as major childhood health initiatives, a reliable information base is critical.

It is essential for the United Nations to disseminate identical estimates on the MDGs, including under-five mortality, in order to enhance proper use of these figures in policy planning or in programme monitoring and evaluation. There is thus an urgent need to develop a system through which the United Nations speaks with a single voice and produces estimates that agree. Four specialized agencies – WHO, the United Nations Children's Fund (UNICEF), the United Nations Population Division, and the World Bank – organized a meeting on child mortality (infant and under-five mortality rates) in May 2004. Meeting participants agreed on the following actions to further explore their joint activities to improve the estimation process on a regular basis: creation of a common database; discussion on the issues of the currently used methods and ways for improvement; and more focus on country capacity building and training to improve data availability and quality.

Accordingly, WHO and UNICEF produced a consistent set of under-five mortality rates by country for the period 1990–2003, which was used as the basis for estimation shown in Annex Tables 1 and 2a. It should be emphasized that such estimates may not be directly derived from reported data. Annex Table 2b summarizes the empirical basis for the estimation of under-five mortality by age group.

WHO is the primary organization to provide estimates on cause-specific mortality. A major problem has been the lack of accurate cause-specific mortality data from developing countries, especially those with higher levels of mortality. In collaboration with its regional offices, WHO headquarters collects cause-of-death data from its 192 Member States. An established agreement between headquarters and the regional offices ensures that there is no duplication of work at the country level to report data to WHO. The WHO Regional Offices for the Americas, Europe and the Eastern Mediterranean deploy simultaneous efforts to ensure that data are received in a regular and timely manner. Data from the African Region are virtually non-existent and account for the major difficulties in assessing the level of cause-specific mortality in that area.

The data submitted by Member States then become part of WHO's unique historical database on causes of death (WHO Mortality Database) which contains data as far back as 1950 *(1)*. During 2000–2003 some 100 Member States provided vital registration data to WHO and captured approximately 18 million deaths. It should be noted, however, that more than two thirds of deaths in the world are not being reported.

These data gaps need to be filled both by stepping up efforts to work with countries and initiatives to obtain more recent mortality data and by collaborating with partners to promote better tools and investment in data collection and analysis. There is also a need for better harmonization of cause-specific mortality estimates within WHO, with other organizations in the United Nations system and with academic institutions.

In 2001, WHO established the Child Health Epidemiology Reference Group (CHERG) to help improve estimates of cause-specific mortality in childhood. This group of independent technical experts has developed and applied rigorous standards for the development of estimates related to the major causes of childhood deaths, and worked closely with WHO and UNICEF to incorporate their results into broader WHO child health estimates at global, regional and when possible country level. Further detail on CHERG methods and products is available elsewhere *(2)*. The results of WHO collaboration with the CHERG and UNICEF are presented in Annex Tables 3 and 4.

These estimates have been reviewed, agreed upon and supported by the WHO Departments of Child and Adolescent Health and Development (CAH) and Measurement and Health Information Systems (MHI), the UNICEF Division of Policy and Planning (DPP) and an independent group of external experts. Initial WHO estimates and technical explanations were sent to Member States for comment. Comments or data provided in response were discussed with them and incorporated where possible. The estimates published here should, however, still be interpreted as the best estimates of WHO rather than the official viewpoint of Member States.

ANNEX TABLE 1

All estimates of population size and structure for 2003 are based on the demographic assessments prepared by the United Nations Population Division *(3)*. These estimates refer to the de facto population, and not the de jure population in each Member State. The annual growth rate, the dependency ratio, the percentage of population aged 60 years and more, and the total fertility rate are obtained from the same United Nations Population Division database.

To assess overall levels of health achievement, it is crucial to develop the best possible assessment of the life table for each country. Life tables have been developed for all 192 Member States for 2003 starting with a systematic review of all available evidence from surveys, censuses, sample registration systems, population laboratories and vital registration on levels and trends in under-five and adult mortality rates. This review benefited greatly from a collaborative assessment of under-five mortality levels for 2003 by WHO and UNICEF. WHO uses a standard method to estimate and project life tables for all Member States using comparable data. This may lead to minor differences compared with official life tables prepared by Member States.

Life expectancy at birth, the probability of dying before five years of age (under-five mortality rate) and the probability of dying between 15 and 60 years of age (adult mortality rate) derive from life tables that WHO has estimated for each Member State. Procedures used to estimate the 2003 life table differed for Member States depending on the data availability to assess child and adult mortality. Because of increasing heterogeneity of patterns of adult and child mortality, WHO has developed a model life table system of two-parameter logit life tables, and with additional age-specific parameters to correct for systematic biases in the application of a two-parameter system, based on about 1800 life tables from vital registration judged to be of good quality *(4)*. This system of model life tables has been used extensively in the development of life tables for those Member States without adequate vital registration and in projecting life tables to 2003 when the most recent data available are from earlier years. Estimates for 2003 have been revised to take into account new data received since publication of *The World Health Report 2004* for many Member States and may not be entirely comparable with those published in the previous reports. The methods used to construct life tables are summarized below and a full detailed overview has been published *(4, 5)*.

For Member States with vital registration and sample vital registration systems, demographic techniques (Preston–Coale method, Brass Growth–Balance method, Generalized Growth–Balance method and Bennett–Horiuchi method) were first applied to assess the level of completeness of recorded mortality data in the population above five years of age and then those mortality rates were adjusted accordingly *(6)*. Where vital registration data for 2003 were available, these were used directly to construct the life table. For other countries where the system provided a time series of annual life tables, the parameters (l_5, l_{60}) were projected using a weighted regression model giving more weight to recent years (using an exponential weighting scheme such that the weight for each year t was 25% less than that for year $t+1$). For countries with a total population of less than 750 000 or where the root mean square error from the regression was greater than or equal to 0.011, a shorter-term trend was estimated by applying a weighting factor with 50% annual exponential decay. Projected values of the two life table parameters were then applied to a modified logit life table model, using the most recent national data as the standard, which allows the capture of the most recent age pattern, to predict the full life table for 2003.

For all Member States, other data available for child mortality, such as surveys and censuses, were assessed and adjusted to estimate the probable trend over the past few decades in order to predict the child mortality in 2003. A standard approach to predicting child mortality was employed to obtain the estimates for 2003 (see Annex Table 2a for more details) *(7)*. Those estimates are, on the one hand, used to replace the under-five mortality rate in life tables of the countries that have a vital registration or sample vital registration system, but with incomplete registration of numbers of deaths under the age of five years. On the other hand, for countries without exploitable vital registration systems, which are mainly those with high mortality, the predicted under-five mortality rates are used as one of the inputs to the modified logit system. Adult mortality rates were derived from either surveys or censuses where available; otherwise the most likely corresponding level of adult mortality was estimated based on regression models of child versus adult mortality as observed in the set of approximately 1800 life tables. These estimated child and adult mortality rates were then applied to a global standard, defined as the average of all the life tables, using the modified logit model to derive the estimates for 2003.

It should be noted that the logit model life table system using the global standard does not capture high HIV/AIDS epidemic patterns, because the observed underlying life tables do not come from countries with the epidemic. Similarly, war deaths are not captured because vital registration systems often break down in periods of war *(8)*. For these reasons, for affected countries, mortality without deaths attributable to HIV/AIDS and war was estimated and separate estimates of deaths caused by HIV/AIDS and war in 2003 were added.

The main results in Annex Table 1 are reported with uncertainty intervals in order to communicate to the user the plausible range of estimates for each country on each measure. For the countries with vital registration data projected using time series regression models on the parameters of the logit life table system, uncertainty around the regression coefficients has been accounted for by taking 1000 draws of the parameters using the regression estimates and variance covariance matrix of the estimators. For each of the draws, a new life table was calculated. In cases where additional sources of information provided plausible ranges around under-five and adult mortality rates the 1000 draws were constrained such that each life table produced estimates within these specified ranges. The range of 1000 life tables produced by these multiple draws reflects some of the uncertainty around the projected trends in mortality, notably the imprecise quantification of systematic changes in the logit parameters over the time period captured in available vital registration data.

For Member States where complete death registrations were available for the year 2003 and projections were not used, the life table uncertainty reflects the event count uncertainty, approximated by the Poisson distribution, in the estimated age-specific death rates arising from the observation of a finite number of deaths in a fixed time interval of one year.

For countries that did not have time series data on mortality by age and sex, the following steps were undertaken. First, point estimates and ranges around under-five and adult mortality rates for males and females were developed on a country-by-country basis *(5)*. In the modified logit life table system described *(4)*, values on these two parameters may be used to identify a range of different life tables in relation to a global standard life table. Using the Monte Carlo simulation methods, 1000 random life tables were generated by drawing samples from normal distributions around these inputs with variances defined according to ranges of uncertainty. In countries where uncertainty around under-five and adult mortality rates was considerable because of a paucity of survey or surveillance information, wide distributions were sampled but the results were constrained based on estimates of the maximum and minimum plausible values for the point estimates.

For 55 countries, mainly in sub-Saharan Africa, estimates of life tables were made by constructing counterfactual life tables excluding the mortality impact of the HIV/AIDS epidemic and then combining these life tables with exogenous estimates of the excess mortality rates attributable to HIV/AIDS. The estimates were based on back-calculation models developed as part of collaborative efforts between WHO and the Joint United Nations Programme on HIV/AIDS (UNAIDS) to derive country-level epidemiological estimates for HIV/AIDS. In countries with substantial numbers of war deaths, estimates of their uncertainty range were also incorporated into the life table uncertainty analysis.

ANNEX TABLE 2A

Estimates of child mortality are regularly published by various international organizations, including WHO. Footnotes are used to explain the underlying methodology and sometimes include information on the availability of empirical data that underlie the estimates. More frequently, however, the reader of the tables is not informed about the source of information. In the current set of tables WHO has made a first attempt to share a brief summary of the underlying empirical information. This should allow the reader to obtain an idea of how much the estimate is based on real data versus assumptions. At this point the tables do not include an assessment of the quality of the data. The estimation process does take the quality of the empirical data into account.

In the context of the Millennium Development Goals (MDGs), particular attention is paid to the measurement of progress towards reaching Goal 4, "to reduce by two thirds the mortality rate among children under five between 1990 and 2015". At country level this implies government commitment not only to implement initiatives to improve child health but also to set up a reliable system to monitor such progress. Such a system, if implemented, should be able to provide the number of deaths of children under five years of age by sex, age and cause. However, countries with high levels of child mortality are those where there is very little information or none at all, especially on trends.

Annex Table 2a presents the sources and results of information on under-five mortality rates during the last 25 years which are available at WHO. All efforts were made to ensure completeness and accuracy of the information presented, but the table does not intend to be exhaustive. Data collection efforts are summarized for three periods: 1980–1989, 1990–1999 and 2000–2003. Only data collected in the most recent period provide new information on the trend in child mortality in the new millennium. In all other cases, the estimates for the MDGs are drawn entirely from projections based on trends derived from empirical data points prior to the year 2000.

There are four primary sources of empirical under-five mortality data: vital registration (VR), sample registration system (SRS), surveys and censuses. The vital registration or sample registration system provides numbers of deaths by age and sex obtained by direct observation and reporting of individual deaths. These are prospectively collected data. In the case of a survey or a census, the empirical data are based on retrospective data. Interviews with mostly the mother or caregiver or head of household provide information on the survival history of children in the household.

This may be through gathering mortality information for a specific period prior to the census or survey interview, through a birth history or through questions on children ever born and children still alive ("indirect" Brass questions) *(9)*.

The sources of information as listed in the Annex Table 2a were used to derive the estimated trends and projections of rates for under-five-year-olds for the year 2003 shown in both Annex Tables 1 and 2a. A standard approach to predicting the most recent child mortality was employed to ensure comparability between countries and may lead to minor differences compared with official statistics prepared by Member States *(7)*. For each country, estimates of under-five mortality rate are derived from weighted least squares regression of under-five mortality rate on their reference dates. Explanatory variables include date, as well as those that capture rates of change of under-five mortality across periods of time. The weights assigned to each data point reflect its quality or consistency with all other data points. In other cases, additional sources were used as inputs in the standard regression model.

Vital registration can be considered as the gold standard for the collection of mortality data, as it allows the registration of deaths by age and sex. Vital registration systems with high levels of completeness are commonplace in developed countries. Although several developing countries are improving their vital registration systems, in many other countries – especially countries with high levels of mortality – such a system is non-existent. Another source of mortality data is the sample vital registration system which assesses vital events at the national level from information collected in sample areas. These two sources, in principle, provide data on a regular yearly basis.

The column "VR/SRS" in Annex Table 2a – vital registration/sample registration system shows the number of years of data from either system available at WHO. In the absence of a prospective data collection system in a country, household surveys will provide direct or indirect estimates of the level of under-five mortality, primarily using birth history questionnaires in which mothers are asked to provide information about their children, those still living as well as those who did not survive. Similarly, census questionnaires may include a module on mortality, which may refer to recent deaths in the household or use "indirect" Brass questions to estimate child mortality. It should be noted that one single survey or census can generate more than one estimate of under-five mortality for different periods of time. However, the "Survey/Census" column of Annex Table 2a shows the number of the surveys or censuses available at WHO. Furthermore, when a survey was carried over from one year to the next, only the starting year was taken into account.

It is worth noting the efforts of WHO regional offices in collecting vital registration data from Member States. International agencies such as the United Nations and UNICEF also maintain historical databases on under-five mortality rates, which have been generously shared and incorporated in our analyses. Other sources of information include data from national censuses or surveys, or from specialist surveys such as the Demographic and Health Survey (DHS) undertaken by ORC Macro and the Multiple Indicator Cluster Survey (MICS) conducted by UNICEF. Finally, national statistical documents such as statistical yearbooks, reports from specialized agencies and periodical paper findings were also incorporated into the database.

ANNEX TABLE 2B

Whereas Annex Table 2a presents the estimates on under-five mortality rates, Annex Table 2b presents an empirical basis of detailed age-specific mortality rates directly obtained from the most readily available sources on the subject, namely,

Demographic and Health Survey (DHS) and vital registration (VR). In addition to the familiar breakdown of infants under the age of one year into neonatal (0–27 days) and postneonatal (28 days–11 months) periods *(10)*, the latter age group was further divided into two intervals, 28 days–5 months and 6–11 months. Similarly, the child period between the first and fifth birthday was divided into 12–23 and 24–59 months. The table here summarizes the definitions of the age breakdown.

The mortality rates presented in Annex Table 2b are expressed as the probability of dying during each period, for those who have survived until the beginning of that period. Therefore the totals are not equivalent to the sum of the rates of the component age groups.

From DHS raw data sets, UNICEF collaborated in re-analysing them to compute detailed age-specific death rates, following the DHS approach, using synthetic cohort probabilities of death *(11)*. In order to obtain sufficient robustness in the estimates, these represent the period of five years prior to the surveys. No adjustments have been made for reporting issues such as heaping in these calculations.

VR data reported by Member States *(1)* are the other source where age-specific mortality can be computed, although the current under-one mortality age split that WHO requests does not allow detail within the postneonatal mortality rate. Thus, only neonatal and postneonatal mortality rates are presented in Annex Table 2b. For these two rates, we applied the following formula based on live births *(12)*:

Neonatal mortality rate = neonatal deaths / live births
Postneonatal mortality rate = postneonatal deaths / (live births − neonatal deaths)

For the other age groups, we applied a standard formula from the abridged lifetable:

$$_nq_x = \frac{n \, _nM_x}{1 + n(1 - \, _na_x) \, _nM_x}$$

where

$_nq_x$ is the probability of dying between exact ages x and $x+n$;
n is the interval of the age group expressed in years;
x is the exact age at the beginning of the age group;
$_nM_x$ is the age-specific death rate of the age group between x and $x+n$; and
$_na_x$ is the fraction of last age interval of life.

In this table we relied as much as possible on empirical data; for the denominators (live births and population of age-specific death rates) national data were given priority, otherwise the estimates from the United Nations Population Division were used *(3)*.

Comparisons across countries should be made with great caution as the results are not directly comparable since the method of calculation varies depending on sources and there are different degrees of completeness of vital registration data submitted by Member States.

Those DHS and VR data that can be supplemented by other sources of information would serve as the basis of the analysis between the age groups, by country or by region. This insight into the level of mortality would possibly lead to identification of some cause-specific pattern for a better understanding of the epidemiological transition within childhood mortality.

Definition		Interval[a]
0.	Under-five	0–4 years
1.	Infant	0–11 months
1.1	Neonatal	0–27 days
1.2	Postneonatal	28 days–11 months
1.2.1	Early postneonatal	28 days–5 months
1.2.2	Late postneonatal	6–11 months
2.	Child	1–4 years
2.1	Toddler	12–23 months
2.2	Early childhood	24–59 months

[a] The upper limit of the interval refers to completed days, months or years.

ANNEX TABLE 3

Before estimating the number of deaths for individual causes, the first step is to obtain an estimated number of deaths from all causes combined, which will constitute an "envelope" to make sure that the sum of all cause-specific mortality does not exceed the estimated number of deaths in each country. The envelope itself is derived from the mortality rates from abridged life tables *(4, 5)* and applying them to the population estimates obtained from the United Nations Population Division *(3)*. The current mortality envelope was based on the joint work by WHO and UNICEF for the period 1990–2003.

Countries with a sound vital registration system (VR) with a relatively high coverage would capture the representative pattern of causes of death at the national level. In addition to the levels of coverage, it is important to analyse carefully the quality of the coding pratices which should follow the rules of the International Statistical Classification of Diseases and Related Health Problems (ICD) *(6, 8, 10)*. In some countries, improper completion of death certificates or systematic biases in diagnosis are quite frequent.

For 72 countries where the VR coverage is over 85%, WHO considers VR as the gold standard and uses the pattern directly derived from VR, after adjusting for the ill-defined categories (e.g. ICD-9 Chapter XVI, ICD-10 Chapter XVIII; unspecified cardiovascular diseases; cancers of unknown sites; unspecified external causes) and checking cause-specific trends for the most recent years available. When estimating death rates for very small countries whereby a small change in the number of deaths substantially affects the overall cause-of-death pattern, an average of the last three years of data from their VR is used to avoid spurious trends. In the absence of a

Data and methods used for estimating under-five causes of death

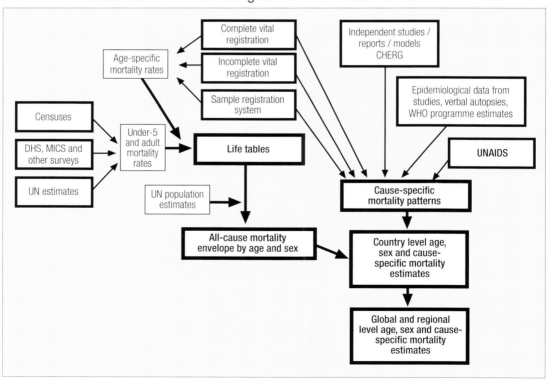

complete VR system for obtaining cause-of-death information, sample registration systems are now implemented in a few countries such as China and India to obtain representative cause-of-death patterns *(8)*.

In many countries, however, VR systems are only operating in specific areas (selected provinces or urban/rural areas) and there are virtually none in the majority of countries with high child mortality. Estimates on cause-of-death patterns should be based on both limited sets of available data and extensive use of models.

Since areas not covered by the VR system are often rural and marginalized regions with a lower socioeconomic status than the covered ones, mortality patterns in both areas are likely to be different. A statistical model to make such an inference has been developed *(13)*, based on the historical VR data for selected countries since 1950 that register at least 95% of all deaths. Although a few developing countries are included, most countries reporting complete VR data to WHO are from developed regions and the countries included are mostly in the WHO European Region and the Region of the Americas.

This model assumes that the broader cause-of-death pattern in high-mortality countries would follow the historical health transitions previously observed in the current high-income and middle-income countries in the absence of major epidemics, natural disasters and war. Conditional on the values for all-cause mortality and income per capita, the model predicts the cause-of-death pattern for the three broader cause categories: communicable diseases; noncommunicable diseases; and external causes (injuries). This model was applied for assigning the under-five mortality envelope to the three broader causes in many high-mortality countries where no reliable information on cause-of-death patterns is available. Information drawn from neighbouring countries within the same region was also used to check the plausibility of model outputs *(8)*.

Once the allocation of the all-cause under-five mortality envelope into the three broader causes is done, the final step is to obtain the distribution of deaths from individual diseases or external causes within each of the three broad groups. For communicable diseases, from which the majority of children under five years of age die, estimates on specific diseases from the Child Health Epidemiology Reference Group (CHERG) *(2)*, WHO technical programmes and UNAIDS are taken into account when making final estimates. The results of this joint work were then incorporated into the all-cause under-five mortality envelope, including deaths from remaining communicable and noncommunicable diseases, and injuries representing 10% and 3% of global deaths, respectively. Because 2000 was the baseline year for the calculation of the estimates of the majority of the cause distribution, except for HIV/AIDS which is updated annually, cause-of-death distribution for 2000 was applied to the average under-five mortality envelope for 2000–2003 to obtain the average annual number of deaths from each cause.

The recent WHO work on neonatal mortality provided a sub-envelope of deaths during the neonatal period out of the total under-five mortality envelope *(14)*. Deaths attributable to HIV/AIDS were allocated based on annual mortality estimates produced by UNAIDS and WHO *(15)*. For pneumonia, diarrhoea, malaria, and measles, the CHERG estimates derived from single-cause models *(16–18)*, as well as estimates from WHO technical programmes *(19)* and other published literature, were then triangulated with the results of the multi-cause proportional mortality model, which takes into account the major causes of death simultaneously *(20)*, to produce the new set of cause-specific mortality proportions.

Estimates of mortality due to acute lower respiratory infections (ARI), which correspond mainly to pneumonia deaths, were based on the relationship between ARI proportional mortality and all-cause mortality among children under-five years of age. Forty-nine observations were included in the final analysis, which consisted in the fitting of a log-linear curve for ARI proportional mortality against total under-five mortality (18). There was a high degree of consistency at country level between results from this single-proportional model and those from the multi-cause proportional model (20).

The estimated number of deaths from diarrhoea varies substantially, ranging from 1.6 million (16) to 2.6 million total deaths (21). The CHERG single-cause model used to estimate deaths attributable to diarrhoeal diseases included 77 observations. Results of this model (16) were triangulated with the results of the multi-cause proportional model (20) as well as with other available estimates published in the literature (21, 22).

Malaria mortality in sub-Saharan Africa was estimated from an innovative method based on sub-regional mapping of intensity of malaria transmission and risks for dying from malaria (17, 23). The literature review identified 31 studies from 14 countries in middle Africa and 17 studies and reports from four countries in southern Africa. Estimated malaria mortality among children under five years old in sub-Saharan Africa in the year 2000 was between 700 000 and 900 000 deaths. Nearly all malaria deaths occurred in populations exposed to high-intensity transmission in middle Africa. For regions outside Africa, the outputs from the multi-cause model were used to derive the proportion of under-five deaths from malaria (20).

There was a wide discrepancy between CHERG and WHO programme estimates for under-five deaths attributable to measles (19, 20). It was suggested that the CHERG multi-cause model may underestimate causes representing only a small proportion of deaths, and that WHO's natural history model based on incidence, vaccine coverage and case-fatality rate may overestimate measles deaths, because of its reliance on inputs on case-fatality rates of questionable validity (24). WHO convened an expert panel on this issue, resulting in a comparison of the two estimates for the 20 countries with largest absolute discrepancies. Efforts to improve the estimation methodology for measles mortality are ongoing, and WHO has adopted an interim estimate of about 400 000 annual deaths, or 4% of total deaths of children under five years of age worldwide.

In the majority of countries, no further adjustments were made; since some estimates of each cause have been done separately from the multi-cause model, however, the sum of each individual cause could exceed the envelope for a very few countries. In such cases, thorough review of the estimates of each individual cause has been undertaken to resolve the "envelope" violation. Adjustments of the estimated number of deaths by cause were made within the plausible ranges estimated for each cause.

ANNEX TABLE 4

For the first time, WHO is publishing a table on the annual number of deaths by cause for neonates for the period 2000–2003. Neonatal deaths, deaths among live births (0–27 days) may be subdivided into early neonatal deaths (0–6 days) and late neonatal deaths (7–27 days). Annex Table 4 shows only the total neonatal deaths by cause, with no distinction of early or late neonatal deaths.

The total estimated number of deaths of neonates has been derived from the envelope of under-five mortality as described above. Where vital registration (VR) data exist, countries reporting data to WHO sometimes include neonatal deaths; this accounts for only 82 countries. For countries where no such information exists, modelling techniques have been used.

Less than 3% of the world's neonatal deaths occur in countries with VR data that are reliable for cause-of-death analysis. Population-based information in high-mortality settings is often dependent on verbal autopsy tools of variable quality. The Child Health Epidemiology Reference Group (CHERG) undertook an extensive exercise to derive global estimates for programme-relevant causes of neonatal death, including preterm birth, asphyxia, severe infection, neonatal tetanus, diarrhoea, and other causes comprising specific but less prevalent causes (e.g. jaundice). These estimates were compared with existing high quality data such as those from confidential enquiries and found to match closely.

For low-mortality countries, an analysis was performed using VR data from 45 countries with full VR coverage (cumulative sample size of N = 96 797). For high-mortality countries, studies were identified through extensive systematic searches, and a meta-analysis was performed after applying inclusion criteria and using standard case definitions (56 studies, cumulative sample size of N = 13 685). Multinomial models were developed to estimate simultaneously the distribution of seven causes of death by country. The inputs, methods and results are described in detail elsewhere *(25)*.

Issues surrounding uncertainties in cause of death

All estimates reported in Annex Tables 3 and 4 have uncertainty associated with them. WHO and its technical partners have developed measures of uncertainty for many of the disease-specific or cause-specific estimates that form the basis for their estimates. However, the specific procedures used for the individual cause estimates are not identical and therefore do not produce measures of uncertainty that are comparable across diseases. Rather than reporting measures of uncertainty for different diseases or causes that are uncomparable, it was decided that no measure of uncertainty would be used for this year's report.

WHO, UNICEF and their partners have begun developing a common approach and metric of uncertainty that can be used in future estimates of causes of death. The process builds on previous work by various groups and organizations and will produce a set of guidelines and standards for calculating uncertainty associated with an estimate that will be comparable across cause and estimation methods. More details on the various approaches to quantifying uncertainty can be found in some of the work that has been done on disease-specific estimates *(17, 23, 26)*.

ANNEX TABLE 5

National health accounts (NHA) are a synthesis of the financing and spending flows recorded in the operation of a health system, with the potential to monitor all transactions from funding sources to the distribution of benefits across geographical, demographic, socioeconomic and epidemiological dimensions. NHA are related to the macroeconomic and macrosocial accounts whose methodological approach they borrow.

Annex Table 5 provides the best figures that were available to WHO up to December 2004 for each of its 192 Member States. Any subsequent updates will be made available on the WHO NHA website at http://www.who.int/nha/en/. Although more and more countries collect health expenditure data, only about 95 either produce full national health accounts (some of them have done so only once) or report expenditure on health to OECD. Nationally and internationally available information has been identified and compiled for each country. Standard accounting estimation and extrapolation techniques have been used to provide time series. A policy-relevant breakdown of the data (for example, general government/private expenditure) is also provided. Each year draft templates are sent to ministers of health seeking comments and their assistance in obtaining additional information should that be necessary. The constructive responses from ministries and other government agencies such as statistical offices have provided valuable information for the NHA estimates reported here. WHO staff at headquarters and in regional and country offices participated in this process.

An important methodological contribution to producing national health accounts is available in the *Guide to producing national health accounts with special applications for low-income and middle-income countries (27)*. This guide is based on the Organisation for Economic Co-operation and Development (OECD) *System of health accounts (28)*. Both documents were built on the principles of the *United Nations System of national accounts* (commonly referred to as SNA93) *(29)*.

The principal international references used to produce the tables are the International Monetary Fund (IMF) *Government finance statistics yearbook, 2003 (30)*, *International financial statistics yearbook, 2003 (31)* and *International financial statistics* (November 2004) *(32)*; the Asian Development Bank *Key indicators 2004 (33)*; OECD *health data 2004 (34)* and *International development statistics (35)*; and the United Nations *National accounts statistics: main aggregates and detailed tables, 2001 (36)*. The organizations charged with producing these reports facilitated the supply of advance copies to WHO and gave additional related information, and their contributions are acknowledged here with gratitude.

National sources include: national health accounts reports, public expenditure reports, statistical yearbooks and other periodicals, budgetary documents, national accounts reports, statistical data on official web sites, central bank reports, nongovernmental organization reports, academic studies, and reports and data provided by central statistical offices, ministries of health, ministries of finance and economic development, planning offices, and professional and trade associations.

Annex Table 5 provides both updated and revised figures for 1998–2002. Figures have been updated when new information that changes the original estimates has become available (e.g. for India, details of expenditure on social security, private insurance, by firms and by other ministries became available this year which led to a revision of the ratios published in *The World Health Report 2004*). This includes benchmarking revisions, whereby an occasional wholesale revision is made by a country owing to a change in methodology, when a more extensive NHA effort is undertaken, or when shifting the main denominator from the *System of national accounts* 1968 version (SNA68) to SNA93. This category includes benchmarking revisions, whereby an occasional wholesale revision is made by a country owing to a change in methodology, when a more extensive NHA effort is undertaken, or when shifting the main denominator from the *System of national accounts* 1968 version (SNA68) to SNA93.

Total expenditure on health has been defined as the sum of general government health expenditure (GGHE, commonly called public expenditure on health), and private health expenditure (PvtHE). All estimates are calculated in millions of national currency units (million NCU) in current prices. The estimates are presented as ratios to gross domestic product (GDP), to total health expenditure (THE), to total general government expenditure (GGE), to general government health expenditure (GGHE), or to total private health expenditure (PvtHE).

GDP is the value of all goods and services provided in a country by residents and non-residents without regard to their allocation among domestic and foreign claims. This (with small adjustments) corresponds to the total sum of expenditure (consumption and investment) of the private and government agents of the economy during the reference year. The United Nations *National accounts statistics: main aggregates and detailed tables, 2001 (36)*, Table 1.1, was the main source of GDP estimates. Updated 2002 unpublished figures were obtained for most countries. For most Member countries of the OECD, the macroeconomic accounts have been imported from the OECD health data 2004 *(34)*. Updates for some countries (e.g. Australia) that had not yet been transmitted to the OECD were provided by the country. For non-OECD countries, collaborative arrangements between WHO and the United Nations Statistics Division and the Economic Commission for Europe of the United Nations have permitted the receipt of advance information on 2002. For Lebanon and the United Arab Emirates, United Nations Economic and Social Commission for Western Asia data were used. Likewise, the estimates for Liberia, Nauru and Somalia originate from the web site of the United Nations Statistical Department (UNSTAT).

When United Nations data were unavailable, GDP data reported by the IMF (*International financial statistics*, November 2004) have been used. Unpublished data from the IMF Research Department were used for Palau and Suriname. In cases where none of the preceding institutions reported updated GDP information, national series were used. This covers Andorra, Djibouti, Cape Verde, Cook Islands, Georgia, Jamaica, Jordan, the Federated States of Micronesia, Niue, Pakistan, the Russian Federation, Solomon Islands, Sudan, Tonga and Yemen. Figures for Afghanistan, Kiribati, Myanmar, Samoa and Tuvalu were obtained from the Asian Development Bank. The estimates for Comoros, the Democratic Republic of the Congo, the Democratic People's Republic of Korea, Eritrea, Ghana, Guinea, Mauritania, Timor-Leste and Zimbabwe originate from the World Bank (WDI). Estimates for Benin, Cameroon, Côte d'Ivoire, Equatorial Guinea, Gabon, Guinea Bissau, Mali, Niger, Senegal and Togo originate from the Banque des Etats de l'Afrique Centrale (BEAC). Those for Antigua and Barbuda, Barbados and Grenada are taken from the Caribbean Community Secretariat (CARICOM).

The data for China exclude estimates for Hong Kong Special Administrative Region and Macao Special Administrative Region. The public expenditure on health data for Jordan includes contributions from United Nations Relief and Works Agency for Palestine Refugees in the Near East (UNRWA) to Palestinian refugees residing in Jordanian territories. The 1998 health expenditure data for Serbia and Montenegro included the provinces of Kosovo and Metohia; for 1999 to 2002 the data excluded these territories placed under the administration of the United Nations.

General government expenditure (GGE) includes consolidated direct outlays and indirect outlays (for example, subsidies to producers, transfers to households), including capital, of all levels of government (central/federal, provincial/regional/state/district, and municipal/local authorities), social security institutions, autonomous bodies, and other extrabudgetary funds. *OECD health data 2004* and *National accounts of OECD countries: detailed tables 1991/2002, 2004 edition, Volume II*, Table 12, supplies information on GGE for 26 OECD Member countries *(37)*. The IMF *Government finance statistics yearbook* supplies GGE, and IMF *International financial statistics* reports central government disbursement figures. These are complemented by data for local/municipal governments (as well as some social security payments for health data received from the IMF). Several other public finance audits, executed budgets, budget plans, statistical yearbooks, web sites, World Bank and Regional Development Bank reports, and academic studies have been consulted to verify general government expenditure. During the consultative process, national authorities had the opportunity to review the GGE figures for their countries.

GGHE comprises the outlays earmarked for the enhancement of the health status of the population and/or the distribution of medical care goods and services among population by the following financing agents:

- central/federal, state/provincial/regional, and local/municipal authorities;
- extrabudgetary agencies, principally social security schemes;
- parastatals' direct expenditure on health care.

All three can be financed through domestic funds or through external resources (mainly grants passing through the governments or loans channelled through the federal budget).

The figures for social security and extrabudgetary expenditure on health include purchases of health goods and services by schemes that are mandatory and controlled by government. A major hurdle has been the need to verify that no double counting occurs and that no cash benefits for sickness and/or loss of employment are included in the estimates, as these are classified as income maintenance expenditure.

All health expenditures include final consumption, subsidies to producers, and transfers to households (chiefly reimbursements for medical and pharmaceutical bills). General government health expenditures include both recurrent and investment expenditures (including capital transfers) made during the year. The classification of the functions of government, promoted by the United Nations, IMF, OECD and other institutions, sets the boundaries. In many instances, the data contained in the publications are limited to those supplied by ministries of health. Expenditure on health, however, should include expenditure where the primary intent is to improve health regardless of the implementing entity. An effort has been made to obtain data on health expenditure by other ministries, the armed forces, prisons, schools, universities and others, to ensure that all resources accounting for health expenditures are included.

Variations in the boundaries used in the original sources were adjusted to allow a standardized definition. For example, in some countries THE includes expenditure on environmental health, training of health personnel and health research activities whereas others treat these expenses as memorandum items. Inclusion of these have sometimes led to a ratio of THE to GDP that is higher than previously reported, as in case of Togo. Some countries report expenditure on health by parastatal institutions as public whereas others include them as private. Many countries following the OECD *System of health accounts* framework treat environmental health, training and health research as memorandum items. In the tables reported here, the principles outlined in the *Guide to producing national health accounts with special applications for low-income and middle-income countries (27)* were followed.

OECD health data 2004 supplies GGHE and PvtHE entries for its Member countries, with some gaps mainly for the year 2002. The data for 2002 for Japan and Turkey have been projected by WHO and others such as Australia and the Netherlands provided data directly to WHO to fill these gaps. A larger number of health expenditure reports from non-OECD countries were available than in previous years which allowed a more complete estimation than in recent *World health reports*. The IMF *Government finance statistics* reports central government expenditure on health for over 120 countries, and regional government outlays and local government outlays on health for a third of these countries. The entries are not continuous time series for all countries, but the document serves as an indicator that a reporting system exists in those countries allowing a thorough search to be conducted for the relevant national publications. In some cases expenditures reported under the government finance classification were limited to those of the ministry of health rather than all expenditures on health regardless of ministry. In such cases, wherever possible, other series were used to supplement that source. Government finance data, together with statistical yearbooks, public finance reports, and analyses reporting on the implementation of health policies, have led to GGHE estimates for most WHO Member States. Information on Brunei Darussalam, for example, was accessed from national sources, but also from an International Medical Foundation of Japan data compendium *(38)*. This source provided a means for double checking health budget data for seven countries.

Private expenditure on health has been defined as the sum of expenditures by the following entities:

- Prepaid plans and risk-pooling arrangements: the outlays of private and private social (with no government control over payment rates and participating providers but with broad guidelines from government) insurance schemes, commercial and non-profit (mutual) insurance schemes, health maintenance organizations, and other agents managing prepaid medical and paramedical benefits (including the operating costs of these schemes).

- Firms' expenditure on health: outlays by public and private enterprises for medical care and health-enhancing benefits other than payment to social security.

- Non-profit institutions serving mainly households: resources used to purchase health goods and services by entities whose status does not permit them to be a source of income, profit or other financial gain for the units that establish, control or finance them. This includes funding from internal and external sources.

- Household out-of-pocket spending: the direct outlays of households, including gratuities and in-kind payments made to health practitioners and suppliers of pharmaceuticals, therapeutic appliances, and other goods and services, whose primary intent is to contribute to the restoration or to the enhancement of the health status of individuals or population groups. This includes household payments to public services, non-profit institutions or nongovernmental organizations and non-reimbursable cost sharing, deductibles, copayments and fee-for-service. It excludes payments made by enterprises which deliver medical and paramedical benefits, mandated by law or not, to their employees and payments for overseas treatment.

Most of the information on private health expenditures comes from NHA reports, statistical yearbooks and other periodicals, statistical data on official web sites, reports of nongovernmental organizations, household expenditure surveys, academic studies, and relevant reports and data provided by central statistical offices, ministries of health, professional and trade associations and planning councils (eg. for Qatar's out-of-pocket expenditures). For most OECD Member countries they are obtained from *OECD health data 2004*. Standard extrapolation and estimation techniques were used to obtain the figures for missing years.

Information on external resources was received by courtesy of the Development Action Committee of the OECD (DAC/OECD). Some Member States explicitly monitor the external resources entering their health system, information that has been used to validate or amend the order of magnitude derived from the DAC entries which often related to commitments rather than disbursements.

External resources appearing in Annex Table 5 are those entering the system as a financing source, i.e. all external resources whether passing through governments or private entities are included. On the other hand, other institutions and entities under the public or private health expenditures are financing agents. Financing agents include institutions that pool health resources collected from different sources that pay directly for health care from their own resources.

Several quality checks have been used to assess the validity of the data. For example, estimated health expenditure has been compared against in-patient care expenditure, pharmaceutical expenditure data and other records (including programme administration) to ensure that the outlays for which details have been compiled constitute the bulk of the government/private expenditure on health. The estimates obtained are thus plausible in terms of systems' descriptions. For countries where there is a severe scarcity of information (such as Afghanistan, Democratic People's Republic of Korea, Equatorial Guinea, Gabon, Guinea Bissau, Libya, Sao Tome and Principe, Somalia, Sudan and Turkmenistan), indirect estimating methods were used. WHO intends to introduce a grading system in future publications reporting NHA data, after consultation with partners, showing the extent to which data have had to be estimated.

The aggregate governmental health expenditure data have also been compared with total GGE, providing an additional source of verification. It is possible that the GGHE and, therefore, the figures for total health expenditure, may be an underestimate in the cases where it is not possible to obtain data for local government, nongovernmental organizations and insurance expenditures.

ANNEX TABLE 6

Annex Table 6 presents total expenditure on health and general government expenditure on health in per capita terms. The methodology and sources to derive THE and GGHE have been discussed in the notes to Annex Table 5. Ratios are represented in per capita terms by dividing the expenditure figures by population figures. These per capita figures are expressed first in US dollars at an average exchange rate, or the observed annual average number of units at which a currency is traded in the banking system. They are also presented in international dollar estimates, derived by dividing per capita values in local currency units by an estimate of their purchasing power parity (PPP) compared to US dollars, i.e. a rate or measure that minimizes the consequences of differences in price levels existing between countries.

OECD health data 2004 is the major source for population estimates for the 30 OECD Member countries, just as it is for other health expenditure and macroeconomic variables. All estimates of population size and structure, other than for OECD countries, are based on demographic assessments prepared by the United Nations Population Division *(3)*. This report uses the estimates referred to as the de facto population, and not the de jure population, in each Member State. An exception was made for Serbia and Montenegro for 2001 and 2002, because expenditure figures excluded the provinces of Kosovo and Metohia which became territories under the administration of the United Nations. Population figures for Serbia and Montenegro, excluding Kosovo and Metohia, were obtained from the *Statistical pocket book 2004*, Serbia and Montenegro *(39)*, thus ensuring that the basis for the numerator and denominator is consistent.

Three quarters of the exchange rates (average official rate for the year) have been obtained from the IMF's *International financial statistics*, November 2004. Where information was lacking, available data from the United Nations, the World Bank, the Asian Development Bank and donor reports were used. The euro:US dollar rate has been applied for Andorra, Monaco and San Marino. The New Zealand dollar:US dollar rate has been applied for Niue. The Australian dollar:US dollar rate has been applied for Nauru and Palau. The exchange rate regime in the Islamic Republic of Iran changed in March 2002 from multiple exchange rates to a managed floating exchange rate. This year the inter-bank market rate has been used, replacing the lower pre-2002 official exchange rate series used in the previous *World Health Reports*. Ecuador dollarized its economy in 2000, and the entire dataset has been recalculated in dollar terms for the five-year period reported.

For OECD Member countries, the OECD PPP has been used to calculate international dollars. For countries that are part of the UNECE but are not members of OECD, the UNECE PPPs are used. The Spanish euro, French euro, and Italian euro rates have been used for Andorra, Monaco and San Marino, respectively. For other countries international dollars have been estimated by WHO using methods similar to those used by the World Bank.

ANNEX TABLE 7

In an effort to strengthen collaboration and minimize the reporting burden, WHO and UNICEF jointly collect information through a standard questionnaire (the Joint Reporting Form on Vaccine Preventable Diseases) from all Member States. The content of the Joint Reporting Form was developed through a consensus process among staff from UNICEF, WHO, and selected ministries of health. Information collected in the Joint Reporting Form constitute the major source of information for the following indicators.

Information on immunization coverage is used for a variety of purposes: to monitor the performance of immunization services at local, national and international levels; to guide polio eradication, measles control, and neonatal tetanus elimination; to identify areas of weak system performance that may require extra resources and focused attention; and as one consideration when deciding whether to introduce a new vaccine. Country estimates of national immunization coverage are reported in the Joint Reporting Form. Additionally, since 2000 WHO and UNICEF have conducted a review of data available on national immunization coverage to determine the most likely true level of immunization coverage. Based on the data available, consideration of potential biases, and contributions from local experts, the most likely true level of immunization coverage is determined. For BCG, DTP3, Measles, HepB3 and PAB WHO/UNICEF estimates are presented; for Hib3, yellow fever and TT2+ country estimates are presented.

Newborns immunized with BCG in 2003 (%)

A total of 157 Member States have BCG in their national infant vaccination schedule and coverage estimates has been provided only for them. BCG coverage is often used to reflect the proportion of children who are protected against the severe forms of tuberculosis during the first year of life, and also as an indicator of access to health services.

1-year-olds immunized with 3 doses of DTP in 2003 (%)

DTP vaccine is given universally in all Member States, sometimes in combination with other antigens. DTP3 coverage data are used to indicate the proportion of children protected against diphtheria, pertussis and tetanus, and to indicate performance of immunization services and the health system in general. DTP3 figures are also compared with DTP1 or BCG to assess "drop-out" rates – an indicator of the quality of services and managerial capacity at peripheral levels.

Children under 2 years immunized with 1 dose of measles in 2003 (%)

Measles vaccine is given universally in all member states, sometimes in combination with other antigens. Measles coverage is one of the selected critical indicators to monitor the progress towards the achievement of the Millennium Development Goal 4, to reduce child mortality.

1-year-olds immunized with 3 doses of hepatitis B in 2003 (%)

Hepatitis B vaccination is recommended universally but only 147 member states had introduced hepatitis B vaccine in routine infant immunization by the end of 2003. HepB3 coverage data are critical to estimate the impact of the vaccine on chronic infection with hepatitis B and its deadly sequelae (hepatoma and cirrhosis).

1-year-olds immunized with 3 doses of Hib vaccine in 2003 (%)

WHO recommends that *Haemophilus influenzae* type b vaccine (Hib) should be included in routine infant immunization services, as appropriate, given epidemiological evidence of disease burden and national capacities and priorities. As of 2003, 87 countries had included it in national routine infant immunization schedule and two in part of the country.

1-year-olds immunized with yellow fever vaccine in 2003 (%)

WHO recommends that yellow fever vaccine be introduced in countries at risk for outbreaks. These include 31 Member States in the African Region, two Member States in the eastern Mediterranean Region, and 11 in the Region of the Americas. Some 21 Member States have introduced yellow fever vaccine in the national routine immunization schedule and seven have introduced it in high risk areas.

Districts achieving at least 80% DTP3 coverage in 2003 (%)

A district is defined here as a third administrative level. In 2002 at the Special Session of the United Nations General Assembly on Children, the nations of the world committed themselves to achieving the following goal: by 2010 or sooner all countries will have routine immunization coverage at 90% nationally with at least 80% coverage in every district.

Children born in 2003 protected against tetanus by vaccination of their mothers with tetanus toxoid (PAB) (%)

Estimates for protection at birth (PAB) are available for a subset of countries where neonatal tetanus has not yet been eliminated. The data reflect the proportion of mothers protected against tetanus at the moment of child delivery through immunization. This may include protective doses received during campaigns or during previous pregnancies.

Pregnant women immunized with two or more doses of tetanus toxoid in 2003 (%)

Tetanus toxoid (TT) administered to women of childbearing age (including pregnant women) protects against both maternal and neonatal tetanus. In the absence of previous tetanus immunization, at least two doses TT (TT2+) are needed to provide protection. WHO recommends that TT2+ be calculated as the proportion of pregnant women having received the second or superior dose of tetanus toxoid in a given year. The data provided are as reported by Member States, of which 110 have TT in the national immunization schedule.

Number of diseases covered by routine immunization before 24 months in 2003

This describes the number of antigens included in the national immunization schedule for children aged less than 24 months in 2003.

Was a second opportunity for measles immunization provided?

The critical strategy to achieve measles mortality reduction is to provide a second vaccine opportunity. A country should have implemented a two-dose routine measles schedule and/or within the last four years have conducted a national immunization campaign achieving more than 90% coverage of children aged less than five years.

Vitamin A distribution linked with routine immunization in 2003

WHO recommends vitamin A supplementation with measles vaccine in countries where vitamin A deficiency is a problem. The data presented in the table do not include vitamin A distributed through campaigns.

Number of wild polio cases reported in 2004

Number of wild polio cases reported for 2004 as of 25 January 2005.

Country polio eradication status in 2004

In 1988, the polio eradication initiative was launched. By the end of 2004, three WHO regions were certified as polio free (the Region of the Americas, and the European and Western Pacific Regions). Only six countries remained polio endemic, four countries re-established transmission (where circulation of imported poliovirus occurred for a period greater than six months) and seven countries reported importation of wild polio virus.

Use of auto-disable syringes in 2003

In 1999 WHO, UNICEF and the United Nations Population Fund (UNFPA) published a joint statement on the use of auto-disable syringes in immunization services, urging that all countries should use only auto-disable syringes for immunization. By the end of 2003, 46 Member States reported exclusive auto-disable syringe use for immunization and 51 countries reported partial use.

Use of vaccine of assured quality in 2003 *(40)*

The National Regulatory Authority independently controls the quality of the vaccine in accordance with the six regulatory functions defined by WHO (in WHO Technical Report Series, No. 822, 1992). There are no unresolved confirmed reports of quality problems.

Total routine vaccine spending financed using government funds in 2003 (%)

The percentage of all vaccine expenditure in 2003 that was financed using national public funds. In the majority of cases, this excludes any external private and public financing provided to national government for immunization services and used to purchase vaccines, except in the case of countries receiving direct budget support. The data can however include grant portion of development bank loan funds used to purchase vaccines.

ANNEX TABLE 8

Contraceptive prevalence rate (modern methods)

The contraceptive prevalence rate for modern methods is the percentage of women who are practising, or whose sexual partners are practising, any form of contraception. It is measured for married women aged between 15 and 49 years. Modern contraceptive methods include female and male sterilization, injectable or oral hormones, intrauterine devices, diaphragms, spermicides, and condoms. Data sources include Demographic and Health Surveys (ORC Macro and national statistical offices), and *World Contraceptive Use 2003 (41)*.

Antenatal care use

Based on recent research findings, WHO recommends a minimum of four antenatal visits at specific times for all pregnant women. The table provides the most recent statistics on the number of antenatal care contacts for women during their last pregnancy in the five years prior to the most recent survey conducted in that country. The proportion of women who had one or more antenatal care contacts, as well as the proportion of women who had four or more visits during their last pregnancy are given.

For most countries, the main sources of information on antenatal care use are household surveys. Data sources include Demographic and Health Surveys (ORC Macro and national statistical offices), Reproductive Health Surveys (Centers for Disease Control), Multiple Indicator Cluster Surveys (UNICEF), Pan-Arab Maternal and Child Health Surveys (PAPCHILD), Gulf Fertility Surveys, Fertility and Family Surveys (ECE), national surveys, data files of the United Nations Population Division, and from the 2004 Global Estimates Geneva, Monitoring and Evaluation, Department of Reproductive Health and Research, World Health Organization, 2004.

Proportion of births attended by skilled personnel

International agreement on the definition of a skilled attendant has been reached. A skilled attendant is an accredited health professional – such as a midwife, doctor or nurse – who has been educated and trained to proficiency in the skills needed to manage normal (uncomplicated) pregnancies, childbirth and the immediate postnatal period, and in the identification, management and referral of complications in women and newborns *(42)*. Traditional birth attendants, trained or not, are excluded from the category of skilled attendant at birth.

For most countries, the main sources of information on childbirth care are from household surveys. Data sources include Demographic and Health Surveys (ORC Macro and national statistical offices), Reproductive Health Surveys (Centers for Disease Control), Multiple Indicator Cluster Surveys (UNICEF), Pan-Arab Maternal and Child Health Surveys (PAPCHILD), Gulf Fertility Surveys, Fertility and Family Surveys (ECE), national surveys, data files of the United Nations Population Division, and from the 2004 Global Estimates Geneva, Monitoring and Evaluation, Department of Reproductive Health and Research, World Health Organization, 2004.

The use of various sources that use different definitions of a skilled attendant, however, makes the comparability of the data across countries and within countries at different times difficult. Although WHO has defined the specific competencies that the skilled attendant should have, there have been no systematic efforts to ensure that the groups classified under the heading of skilled attendant actually have them.

Proportion of births at a health facility

The table presents the proportion of births that occurred in health facilities. The term health facility includes any hospital or clinic in the public or private sector. Sources are as for the proportion of births attended by skilled personnel.

Proportion of births by caesarean section

The table presents the proportion of women who had a cesarean section in their last birth. For most countries, the main sources of information on childbirth care are from household surveys, originating from similar sources to those for the proportion of births attended by skilled personnel.

Number of midwives and number of births

The table gives, by country, the total number of midwives and the yearly number of births. Data on human resources in countries are often difficult to obtain, incomplete and unreliable. The main sources of data are the WHO Global Atlas, Human Resources for Health, WHO EURO Health for All Database, and from Population Division (DESA) United Nations Population Division.

Maternal mortality ratio

The inclusion of maternal mortality reduction in the Millennium Development Goals stimulated an increase in the attention paid to the issue and created additional demands for information. WHO, UNICEF and UNFPA undertook a process to produce global and national estimates of maternal mortality ratio (MMR) for the year 2000, the results of which are published in this table. The Tenth Revision of the *International Classification of Diseases* (ICD-10) *(10)* defines a maternal death as *the death of a woman while pregnant or within 42 days of termination of pregnancy, irrespective of the duration and site of the pregnancy, from any cause related to or aggravated by the pregnancy or its management but not from accidental or incidental causes.* The MMR is the most commonly used measure of maternal mortality, and it is defined as the number of maternal deaths during a given time period per 100 000 live births during the same time period. This is a measure of the risk of death once a woman has become pregnant. Maternal mortality is difficult to measure, particularly in settings where deaths are not comprehensively reported through the vital registration system and where there is no medical certification of cause of death. Moreover, even where overall levels of maternal mortality are high, maternal deaths are nonetheless relatively rare events and thus prone to measurement error. As a result, all existing estimates of maternal mortality are subject to greater or lesser degrees of uncertainty. Approaches used for obtaining data on levels of maternal mortality in this table vary considerably in terms of methodology, source of data and precision of results. The main approaches are household surveys (including sisterhood surveys), censuses, Reproductive Age Mortality Studies (RAMOS) and statistical modelling.

Neonatal, early neonatal and stillbirth mortality rates

Events related to birth, death, and the perinatal period, as well as the reporting and statistics amenable to international comparison and to reporting requirements for the data from which they are derived, are defined in the chapter on "Standards and reporting requirements related to fetal, perinatal, neonatal and infant mortality" of the *International statistical classification of diseases and related health problems – 10th revision* (ICD-10). Some key issues specifically relevant to neonatal and perinatal mortalities are highlighted below.

The legal requirements for registration of fetal deaths and live births vary from country to country and even within countries. If possible, all fetuses and infants weighing at least 500 g at birth, whether alive or dead, should be included in the statistics. The inclusion of fetuses and infants weighing between 500 g and 1000 g in national statistics is recommended both because of its inherent value and because it improves the coverage of reporting at 1000 g and over. In statistics for international comparison, both the numerator and the denominator of all rates should be restricted to fetuses and infants weighing 1000 g or more. Published ratios and rates should always specify the denominator, i.e. live births or total births (live births plus fetal deaths).

Key issues specifically relevant to neonatal and perinatal mortalities include the following:

- *Perinatal mortality* is death in the perinatal period which includes late pregnancy, birth and the first week of life, and thus includes stillbirths and early neonatal mortality. *Perinatal mortality rates* are calculated per 1000 *total* births (live and stillbirths).
- *Neonatal mortality* relates to the death of live-born infants during the neonatal period, which begins with birth and covers the first four weeks of life. The neonatal period may be subdivided into the early neonatal period, which is the first week of life (and is also part of the perinatal period), and the late neonatal period, which is from the second to the fourth week of life. *Neonatal mortality rates* are calculated per 1000 live births.
- *Early neonatal mortality* relates to the death of live-born infants during the first week of life, which is also part of the perinatal period. *Early neonatal mortality rates* are calculated per 1000 live births.
- *Stillbirth mortality* relates to the fetus of 28 weeks *(10)* gestation that at birth shows no sign of life. *Stillbirth mortality rates* are calculated per 1000 total births (live and stillbirths).

Data for the estimates originated from survey and registration data. The most frequently available early mortality data are for neonatal deaths. The neonatal mortality rate also provides a reliable national survey or registration rate that can be used to derive estimates of the earlier mortality, if required. For only 5% of births, no neonatal mortality data at national level could be identified, as this data was available for 83% of countries and 95% of births. Data for 81% of births (87 countries) came from surveys. Data originating from civil registration were available for 72 countries, or 37% of all countries, which nevertheless only covers 14% of births. Early neonatal mortality and stillbirth data were available for 73% and 53% of countries respectively, covering 76% and 40% of births respectively.

Estimates for countries for which neonatal mortality data were not available were calculated using WHO under-five mortality estimates and applying a regression formula corrected for deaths due to AIDS; early neonatal mortality rates were estimated from the neonatal mortality by regression; and stillbirths were estimated relying on the relationship between early neonatal mortality and stillbirths in 14 mortality regions.

The estimates so derived relate mostly to the second half of the 1990s or the early years of the 21st century. In order to project year-specific mortality estimates, the ratio between WHO's estimated under-five mortality rate for the year 2000 and the under-five mortality rate of each country's estimation dataset was calculated. To obtain the early mortality estimates for the year 2000 this ratio was used to adjust the rates provided by surveys or vital registration data or regression. With this adjustment the distribution of age at death within the overall WHO estimated under-five mortality envelope was maintained.

References

1. *WHO mortality database*. Geneva, World Health Organization, 2004.
2. Bryce J, Boschi-Pinto C, Shibuya K, Black RE and the Child Health Epidemiology Reference Group. New WHO estimates of the causes of child deaths. *Lancet* (submitted).
3. United Nations Population Division. *World population prospects – the 2002 revision*. New York, NY, United Nations, 2003.
4. Murray CJL, Ferguson BD, Lopez AD, Guillot M, Salomon JA, Ahmad O. Modified logit life table system: principles, empirical validation and application. *Population Studies*, 2003, 57:1–18.
5. Lopez AD, Ahmad O, Guillot M, Ferguson B, Salomon J, Murray CJL et al. *World mortality in 2000: life tables for 191 countries*. Geneva, World Health Organization, 2002.
6. Mathers CD, Ma Fat D, Inoue M, Rao C, Lopez AD. Counting the dead and what they died of: an assessment of the global status of cause-of-death data. *Bulletin of the World Health Organization*, 2005 (in press).
7. Hill K, Pande R, Mahy M, Jones G. *Trends in child mortality in the developing world: 1990 to 1996*. New York, NY, United Nations Children's Fund, 1998.
8. Mathers CD, Bernard C, Iburg KM, Inoue M, Ma Fat D, Shibuya K et al. *Global burden of disease in 2002: data sources, methods and results*. Geneva, World Health Organization, 2003 (GPE Discussion Paper No. 54; http://www3.who.int/whosis/menu.cfm?path=ev idence,burden,burden_gbd2000docs,burden_gbd2000docs_DP54&language=english, accessed 4 February 2004).
9. United Nations Department of International Economic and Social Affairs. *Manual x: indirect techniques for demographic estimation*. New York, NY, United Nations, 1983 (Population Studies No. 81; ST/ESA/SER.A/81).
10. *International statistical classification of diseases and related health problems – 10th revision*. Geneva, World Health Organization, 1993.
11. Rutstein SO. *Infant and child mortality: levels, trends, and demographic differentials*. Revised ed. Voorburg, International Statistical Institute, 1984 (WFS Comparative Studies No. 43).
12. Pressat R. *Manuel d'analyse de la mortalité [Mortality Analysis Manual]*. Paris, L'Institut national d'études démographiques, 1985.
13. Salomon JA, Murray CJL. The epidemiologic transition revisited: compositional models for causes of death by age and sex. *Population and Development Review*, 2002, 28:205–228.
14. *Neonatal and perinatal mortality for the year 2000*. Geneva, World Health Organization, 2005 (in press).
15. *AIDS epidemic update 2004*. Geneva, Joint United Nations Programme on HIV/AIDS, 2004.
16. Boschi-Pinto C, Tomaskovic L, Gouws E, Shibuya K. Estimates of the distribution of child deaths due to diarrhoea in developing regions of the world. *International Journal of Epidemiology* (submitted).
17. Rowe AK, Rowe SY, Snow RW, Korenromp EL, Armstrong Schellenberg JRM, Stein C et al. The burden of malaria mortality among African children in the year 2000. *Lancet* (submitted).
18. Williams BG, Gouws E, Boschi-Pinto C, Bryce J, Dye C. Estimates of world-wide distribution of child deaths from acute respiratory infections. *Lancet Infectious Diseases*, 2002, 2:25–32.

19. Stein CE, Birmingham M, Kurian M, Duclos P, Strebel P. The global burden of measles in the year 2000 – a model that uses country-specific indicators. *Journal of Infectious Diseases*, 2003, 187(Suppl. 1):S8–S14.

20. Morris SS, Black RE, Tomaskovic L. Predicting the distribution of under-five deaths by cause in countries without adequate vital registration systems. *International Journal of Epidemiology*, 2003, 32:1041–1051.

21. Kosek M, Bern C, Guerrant R. The global burden of diarrhoeal disease, as estimated from studies published between 1992 and 2000. *Bulletin of the World Heatlh Organization*, 2003, 81:197–204.

22. Parashar UD, Hummelman EG, Bresee JS, Miller MA, Glass RI. Global illness and deaths caused by rotavirus disease in children. *Emerging Infectious Diseases*, 2003, 9:565–572.

23. Mapping Malaria Risk in Africa (MARA) Collaboration. *Towards an atlas of malaria risk in Africa. First technical report of the MARA/ARMA Collaboration*. Durban, Albany Print, 1998.

24. World Health Organization. *Measles mortality review meeting report, 22–23 January 2004* (http://www3.who.int/whosis/mort/text/measles_report.zip, accessed 19 January 2005).

25. Lawn JE, Cousens S, Wilczynska-Ketende K for the CHERG Neonatal Group. *Estimating the causes of 4 million neonatal deaths in 2000. CHERG preliminary report 2004*.

26. Grassly NC, Morgan M, Walker N, Garnett G, Stanecki KA, Stover J et al. Uncertainty in estimates of HIV/AIDS: the estimation and application of plausibility bounds. *Sexually Transmitted Infections*, 2004, 80(Suppl. 1):S31–S38.

27. WHO/World Bank/United States Agency for International Development. *Guide to producing national health accounts with special applications for low-income and middle-income countries*. Geneva, World Health Organization, 2003 (http://whqlibdoc.who.int/publications/2003/9241546077.pdf, accessed 13 October 2003).

28. *A system of health accounts*. Paris, Organisation for Economic Co-operation and Development, 2000 (http://www.oecd.org/dataoecd/41/4/1841456.pdf, accessed 13 October 2003).

29. Organisation for Economic Co-operation and Development/International Monetary Fund/World Bank/United Nations/Eurostat. *System of national accounts 1993*. New York, NY, United Nations, 1994.

30. *Government finance statistics yearbook, 2003*. Washington, DC, International Monetary Fund, 2003.

31. *International financial statistics yearbook, 2003*. Washington, DC, International Monetary Fund, 2003.

32. *International Financial Statistics*, 2004, November.

33. *ADB Key indicators 2003*. Manila, Asian Development Bank, 2004.

34. *OECD health data 2004*. Paris, Organisation for Economic Co-operation and Development 2004.

35. *International development statistics 2004*. Organisation for Economic Co-operation and Development, Development Assistance Committee, 2004 (http://www1.oecd.org/dac/htm/online.htm, accessed 15 October 2004).

36. *National accounts statistics: main aggregates and detailed tables, 2001*. New York, NY, United Nations, 2004.

37. *National accounts of OECD countries: detailed tables 1991/2002, 2004 edition, volume II*. Paris, Organisation for Economic Co-operation and Development, 2004.

38. *Southeast Asian Medical Information Center health statistics 2002*. Tokyo, The International Medical Foundation of Japan, 2003.

39. *Statistical pocket book 2004*. Belgrade, Serbia and Montenegro Statistical Office, 2004.

40. *GPV policy statement. Statement on vaccine quality*. Geneva, World Health Organization, 1997 (WHO/VSQ/GEN/96.02 Rev.1).

41. *World Contraceptive Use 2003*. New York, NY, Department of Economic and Social Affairs, Population Division, United Nations, 2004.

42. *Making pregnancy safer: the critical role of the skilled attendant. A joint statement by WHO, ICM and FIGO*. Geneva, World Health Organization, 2004.

Annex Table 1 Basic indicators for all WHO Member States

Figures computed by WHO to ensure comparability;[a] they are not necessarily the official statistics of Member States, which may use alternative rigorous methods.

		POPULATION ESTIMATES									LIFE EXPECTANCY AT BIRTH (YEARS) Both sexes		PROBABILITY OF DYING Under age 5 years (under-5 mortality) Both sexes	
		Total population (000)	Annual growth rate (%)	Dependency ratio (per 100)		Percentage of population aged 60+ years		Total fertility rate						
	Member State	2003	1993–2003	1993	2003	1993	2003	1993	2003	2003	Uncertainty	2003	Uncerta
1	Afghanistan	23 897	3.4	88	86	4.7	4.7	7.0	6.8	42	36 - 47	257	206 - 3
2	Albania	3 166	-0.3	60	52	8.0	9.7	2.8	2.3	72	72 - 73	21	19 -
3	Algeria	31 800	1.7	80	59	5.7	6.0	4.0	2.8	70	69 - 72	41	31 -
4	Andorra	71	1.7	47	45	20.3	21.8	1.4	1.3	81	80 - 82	5	5 -
5	Angola	13 625	2.9	98	101	4.6	4.3	7.2	7.2	40	31 - 47	260	225 - 2
6	Antigua and Barbuda	73	1.1	62	55	9.2	10.6	1.8	1.6	72	67 - 77	12	9 -
7	Argentina	38 428	1.3	63	59	13.1	13.6	2.8	2.4	74	74 - 75	17	16 -
8	Armenia	3 061	-1.2	57	43	10.7	12.9	2.1	1.1	68	67 - 69	33	29 -
9	Australia	19 731	1.1	50	48	15.7	16.9	1.9	1.7	81	80 - 81	6	5 -
10	Austria	8 116	0.2	48	47	19.8	21.6	1.5	1.3	79	77 - 81	6	4 -
11	Azerbaijan	8 370	1.0	64	55	7.8	9.1	2.8	2.1	65	64 - 66	91	77 - 1
12	Bahamas	314	1.4	58	53	6.9	8.8	2.6	2.3	72	71 - 74	14	11 -
13	Bahrain	724	2.8	51	46	3.7	4.1	3.4	2.6	74	70 - 77	9	8 -
14	Bangladesh	146 736	2.2	80	70	4.8	5.1	4.4	3.4	63	62 - 64	69	65 -
15	Barbados	270	0.4	54	42	14.7	13.1	1.6	1.5	75	69 - 79	13	8 -
16	Belarus	9 895	-0.4	52	45	17.6	19.1	1.6	1.2	68	68 - 69	10	9 -
17	Belgium	10 318	0.2	50	53	21.0	22.3	1.6	1.7	79	78 - 79	5	5 -
18	Belize	256	2.4	90	72	6.0	5.9	4.3	3.1	68	62 - 72	39	31 -
19	Benin	6 736	2.7	105	92	4.5	4.1	6.5	5.6	53	45 - 60	154	139 -
20	Bhutan	2 257	2.5	90	84	6.2	6.5	5.7	5.0	63	58 - 66	85	68 - 7
21	Bolivia	8 808	2.1	81	76	6.1	6.6	4.8	3.8	65	61 - 69	66	60 -
22	Bosnia and Herzegovina	4 161	1.1	43	39	11.5	15.4	1.5	1.3	73	72 - 74	17	15 -
23	Botswana	1 785	1.9	87	74	3.7	4.5	4.4	3.7	36	34 - 39	112	96 - 1
24	Brazil	178 470	1.4	62	50	6.9	8.2	2.6	2.2	69	69 - 70	35	31 -
25	Brunei Darussalam	358	2.5	57	50	4.1	4.5	3.1	2.5	77	76 - 78	6	5 -
26	Bulgaria	7 897	-0.8	50	44	20.4	21.8	1.4	1.1	72	72 - 73	15	14 -
27	Burkina Faso	13 002	2.9	107	106	4.5	4.0	7.1	6.7	45	39 - 49	207	187 - 2
28	Burundi	6 825	1.5	99	96	4.6	4.3	6.8	6.8	42	37 - 48	190	159 - 2
29	Cambodia	14 144	2.7	101	80	4.4	4.7	5.4	4.7	54	51 - 57	140	124 - 1
30	Cameroon	16 018	2.3	93	85	5.5	5.6	5.6	4.6	48	42 - 53	166	148 - 1
31	Canada	31 510	0.9	48	45	15.9	17.4	1.7	1.5	80	79 - 81	6	5 -
32	Cape Verde	463	2.2	101	78	6.6	6.1	4.6	3.3	70	67 - 73	35	30 -
33	Central African Republic	3 865	2.0	88	89	6.1	6.1	5.6	4.9	42	37 - 47	180	156 - 2
34	Chad	8 598	3.1	96	100	5.2	4.8	6.7	6.6	46	41 - 50	200	175 - 2
35	Chile	15 806	1.4	56	54	9.3	10.9	2.5	2.3	77	74 - 80	9	7 -
36	China	1 311 709	0.9	49	43	9.0	10.5	1.9	1.8	71	70 - 72	37	31 -
37	Colombia	44 222	1.8	65	58	6.4	7.2	3.0	2.6	72	72 - 73	21	19 -
38	Comoros	768	2.9	94	81	4.0	4.2	5.8	4.8	64	56 - 73	73	59 -
39	Congo	3 724	3.1	96	100	4.8	4.5	6.3	6.3	54	48 - 61	108	89 - 1
40	Cook Islands	18	-0.3	71	64	6.3	7.3	3.9	3.2	71	70 - 72	21	20 -
41	Costa Rica	4 173	2.3	67	55	7.2	8.0	2.9	2.3	77	77 - 77	10	9 -
42	Côte d'Ivoire	16 631	2.0	93	80	4.4	5.2	5.9	4.7	45	39 - 51	193	161 - 2
43	Croatia	4 428	-0.4	46	50	18.8	21.7	1.5	1.7	75	74 - 75	7	6 -
44	Cuba	11 300	0.4	45	43	12.0	14.8	1.6	1.6	77	76 - 78	7	6 -
45	Cyprus	802	1.1	58	50	14.9	16.4	2.3	1.9	78	78 - 79	6	5 -
46	Czech Republic	10 236	-0.1	49	41	17.9	19.2	1.6	1.2	75	75 - 76	5	4 -
47	Democratic People's Republic of Korea	22 664	0.8	47	48	8.2	10.9	2.3	2.0	66	63 - 70	55	39 -
48	Democratic Republic of the Congo	52 771	2.4	100	98	4.4	4.2	6.7	6.7	44	40 - 48	205	180 - 2
49	Denmark	5 364	0.3	48	51	20.0	20.7	1.7	1.8	77	77 - 78	5	5 -
50	Djibouti	703	2.4	85	86	4.6	5.1	6.2	5.7	55	51 - 58	138	93 - 1
51	Dominica	79	0.7	62	55	9.2	10.6	2.0	1.8	73	72 - 74	12	11 -
52	Dominican Republic	8 745	1.6	69	58	5.8	7.1	3.1	2.7	68	66 - 70	35	29 -
53	Ecuador	13 003	1.7	72	61	6.3	7.5	3.5	2.7	71	70 - 72	27	24 -
54	Egypt	71 931	2.0	79	65	6.4	6.9	4.0	3.3	67	66 - 68	39	36 -
55	El Salvador	6 515	1.8	76	67	6.7	7.6	3.5	2.9	70	69 - 71	36	31 -

LIFE EXPECTANCY AT BIRTH (YEARS)				PROBABILITY OF DYING (PER 1000)							
				Under age 5 years (under-5 mortality rate[b])				Between ages 15 and 60 years (adult mortality rate)			
Males		Females		Males		Females		Males		Females	
2003	Uncertainty	2003	Uncertainty	2003	Uncertainty	2003	Uncertainty	2003	Uncertainty	2003	Uncertainty
41	31 - 52	42	28 - 54	258	179 - 336	256	181 - 332	510	326 - 740	448	196 - 736
69	68 - 71	75	74 - 76	23	20 - 25	19	17 - 20	167	147 - 185	92	82 - 105
69	68 - 70	72	71 - 73	45	36 - 54	36	29 - 44	155	140 - 169	125	111 - 141
78	77 - 79	84	84 - 85	5	5 - 6	4	4 - 5	107	96 - 119	41	37 - 46
38	31 - 44	42	34 - 49	276	245 - 306	243	216 - 271	584	450 - 774	488	304 - 700
70	69 - 71	75	74 - 76	13	7 - 20	11	6 - 17	193	169 - 213	122	110 - 136
71	70 - 71	78	78 - 78	19	18 - 21	16	15 - 17	176	169 - 183	90	88 - 92
65	64 - 66	72	70 - 73	35	32 - 39	31	28 - 34	240	204 - 282	108	91 - 127
78	78 - 78	83	83 - 83	6	6 - 7	5	4 - 5	89	86 - 92	51	49 - 53
76	76 - 76	82	81 - 82	6	5 - 7	5	5 - 6	115	111 - 120	59	56 - 62
62	61 - 63	68	66 - 69	96	77 - 115	85	69 - 101	220	193 - 246	120	100 - 141
69	69 - 70	75	75 - 76	16	13 - 19	13	10 - 15	257	239 - 276	146	138 - 155
73	70 - 76	75	67 - 83	10	9 - 11	8	7 - 9	117	80 - 165	81	28 - 175
63	62 - 64	63	62 - 64	68	61 - 75	70	63 - 77	251	222 - 281	258	231 - 283
71	70 - 72	78	78 - 79	14	11 - 18	12	9 - 14	189	171 - 208	106	95 - 117
63	63 - 63	75	75 - 75	11	10 - 12	8	7 - 9	370	366 - 373	130	127 - 132
75	75 - 76	82	81 - 82	6	5 - 6	5	4 - 5	125	121 - 129	66	64 - 69
65	63 - 67	71	70 - 72	44	35 - 55	34	26 - 41	257	218 - 293	153	136 - 169
52	45 - 57	54	46 - 60	158	142 - 174	150	135 - 164	393	257 - 564	332	196 - 522
61	54 - 68	64	56 - 70	85	67 - 101	85	68 - 100	261	118 - 448	202	94 - 382
63	57 - 70	67	59 - 72	68	61 - 75	64	58 - 71	247	100 - 405	180	83 - 351
69	68 - 71	76	75 - 78	20	15 - 25	15	11 - 19	190	161 - 216	89	76 - 103
37	34 - 40	36	33 - 39	114	96 - 129	111	93 - 127	850	793 - 890	839	777 - 884
66	66 - 67	73	72 - 73	39	33 - 45	32	27 - 36	240	231 - 249	129	121 - 137
75	74 - 77	79	78 - 80	6	5 - 7	5	4 - 6	114	98 - 131	86	76 - 100
69	69 - 69	76	76 - 76	17	15 - 18	13	12 - 14	216	213 - 219	91	89 - 94
44	38 - 48	46	38 - 52	214	194 - 235	200	180 - 220	533	418 - 687	462	324 - 647
40	34 - 46	45	38 - 51	197	157 - 238	183	147 - 221	654	528 - 777	525	395 - 678
50	45 - 56	57	50 - 64	153	137 - 168	127	114 - 139	441	315 - 597	285	161 - 455
47	42 - 52	48	42 - 54	168	152 - 183	164	149 - 179	503	386 - 635	461	331 - 603
78	77 - 78	82	82 - 83	6	6 - 6	5	5 - 5	93	91 - 95	57	56 - 59
67	62 - 71	73	69 - 76	41	32 - 49	29	23 - 35	213	129 - 320	129	80 - 197
42	36 - 47	43	37 - 49	187	155 - 219	172	144 - 199	641	519 - 759	590	457 - 718
44	38 - 50	47	39 - 54	212	176 - 250	188	159 - 219	513	386 - 680	444	305 - 647
74	73 - 74	80	80 - 81	10	9 - 11	9	8 - 9	133	125 - 144	66	62 - 70
70	69 - 70	73	72 - 73	32	29 - 36	43	38 - 47	164	153 - 174	103	94 - 113
68	67 - 69	77	76 - 78	25	22 - 27	18	16 - 20	231	217 - 246	97	87 - 109
62	55 - 69	66	59 - 73	79	62 - 94	67	53 - 80	254	103 - 432	182	80 - 340
53	47 - 59	55	48 - 62	113	85 - 142	103	79 - 128	434	295 - 585	381	264 - 534
68	67 - 70	74	74 - 75	24	22 - 25	19	18 - 20	166	147 - 186	112	102 - 124
75	74 - 75	80	79 - 80	11	10 - 13	9	8 - 10	129	121 - 138	76	71 - 81
42	35 - 49	49	42 - 55	223	172 - 272	160	126 - 193	558	427 - 726	450	324 - 604
71	71 - 72	78	78 - 79	8	7 - 10	6	5 - 7	173	164 - 181	70	66 - 74
75	75 - 76	79	79 - 80	8	7 - 9	6	6 - 7	137	130 - 144	87	84 - 90
76	76 - 77	81	79 - 82	5	5 - 6	6	5 - 8	99	91 - 108	47	37 - 59
72	72 - 72	79	79 - 79	5	5 - 6	4	4 - 5	166	164 - 169	74	72 - 76
65	58 - 72	68	59 - 75	56	30 - 83	54	28 - 81	231	95 - 390	168	69 - 345
42	36 - 47	47	40 - 53	217	185 - 248	192	163 - 220	578	441 - 720	452	302 - 618
75	75 - 75	80	80 - 80	6	5 - 7	5	4 - 5	121	117 - 124	73	71 - 76
53	47 - 59	56	48 - 62	144	121 - 166	132	110 - 154	376	243 - 544	311	190 - 483
71	70 - 71	76	74 - 77	12	10 - 14	13	9 - 18	210	192 - 231	118	92 - 151
65	64 - 66	72	71 - 73	38	34 - 42	32	29 - 35	250	215 - 285	147	123 - 172
68	68 - 69	74	73 - 75	29	24 - 33	25	21 - 29	212	199 - 225	127	116 - 138
65	64 - 66	69	67 - 71	39	35 - 43	40	36 - 44	242	208 - 280	157	119 - 201
67	65 - 68	73	72 - 74	39	33 - 45	33	28 - 39	248	218 - 284	138	126 - 150

Annex Table 1 Basic indicators for all WHO Member States

Figures computed by WHO to ensure comparability;[a] they are not necessarily the official statistics of Member States, which may use alternative rigorous methods.

		POPULATION ESTIMATES									LIFE EXPECTANCY AT BIRTH (YEARS)		PROBABILITY OF DYING (	
		Total population (000)	Annual growth rate (%)	Dependency ratio (per 100)		Percentage of population aged 60+ years		Total fertility rate			Both sexes		Under age 5 years (under-5 mortality r	
											Both sexes		Both sexes	
	Member State	2003	1993–2003	1993	2003	1993	2003	1993	2003	2003	Uncertainty	2003	Uncertai
56	Equatorial Guinea	494	2.6	88	91	6.3	5.9	5.9	5.9	51	48 - 54	146	121 - 1
57	Eritrea	4 141	2.8	93	90	3.6	3.6	6.1	5.4	59	56 - 63	85	70 - 1(
58	Estonia	1 323	-1.3	52	47	18.3	21.6	1.6	1.2	71	70 - 72	8	7 -
59	Ethiopia	70 678	2.7	94	94	4.4	4.6	6.8	6.1	50	46 - 54	169	133 - 2(
60	Fiji	839	1.2	66	56	5.0	6.2	3.3	2.9	68	67 - 69	20	17 -
61	Finland	5 207	0.3	50	49	18.8	20.6	1.8	1.7	79	77 - 80	4	3 -
62	France	60 144	0.4	53	53	19.7	20.5	1.7	1.9	80	79 - 81	5	4 -
63	Gabon	1 329	2.4	92	82	7.3	6.2	5.1	3.9	58	52 - 63	91	82 - 1(
64	Gambia	1 426	3.2	84	79	5.2	5.8	5.6	4.7	57	54 - 61	123	105 - 1
65	Georgia	5 126	-0.5	53	49	15.8	18.8	1.8	1.4	71	69 - 72	45	40 -
66	Germany	82 476	0.2	46	48	20.5	24.4	1.3	1.4	79	79 - 79	5	4 -
67	Ghana	20 922	2.3	91	76	4.7	5.2	5.2	4.1	58	55 - 62	95	85 - 1(
68	Greece	10 976	0.6	48	49	21.0	24.0	1.4	1.3	79	78 - 79	6	5 -
69	Grenada	80	-0.5	62	55	9.2	10.6	3.9	3.5	67	66 - 69	23	17 -
70	Guatemala	12 347	2.7	95	86	5.2	5.3	5.4	4.4	66	65 - 68	47	40 -
71	Guinea	8 480	2.2	92	88	4.4	4.6	6.4	5.8	52	49 - 55	160	145 - 1
72	Guinea-Bissau	1 493	2.9	96	101	5.3	4.8	7.1	7.1	47	43 - 49	204	183 - 2
73	Guyana	765	0.4	65	53	6.8	7.1	2.5	2.3	62	57 - 67	69	42 -
74	Haiti	8 326	1.4	90	74	5.7	6.0	4.7	3.9	53	50 - 57	119	102 - 1
75	Honduras	6 941	2.7	90	78	4.7	5.4	4.9	3.7	67	64 - 70	41	36 -
76	Hungary	9 877	-0.4	49	45	19.3	20.2	1.7	1.2	73	72 - 74	9	7 -
77	Iceland	290	1.0	55	52	14.9	15.5	2.2	1.9	80	79 - 82	3	3 -
78	India	1 065 462	1.7	68	61	7.0	7.8	3.8	3.0	62	61 - 62	87	76 -
79	Indonesia	219 883	1.4	63	53	6.6	8.0	3.0	2.3	67	66 - 67	41	32 -
80	Iran, Islamic Republic of	68 920	1.3	92	56	6.0	6.4	4.2	2.3	69	69 - 70	39	31 -
81	Iraq	25 175	2.9	87	78	4.4	4.7	5.7	4.7	55	52 - 58	125	96 - 1
82	Ireland	3 956	1.1	59	47	15.3	15.5	2.0	1.9	78	78 - 79	6	5 -
83	Israel	6 433	2.5	66	61	12.8	13.0	2.9	2.7	80	80 - 80	6	6 -
84	Italy	57 423	0.1	46	49	21.9	24.7	1.3	1.2	81	79 - 83	5	4 -
85	Jamaica	2 651	0.9	72	60	9.9	9.6	2.7	2.3	73	71 - 74	20	17 -
86	Japan	127 654	0.2	43	49	19.3	25.0	1.5	1.3	82	82 - 82	4	4 -
87	Jordan	5 473	3.6	86	69	4.3	4.9	4.8	3.5	71	70 - 72	28	22 -
88	Kazakhstan	15 433	-0.8	58	49	9.4	11.5	2.4	1.9	61	60 - 65	73	56 -
89	Kenya	31 987	2.1	102	80	4.1	4.2	5.3	3.9	50	47 - 53	123	108 - 1
90	Kiribati	88	1.5	70	67	6.3	7.1	4.6	4.0	65	58 - 71	66	58 -
91	Kuwait	2 521	3.2	52	38	2.1	2.9	3.2	2.6	77	77 - 78	12	11 -
92	Kyrgyzstan	5 138	1.4	75	62	8.4	8.5	3.4	2.6	63	62 - 65	68	53 -
93	Lao People's Democratic Republic	5 657	2.4	91	82	5.7	5.4	5.8	4.7	59	57 - 60	91	81 -
94	Latvia	2 307	-1.2	52	47	18.7	22.0	1.6	1.1	71	69 - 73	13	10 -
95	Lebanon	3 653	2.1	65	54	8.3	8.5	2.8	2.2	70	69 - 71	31	27 -
96	Lesotho	1 802	1.0	93	80	6.8	6.9	4.7	3.8	38	37 - 40	84	74 -
97	Liberia	3 367	5.1	97	96	3.9	3.6	6.9	6.8	41	37 - 45	235	177 - 3
98	Libyan Arab Jamahiriya	5 551	2.0	79	53	4.6	6.2	4.0	3.0	73	70 - 75	16	14 -
99	Lithuania	3 444	-0.6	52	50	17.2	19.9	1.7	1.3	72	72 - 72	9	7 -
100	Luxembourg	453	1.4	45	49	18.2	18.3	1.7	1.7	79	79 - 79	4	4 -
101	Madagascar	17 404	2.9	92	91	4.8	4.7	6.2	5.7	57	54 - 61	126	109 - 1
102	Malawi	12 105	2.1	92	100	5.0	5.2	6.7	6.1	42	39 - 44	178	157 - 2(
103	Malaysia	24 425	2.4	66	60	5.9	6.7	3.6	2.9	72	72 - 73	7	6 -
104	Maldives	318	3.0	98	85	5.4	5.2	6.1	5.3	65	64 - 66	72	63 -
105	Mali	13 007	2.9	103	107	3.9	3.8	7.0	7.0	45	41 - 48	220	180 - 2(
106	Malta	394	0.6	51	47	15.4	17.8	2.0	1.8	79	78 - 79	6	5 -
107	Marshall Islands	53	1.3	70	67	6.3	7.1	6.2	5.4	61	56 - 66	61	50 -
108	Mauritania	2 893	2.9	89	87	5.3	5.3	6.1	5.8	51	47 - 54	184	161 - 2(
109	Mauritius	1 221	1.1	52	46	8.4	9.1	2.3	1.9	72	70 - 74	17	11 -
110	Mexico	103 457	1.6	70	60	6.1	7.4	3.1	2.5	74	74 - 75	28	24 -

LIFE EXPECTANCY AT BIRTH (YEARS)				PROBABILITY OF DYING (PER 1000)							
				Under age 5 years (under-5 mortality rate[b])				Between ages 15 and 60 years (adult mortality rate)			
Males		Females		Males		Females		Males		Females	
2003	Uncertainty	2003	Uncertainty	2003	Uncertainty	2003	Uncertainty	2003	Uncertainty	2003	Uncertainty
50	44 - 55	52	46 - 58	152	129 - 173	139	121 - 157	464	331 - 625	404	272 - 554
58	52 - 64	61	54 - 66	91	82 - 99	78	71 - 87	359	219 - 507	301	190 - 445
65	65 - 66	77	76 - 78	10	8 - 11	6	4 - 9	319	294 - 344	114	100 - 129
49	42 - 55	51	44 - 57	177	142 - 210	160	133 - 186	450	305 - 606	386	252 - 562
66	65 - 67	71	70 - 72	21	19 - 24	19	17 - 21	275	249 - 301	173	153 - 193
75	75 - 75	82	82 - 82	5	4 - 5	4	3 - 4	134	131 - 138	57	55 - 60
76	76 - 77	84	83 - 84	5	5 - 6	4	4 - 5	132	128 - 137	59	57 - 62
55	50 - 62	60	54 - 66	102	92 - 112	80	71 - 88	397	250 - 533	323	209 - 464
56	49 - 62	59	52 - 65	130	111 - 150	116	99 - 132	332	189 - 510	262	146 - 434
67	66 - 68	75	73 - 76	50	45 - 54	39	35 - 42	195	170 - 223	76	59 - 96
76	76 - 76	82	82 - 82	5	5 - 5	4	4 - 4	115	111 - 119	59	58 - 60
57	51 - 63	60	54 - 66	99	84 - 111	92	81 - 104	352	209 - 513	295	187 - 433
76	76 - 76	81	81 - 82	6	6 - 7	5	4 - 6	118	115 - 120	48	45 - 50
66	65 - 67	69	68 - 70	24	19 - 31	21	15 - 26	258	234 - 281	220	203 - 239
64	62 - 65	69	68 - 71	50	45 - 55	44	39 - 48	289	246 - 332	165	132 - 202
51	45 - 56	53	46 - 59	165	151 - 180	154	141 - 170	403	269 - 572	342	201 - 516
45	39 - 50	48	40 - 55	213	190 - 232	195	174 - 215	479	354 - 650	405	254 - 605
61	58 - 64	64	61 - 67	75	39 - 111	62	32 - 91	290	254 - 330	255	214 - 296
52	46 - 58	54	48 - 61	123	107 - 140	114	98 - 129	450	307 - 598	385	257 - 525
65	61 - 69	69	66 - 72	42	39 - 46	40	36 - 44	248	170 - 348	181	126 - 248
68	68 - 68	77	77 - 77	9	9 - 10	8	7 - 9	257	254 - 261	111	109 - 113
78	78 - 79	82	82 - 83	4	4 - 4	2	2 - 2	81	73 - 89	53	49 - 57
60	60 - 61	63	62 - 64	85	76 - 93	90	81 - 98	283	261 - 305	213	194 - 235
65	64 - 66	68	67 - 69	45	40 - 49	37	33 - 40	241	224 - 259	204	191 - 219
67	66 - 68	72	71 - 73	42	33 - 51	36	29 - 43	201	182 - 219	125	114 - 136
50	45 - 56	61	57 - 65	130	77 - 180	120	76 - 170	466	350 - 559	205	175 - 235
76	76 - 76	81	80 - 81	7	6 - 8	5	4 - 6	100	96 - 104	60	57 - 63
78	77 - 78	82	82 - 82	7	6 - 7	6	5 - 6	92	89 - 95	51	49 - 54
78	77 - 78	84	83 - 84	5	5 - 6	4	4 - 5	93	90 - 97	47	46 - 49
71	70 - 72	74	73 - 75	21	17 - 25	19	15 - 22	165	144 - 187	123	109 - 137
78	78 - 79	85	85 - 85	4	4 - 4	4	4 - 4	96	95 - 96	45	45 - 45
69	67 - 70	73	72 - 74	29	21 - 36	27	20 - 33	189	170 - 207	120	111 - 129
56	55 - 62	67	66 - 68	83	63 - 104	62	47 - 78	419	404 - 434	187	166 - 207
50	45 - 56	49	44 - 55	126	114 - 138	120	108 - 132	495	369 - 626	521	396 - 643
62	61 - 63	67	66 - 69	73	63 - 83	59	49 - 68	304	270 - 338	191	165 - 218
76	76 - 77	79	78 - 79	12	11 - 14	12	10 - 13	73	69 - 78	53	47 - 59
59	59 - 60	68	67 - 68	73	58 - 88	63	50 - 75	339	318 - 358	160	143 - 177
58	55 - 61	60	57 - 62	96	75 - 113	85	68 - 104	335	279 - 394	303	270 - 339
66	65 - 66	76	76 - 76	14	12 - 16	11	9 - 13	306	299 - 314	120	115 - 124
68	67 - 69	72	71 - 73	34	30 - 37	28	25 - 30	199	175 - 225	138	123 - 152
35	33 - 38	40	37 - 44	87	73 - 99	82	69 - 95	912	860 - 945	781	710 - 834
40	33 - 46	43	35 - 51	246	198 - 291	224	178 - 265	590	445 - 752	484	316 - 683
71	67 - 74	76	73 - 78	16	14 - 19	15	13 - 18	172	105 - 258	101	64 - 151
66	66 - 67	78	78 - 78	10	8 - 11	7	6 - 9	302	296 - 309	106	102 - 110
76	76 - 76	82	81 - 82	5	4 - 6	4	4 - 6	115	109 - 121	63	57 - 70
55	49 - 61	59	51 - 65	135	118 - 151	117	104 - 132	337	190 - 510	260	143 - 456
41	37 - 46	42	37 - 47	182	165 - 199	175	160 - 191	652	546 - 757	615	501 - 731
70	70 - 71	75	74 - 75	8	7 - 9	7	6 - 7	195	185 - 206	108	102 - 114
66	65 - 67	64	64 - 65	67	58 - 74	77	68 - 88	165	144 - 186	146	126 - 166
44	38 - 50	46	38 - 53	225	202 - 248	216	195 - 237	486	359 - 657	427	247 - 624
76	76 - 77	81	81 - 82	7	6 - 8	5	4 - 7	84	79 - 90	49	45 - 53
60	58 - 62	63	62 - 65	68	51 - 86	53	40 - 67	333	306 - 361	280	260 - 302
48	41 - 54	53	45 - 60	200	169 - 231	167	143 - 191	408	278 - 601	312	160 - 506
69	68 - 69	76	75 - 76	19	15 - 24	14	11 - 18	218	199 - 238	115	107 - 123
72	71 - 72	77	77 - 77	31	27 - 35	25	22 - 28	166	157 - 174	95	90 - 101

Annex Table 1 Basic indicators for all WHO Member States

Figures computed by WHO to ensure comparability;[a] they are not necessarily the official statistics of Member States, which may use alternative rigorous methods.

	POPULATION ESTIMATES										**LIFE EXPECTANCY AT BIRTH (YEARS)**		**PROBABILITY OF DYING (**
	Total population (000)	Annual growth rate (%)	Dependency ratio (per 100)		Percentage of population aged 60+ years		Total fertility rate		Both sexes		Under age 5 years (under-5 mortality r	
												Both sexes	
Member State	2003	1993–2003	1993	2003	1993	2003	1993	2003	2003	Uncertainty	2003	Uncerta
111 Micronesia, Federated States of	109	0.5	91	73	5.5	5.0	4.8	3.8	70	66 - 74	23	18 -
112 Monaco	34	1.0	53	53	19.7	20.5	1.7	1.8	81	81 - 82	4	4 -
113 Mongolia	2 594	1.1	79	56	5.8	5.7	3.3	2.4	65	64 - 66	68	54 -
114 Morocco	30 566	1.7	71	56	6.1	6.5	3.5	2.7	71	67 - 76	39	32 -
115 Mozambique	18 863	2.4	94	89	5.1	5.1	6.2	5.6	45	41 - 48	158	142 - 1
116 Myanmar	49 485	1.5	68	58	6.7	7.0	3.8	2.8	59	56 - 63	106	80 - 1
117 Namibia	1 987	2.5	87	88	5.4	5.7	5.6	4.5	51	49 - 54	65	54 -
118 Nauru	13	2.5	70	67	6.3	7.1	4.4	3.8	61	53 - 68	30	26 -
119 Nepal	25 164	2.3	81	78	5.6	5.9	4.9	4.2	61	60 - 61	82	69 -
120 Netherlands	16 149	0.6	46	48	17.6	18.7	1.6	1.7	79	79 - 79	6	5 -
121 New Zealand	3 875	1.0	53	52	15.3	16.1	2.1	2.0	79	73 - 86	6	5 -
122 Nicaragua	5 466	2.7	94	81	4.4	4.7	4.8	3.7	70	69 - 71	38	32 -
123 Niger	11 972	3.5	108	109	3.5	3.2	8.0	8.0	41	37 - 45	262	219 - 3
124 Nigeria	124 009	2.8	96	90	4.7	4.8	6.3	5.4	45	42 - 48	198	173 - 2
125 Niue	2	-1.2	71	64	6.3	7.3	3.5	2.9	71	67 - 74	33	14 -
126 Norway	4 533	0.5	55	53	20.4	19.8	1.9	1.8	79	79 - 80	4	4 -
127 Oman	2 851	3.2	79	65	3.0	3.6	6.4	4.9	74	71 - 76	12	11 -
128 Pakistan	153 578	2.6	87	82	5.6	5.7	5.8	5.0	62	61 - 63	103	90 - 1
129 Palau	20	2.3	70	67	6.3	7.1	2.8	2.4	68	66 - 70	28	22 -
130 Panama	3 120	2.0	64	58	7.3	8.4	2.9	2.7	75	75 - 76	24	21 -
131 Papua New Guinea	5 711	2.5	79	77	4.1	4.0	5.0	4.0	60	55 - 65	93	76 - 1
132 Paraguay	5 878	2.5	84	73	5.2	5.5	4.5	3.8	72	70 - 74	29	23 -
133 Peru	27 167	1.7	70	62	6.3	7.5	3.7	2.8	70	70 - 71	34	31 -
134 Philippines	79 999	2.0	76	66	5.0	5.9	4.1	3.1	68	67 - 68	36	29 -
135 Poland	38 587	0.0	53	43	15.4	16.6	1.8	1.3	75	75 - 75	8	7 -
136 Portugal	10 061	0.2	49	49	19.6	21.2	1.5	1.4	77	77 - 78	6	5 -
137 Qatar	610	1.9	38	39	2.2	3.3	4.1	3.2	74	73 - 75	13	10 -
138 Republic of Korea	47 700	0.8	42	39	8.5	12.1	1.7	1.4	76	76 - 76	5	4 -
139 Republic of Moldova	4 267	-0.2	57	43	13.0	13.8	2.0	1.4	67	66 - 68	32	24 -
140 Romania	22 334	-0.3	50	44	16.7	18.9	1.5	1.3	71	71 - 72	20	19 -
141 Russian Federation	143 246	-0.4	50	41	16.4	18.0	1.5	1.1	65	64 - 65	16	16 -
142 Rwanda	8 387	4.2	98	91	3.8	4.1	6.7	5.7	45	41 - 47	203	183 - 22
143 Saint Kitts and Nevis	42	-0.2	62	55	9.2	10.6	2.6	2.3	70	70 - 71	22	19 -
144 Saint Lucia	149	0.9	73	56	8.4	7.8	3.1	2.3	72	71 - 72	14	12 -
145 Saint Vincent and the Grenadines	120	0.6	79	59	8.7	9.2	2.8	2.2	70	69 - 71	22	19 -
146 Samoa	178	0.9	81	80	6.3	6.5	4.7	4.1	68	62 - 73	24	21 -
147 San Marino	28	1.3	46	49	21.9	24.7	1.3	1.2	81	80 - 83	4	3 -
148 Sao Tome and Principe	161	2.6	102	83	6.6	6.2	4.9	3.9	59	55 - 63	118	95 - 14
149 Saudi Arabia	24 217	3.0	80	71	3.3	4.4	5.7	4.5	71	68 - 73	27	23 -
150 Senegal	10 095	2.4	94	84	4.1	4.1	6.0	4.9	56	52 - 59	137	118 - 15
151 Serbia and Montenegro	10 527	0.1	50	49	16.4	18.4	1.9	1.6	73	72 - 73	14	13 -
152 Seychelles	81	1.0	52	46	8.4	9.1	2.1	1.8	72	71 - 73	15	12 -
153 Sierra Leone	4 971	2.0	87	89	4.9	4.7	6.5	6.5	38	33 - 42	283	240 - 33
154 Singapore	4 253	2.6	38	40	8.9	11.4	1.7	1.3	80	79 - 80	3	3 -
155 Slovakia	5 402	0.1	53	42	15.1	15.7	1.8	1.3	74	74 - 75	8	7 -
156 Slovenia	1 984	0.1	44	42	17.5	20.1	1.3	1.1	77	76 - 77	5	3 -
157 Solomon Islands	477	3.1	92	83	4.4	4.4	5.5	4.4	70	65 - 76	22	18 -
158 Somalia	9 890	3.2	101	102	4.1	3.8	7.3	7.2	44	40 - 48	225	181 - 28
159 South Africa	45 026	1.4	69	58	5.3	6.3	3.4	2.6	49	47 - 51	66	58 -
160 Spain	41 060	0.3	47	45	20.3	21.8	1.3	1.2	80	79 - 80	5	4 -
161 Sri Lanka	19 065	0.9	57	46	8.9	10.3	2.4	2.0	71	70 - 72	15	13 -
162 Sudan	33 610	2.3	81	76	5.1	5.7	5.3	4.3	59	56 - 63	93	81 - 10
163 Suriname	436	0.7	66	57	7.2	8.0	2.5	2.4	66	65 - 68	39	35 -
164 Swaziland	1 077	1.8	97	88	4.6	5.2	5.6	4.5	35	33 - 37	153	140 - 16
165 Sweden	8 876	0.2	57	54	22.2	23.2	2.0	1.6	81	80 - 81	4	3 -

	LIFE EXPECTANCY AT BIRTH (YEARS)				PROBABILITY OF DYING (PER 1000)							
					Under age 5 years (under-5 mortality rate[b])				Between ages 15 and 60 years (adult mortality rate)			
	Males		Females		Males		Females		Males		Females	
	2003	Uncertainty	2003	Uncertainty	2003	Uncertainty	2003	Uncertainty	2003	Uncertainty	2003	Uncertainty
	68	67 - 70	71	70 - 73	25	18 - 32	20	14 - 27	206	181 - 231	172	150 - 196
	78	78 - 78	85	84 - 85	5	4 - 5	3	3 - 5	110	109 - 112	47	44 - 50
	62	61 - 62	69	68 - 70	72	57 - 87	64	51 - 77	310	285 - 332	179	157 - 203
	69	68 - 70	73	72 - 74	40	31 - 48	38	30 - 46	159	148 - 170	103	90 - 114
	44	39 - 48	46	41 - 52	163	144 - 182	154	134 - 171	621	510 - 735	543	427 - 667
	56	49 - 64	63	54 - 69	117	82 - 153	93	65 - 123	337	179 - 507	222	113 - 399
	50	46 - 54	53	49 - 57	66	57 - 76	63	54 - 72	619	534 - 686	529	444 - 596
	58	52 - 63	65	60 - 70	35	28 - 43	24	19 - 30	448	311 - 611	303	192 - 419
	60	59 - 62	61	59 - 62	80	68 - 91	85	73 - 98	290	266 - 310	284	264 - 303
	76	76 - 76	81	81 - 81	6	6 - 7	5	4 - 5	93	92 - 95	66	64 - 67
	77	77 - 77	82	81 - 82	7	6 - 8	6	5 - 7	98	95 - 102	65	61 - 67
	68	67 - 69	73	72 - 73	41	35 - 48	35	30 - 41	209	196 - 223	138	121 - 157
	42	32 - 49	41	31 - 50	258	208 - 311	265	213 - 317	508	363 - 734	477	251 - 717
	45	39 - 50	46	39 - 52	200	177 - 225	197	174 - 222	511	386 - 668	470	337 - 647
	68	64 - 71	74	71 - 77	43	16 - 104	22	11 - 44	189	123 - 258	133	90 - 183
	77	76 - 77	82	82 - 82	4	4 - 5	4	4 - 5	96	91 - 102	58	56 - 60
	71	68 - 75	77	74 - 79	12	11 - 14	12	10 - 13	163	98 - 239	91	60 - 137
	62	60 - 63	62	60 - 64	98	83 - 113	108	92 - 124	225	199 - 250	199	174 - 225
	66	66 - 67	70	68 - 72	29	22 - 37	26	18 - 35	226	209 - 241	205	174 - 241
	73	72 - 74	78	77 - 79	26	23 - 29	22	20 - 24	146	134 - 159	84	75 - 94
	59	57 - 60	62	60 - 64	96	77 - 116	90	72 - 108	309	284 - 335	246	224 - 268
	69	68 - 70	75	74 - 76	33	28 - 38	26	22 - 30	171	156 - 186	119	106 - 133
	68	67 - 69	73	72 - 73	36	31 - 42	32	27 - 37	193	169 - 214	133	117 - 152
	65	64 - 65	71	70 - 72	39	33 - 45	33	27 - 38	271	259 - 282	149	132 - 170
	71	70 - 71	79	79 - 79	9	8 - 9	7	6 - 8	202	196 - 208	81	78 - 84
	74	73 - 74	81	81 - 81	7	6 - 7	5	5 - 6	150	143 - 157	63	60 - 66
	75	74 - 76	74	72 - 76	14	11 - 18	11	10 - 14	93	85 - 102	76	60 - 96
	73	72 - 73	80	79 - 80	5	5 - 6	5	4 - 5	155	145 - 165	61	59 - 63
	63	63 - 64	71	70 - 71	36	27 - 46	27	20 - 34	303	283 - 326	152	139 - 165
	68	67 - 68	75	74 - 76	22	21 - 23	18	17 - 19	239	220 - 258	107	97 - 117
	58	58 - 58	72	72 - 72	18	18 - 18	14	14 - 14	480	474 - 481	182	177 - 184
	43	37 - 48	46	39 - 52	213	193 - 232	193	175 - 213	541	425 - 694	455	320 - 633
	69	68 - 69	72	71 - 73	21	18 - 25	23	20 - 27	200	185 - 214	145	119 - 172
	69	68 - 69	75	74 - 76	15	11 - 19	14	12 - 16	224	215 - 233	131	118 - 145
	68	67 - 69	72	71 - 73	25	21 - 30	20	14 - 28	233	202 - 266	192	167 - 218
	67	66 - 68	70	69 - 71	27	23 - 31	21	17 - 27	235	219 - 252	203	188 - 219
	78	76 - 79	84	83 - 86	5	4 - 8	2	2 - 2	73	61 - 86	32	26 - 37
	58	51 - 65	60	51 - 66	116	89 - 144	120	91 - 151	295	137 - 479	244	124 - 440
	68	64 - 72	74	70 - 77	29	22 - 36	24	18 - 31	196	120 - 293	119	75 - 183
	54	48 - 60	57	50 - 63	142	124 - 160	132	115 - 147	350	211 - 511	280	155 - 477
	70	70 - 71	75	75 - 76	16	14 - 17	12	11 - 13	186	176 - 196	99	94 - 104
	67	67 - 68	77	76 - 79	12	9 - 16	19	14 - 23	235	209 - 258	92	74 - 114
	37	28 - 44	39	29 - 48	297	250 - 341	270	229 - 310	597	443 - 809	517	303 - 762
	78	77 - 78	82	82 - 82	3	3 - 3	3	3 - 3	87	81 - 93	51	48 - 53
	70	70 - 71	78	78 - 79	9	7 - 10	8	6 - 10	204	195 - 214	77	72 - 82
	73	72 - 73	81	80 - 81	5	4 - 7	4	3 - 6	165	159 - 171	69	65 - 73
	69	66 - 73	73	69 - 77	24	20 - 28	21	16 - 26	196	123 - 265	145	81 - 212
	43	36 - 50	45	37 - 52	222	202 - 244	228	205 - 250	518	363 - 672	431	254 - 635
	48	46 - 51	50	47 - 54	70	61 - 79	61	53 - 70	642	585 - 691	579	517 - 633
	76	76 - 77	83	83 - 84	5	5 - 5	4	4 - 5	116	109 - 124	46	45 - 48
	68	66 - 70	75	74 - 76	17	14 - 19	13	11 - 15	235	190 - 284	120	106 - 136
	57	51 - 64	62	55 - 68	95	86 - 104	90	82 - 99	348	200 - 508	248	142 - 406
	63	61 - 65	69	68 - 71	43	38 - 48	36	31 - 40	306	264 - 347	180	153 - 208
	33	30 - 36	36	33 - 41	159	140 - 179	147	129 - 166	894	829 - 933	790	704 - 856
	78	78 - 78	83	83 - 83	5	4 - 5	3	3 - 4	79	77 - 81	50	48 - 52

Annex Table 1 Basic indicators for all WHO Member States

Figures computed by WHO to ensure comparability;[a] they are not necessarily the official statistics of Member States, which may use alternative rigorous methods.

| | | POPULATION ESTIMATES | | | | | | | | LIFE EXPECTANCY AT BIRTH (YEARS) | | PROBABILITY OF DYING (F | |
| | | Total population (000) | Annual growth rate (%) | Dependency ratio (per 100) | | Percentage of population aged 60+ years | | Total fertility rate | | Both sexes | | Under age 5 years (under-5 mortality ra Both sexes | |
	Member State	2003	1993–2003	1993	2003	1993	2003	1993	2003	2003	Uncertainty	2003	Uncertai
166	Switzerland	7 169	0.2	46	48	19.6	22.6	1.5	1.4	81	81 - 81	5	4 -
167	Syrian Arab Republic	17 800	2.5	95	68	4.2	4.6	4.5	3.3	72	71 - 73	18	16 - 1
168	Tajikistan	6 245	1.1	89	70	6.3	6.6	4.4	3.0	61	60 - 62	118	100 - 13
169	Thailand	62 833	1.1	52	46	6.9	9.0	2.1	1.9	70	69 - 71	26	23 - 2
170	The former Yugoslav Republic of Macedonia	2 056	0.6	50	48	12.6	14.9	1.8	1.9	72	71 - 73	12	11 - 1
171	Timor-Leste	778	-0.6	77	65	3.7	5.3	4.7	3.8	58	54 - 61	125	104 - 14
172	Togo	4 909	2.9	93	88	4.8	4.9	6.2	5.3	52	49 - 55	140	124 - 15
173	Tonga	104	0.4	79	73	7.5	8.2	4.5	3.7	71	66 - 75	19	16 - 2
174	Trinidad and Tobago	1 303	0.5	62	42	8.8	10.2	2.1	1.6	70	69 - 71	20	17 - 2
175	Tunisia	9 832	1.3	69	51	7.5	8.5	3.0	2.0	72	71 - 73	24	21 - 2
176	Turkey	71 325	1.6	66	56	7.3	8.2	3.1	2.4	70	70 - 71	39	37 - 4
177	Turkmenistan	4 867	2.0	79	62	6.2	6.4	3.9	2.7	60	60 - 61	102	93 - 11
178	Tuvalu	11	1.4	71	64	6.3	7.3	3.4	2.8	61	56 - 66	51	39 - 6
179	Uganda	25 827	3.1	106	111	4.1	3.9	7.1	7.1	49	38 - 58	140	113 - 16
180	Ukraine	48 523	-0.7	52	45	18.4	20.8	1.6	1.2	67	67 - 68	20	18 - 2
181	United Arab Emirates	2 995	2.6	42	36	1.8	2.5	3.7	2.8	73	72 - 74	8	6 - 1
182	United Kingdom	59 251	0.3	54	52	21.0	20.8	1.8	1.6	79	78 - 79	6	5 -
183	United Republic of Tanzania	36 977	2.5	96	90	3.7	3.9	6.1	5.1	45	42 - 48	165	149 - 18
184	United States of America	294 043	1.1	52	51	16.3	16.3	2.1	2.1	77	77 - 78	8	7 -
185	Uruguay	3 415	0.7	60	60	16.8	17.4	2.5	2.3	75	70 - 79	15	13 - 1
186	Uzbekistan	26 093	1.8	81	63	6.5	6.9	3.5	2.4	66	65 - 67	69	63 - 7
187	Vanuatu	212	2.7	90	78	5.3	4.9	4.8	4.1	68	62 - 74	38	29 - 4
188	Venezuela, Bolivarian Republic of	25 699	2.1	69	59	6.0	7.0	3.3	2.7	74	73 - 75	21	19 - 2
189	Viet Nam	81 377	1.5	75	57	7.3	7.4	3.2	2.3	71	70 - 72	23	20 - 2
190	Yemen	20 010	3.8	113	103	3.7	3.6	7.8	7.0	59	56 - 63	113	88 - 13
191	Zambia	10 812	2.0	94	99	4.4	4.7	6.2	5.6	39	35 - 43	182	154 - 21
192	Zimbabwe	12 891	1.4	95	86	4.5	5.2	5.0	3.9	37	35 - 38	126	111 - 14

[a] See explanatory notes for sources and methods.

[b] Under-five mortality rate is the probability (expressed as per 1000 live births) of a child born in a specific year dying before reaching five years of age, if subjected to current age-specific mortality rates

LIFE EXPECTANCY AT BIRTH (YEARS)				PROBABILITY OF DYING (PER 1000)							
				Under age 5 years (under-5 mortality rate[b])				Between ages 15 and 60 years (adult mortality rate)			
Males		Females		Males		Females		Males		Females	
2003	Uncertainty	2003	Uncertainty	2003	Uncertainty	2003	Uncertainty	2003	Uncertainty	2003	Uncertainty
78	78 - 78	83	83 - 83	5	4 - 6	5	4 - 6	90	88 - 93	50	48 - 52
69	69 - 70	74	74 - 75	20	18 - 22	15	14 - 17	188	175 - 202	126	117 - 136
59	58 - 61	63	60 - 65	121	86 - 156	115	83 - 147	225	182 - 268	169	149 - 211
67	66 - 68	73	72 - 74	29	24 - 33	24	20 - 27	267	245 - 288	153	134 - 176
69	68 - 70	75	75 - 76	13	12 - 14	11	10 - 13	202	187 - 218	86	79 - 93
55	48 - 62	61	53 - 68	141	114 - 168	107	84 - 129	324	170 - 513	228	111 - 407
50	44 - 55	54	47 - 59	151	131 - 171	128	112 - 144	448	319 - 612	377	262 - 545
71	70 - 71	71	70 - 72	24	20 - 27	15	12 - 18	155	150 - 159	188	181 - 195
67	66 - 68	73	73 - 74	24	21 - 28	16	13 - 18	249	223 - 277	155	139 - 171
70	69 - 71	74	74 - 75	27	24 - 29	21	18 - 23	167	155 - 180	113	101 - 126
68	68 - 69	73	72 - 74	40	36 - 44	38	34 - 42	176	164 - 188	111	98 - 124
56	55 - 56	65	64 - 66	116	105 - 128	87	78 - 96	352	331 - 373	171	150 - 196
61	59 - 62	62	60 - 64	57	42 - 70	44	33 - 55	313	261 - 373	274	223 - 338
47	43 - 53	50	44 - 55	146	133 - 160	133	121 - 146	533	412 - 662	459	347 - 598
62	61 - 62	73	72 - 74	23	21 - 25	18	16 - 19	384	364 - 403	142	126 - 160
72	71 - 73	75	75 - 76	8	7 - 9	8	7 - 9	168	149 - 186	121	110 - 133
76	76 - 77	81	81 - 81	7	6 - 7	5	5 - 6	103	100 - 106	64	62 - 65
44	42 - 46	46	43 - 48	176	161 - 190	153	140 - 167	587	543 - 629	550	502 - 595
75	74 - 75	80	80 - 80	9	8 - 9	7	7 - 7	139	133 - 147	82	81 - 84
71	71 - 72	80	79 - 80	17	14 - 20	12	11 - 13	180	171 - 190	87	83 - 91
63	62 - 64	69	68 - 70	81	73 - 88	57	51 - 63	226	207 - 245	142	123 - 161
67	63 - 71	69	66 - 73	38	27 - 49	38	27 - 47	214	145 - 284	173	116 - 231
71	70 - 72	77	77 - 77	24	21 - 26	19	17 - 21	181	168 - 195	97	91 - 103
68	67 - 69	74	73 - 74	26	23 - 29	20	18 - 23	205	190 - 220	129	117 - 140
57	51 - 64	61	53 - 67	119	105 - 134	106	94 - 119	298	154 - 473	227	112 - 411
39	35 - 43	39	35 - 44	191	169 - 213	173	153 - 193	719	618 - 808	685	579 - 782
37	34 - 40	36	34 - 40	133	121 - 145	119	107 - 129	830	776 - 874	819	754 - 864

Annex Table 2a Under-five mortality rates: estimates for 2003,[a] annual average percent change 1990–2003, and availability of data 1980–2003

Figures computed by WHO to ensure comparability; they are not necessarily the official statistics of Member States, which may use alternative rigorous methods.

| | Member State | Under-5 mortality rate (both sexes)[a] | | | | | Data from available sources | | | | | | | |
| | | per 1000 live births | | Annual average percent change | | | 1980–1989 | | 1990–1999 | | 2000–2003 | | Latest available year | |
		2003	Uncertainty	1990–1994	1995–1999	2000–2003	VR/SRS[b]	Survey/Census[c]	VR/SRS[b]	Survey/Census[c]	VR/SRS[b]	Survey/Census[c]	VR/SRS	Survey/Census
1	Afghanistan	257	206 - 308	-0.2	0.0	0.0	0	0	0	0	0	1	...	2000
2	Albania	21	19 - 23	-5.5	-5.9	-6.0	7	0	10	0	4	1	2003	2000
3	Algeria	41	31 - 49	-4.4	-3.9	-3.2	6	1	1	2	1	1	2000	2000
4	Andorra	5	5 - 6	...	...	...	0	0	6	0	1	0	2000	...
5	Angola	260	225 - 293	0.0	0.0	0.0	0	0	0	1	0	1	...	2000
6	Antigua and Barbuda	12	9 - 16	...	-6.5	-6.5	6	0	10	0	0	0	1999	...
7	Argentina	17	16 - 19	-3.9	-4.5	-3.5	10	1	10	1	3	0	2002	1991
8	Armenia	33	29 - 38	-4.0	-5.5	-3.3	10	0	10	0	4	1	2003	2000
9	Australia	6	5 - 6	-6.1	-2.2	-3.6	10	0	10	0	2	0	2001	..
10	Austria	6	4 - 7	-7.1	-2.9	-1.1	10	0	10	0	4	0	2003	...
11	Azerbaijan	91	77 - 104	-1.4	-1.0	-0.9	10	0	10	0	3	2	2002	2001
12	Bahamas	14	11 - 18	-4.5	-5.9	-5.9	10	0	10	0	1	0	2000	...
13	Bahrain	9	8 - 10	-1.7	-1.7	-17.3	9	1	10	1	3	0	2002	1995
14	Bangladesh	69	65 - 75	-4.2	-6.7	-5.7	6	4	0	13	0	2	1987	2001
15	Barbados	13	8 - 18	0.0	-2.6	-2.6	10	0	10	0	2	0	2001	...
16	Belarus	10	9 - 11	1.7	-5.1	-7.0	9	0	10	0	4	0	2003	...
17	Belgium	5	5 - 6	-5.3	-4.0	-5.6	10	0	10	0	2	0	2001	...
18	Belize	39	31 - 48	-2.2	-1.4	-1.4	10	0	10	1	1	0	2000	1991
19	Benin	154	139 - 169	-1.7	-1.2	-1.2	0	2	0	2	0	1	...	2000
20	Bhutan	85	68 - 101	-4.3	-5.5	-5.3	0	1	0	1	0	1	...	2000
21	Bolivia	66	60 - 73	-5.2	-4.0	-4.0	0	3	0	3	0	1	...	2000
22	Bosnia and Herzegovina	17	15 - 20	-2.9	-1.1	-1.1	5	0	3	0	0	0	1999	...
23	Botswana	112	96 - 128	2.6	8.9	3.5	0	3	0	2	0	1	...	2000
24	Brazil	35	31 - 40	-4.4	-4.1	-3.2	10	4	10	1	1	0	2000	1996
25	Brunei Darussalam	6	5 - 6	-4.0	-5.7	-5.8	8	0	10	0	1	0	2000	...
26	Bulgaria	15	14 - 16	-0.3	-1.5	-2.8	10	0	10	0	4	0	2003	...
27	Burkina Faso	207	187 - 227	-0.3	0.0	0.0	0	1	0	5	0	0	...	1999
28	Burundi	190	159 - 222	0.0	0.0	0.0	0	1	0	1	0	1	...	2000
29	Cambodia	140	124 - 158	0.9	2.4	1.2	0	0	0	2	0	1	...	2000
30	Cameroon	166	148 - 184	2.3	1.3	0.0	0	0	0	2	0	1	...	2000
31	Canada	6	5 - 6	-3.1	-3.5	-2.1	10	0	10	0	2	0	2001	...
32	Cape Verde	35	30 - 40	-3.5	-4.4	-4.4	4	0	3	1	0	0	1998	1998
33	Central African Republic	180	156 - 204	0.0	0.0	0.0	0	1	0	1	0	1	...	2000
34	Chad	200	175 - 227	-0.3	0.0	0.0	0	0	0	2	0	1	...	2000
35	Chile	9	7 - 12	-5.9	-3.0	-7.8	10	1	10	1	3	0	2002	1992
36	China	37	31 - 44	-1.3	-2.8	-2.5	2	5	10	22	1	1	2000	2000
37	Colombia	21	19 - 24	-4.2	-3.7	-3.7	8	3	10	2	3	1	2002	2000
38	Comoros	73	59 - 85	-3.6	-3.9	-3.9	0	1	0	1	0	1	...	2000
39	Congo	108	89 - 128	-0.4	0.0	0.0	0	0	0	0	0	0	...	...
40	Cook Islands	21	20 - 23	-2.0	-3.7	-3.7	10	0	10	0	2	0	2001	...
41	Costa Rica	10	9 - 11	-1.2	-5.6	-5.6	10	3	10	0	3	0	2002	1986
42	Côte d'Ivoire	193	161 - 223	2.2	1.5	0.7	0	2	0	3	0	0	...	1998
43	Croatia	7	6 - 8	-4.7	-4.1	-2.4	8	0	10	0	4	0	2003	...
44	Cuba	7	6 - 9	-3.0	-4.9	-6.8	10	2	10	0	3	0	2002	1987
45	Cyprus	6	5 - 6	-6.0	-6.6	-3.7	10	0	10	0	3	0	2002	...
46	Czech Republic	5	4 - 5	-6.9	-9.8	-2.2	8	0	10	0	4	0	2003	...
47	Democratic People's Republic of Korea	55	39 - 72	0.0	0.0	0.0	0	0	0	1	0	0	...	1993
48	Democratic Republic of the Congo	205	180 - 229	0.0	0.0	0.0	0	1	0	2	0	1	...	2001
49	Denmark	5	5 - 6	-7.2	-1.5	-1.7	10	0	10	0	4	0	2003	...
50	Djibouti	138	93 - 183	-1.8	-1.8	-1.8	0	0	0	1	0	0	...	1991

	Member State	Under-5 mortality rate (both sexes)[a]					Data from available sources							
		per 1000 live births		Annual average percent change			1980–1989		1990–1999		2000–2003		Latest available year	
		2003	Uncertainty	1990–1994	1995–1999	2000–2003	VR/SRS[b]	Survey/Census[c]	VR/SRS[b]	Survey/Census[c]	VR/SRS[b]	Survey/Census[c]	VR/SRS	Survey/Census
51	Dominica	12	11 - 14	-2.6	-2.5	-2.3	10	0	10	0	0	0	1999	…
52	Dominican Republic	35	29 - 40	-4.0	-5.5	-4.7	10	4	9	3	0	1	1999	2002
53	Ecuador	27	24 - 30	-5.5	-5.7	-5.7	10	4	10	3	1	0	2000	1999
54	Egypt	39	36 - 43	-7.3	-7.1	-7.0	9	4	10	4	1	1	2000	2000
55	El Salvador	36	31 - 42	-4.8	-3.2	-3.2	10	2	9	6	0	1	1999	2002
56	Equatorial Guinea	146	121 - 169	-3.2	-2.3	-2.3	0	1	0	0	0	0	…	1983
57	Eritrea	85	70 - 100	-3.7	-4.5	-4.5	0	0	0	1	0	2	…	2002
58	Estonia	8	7 - 9	3.2	-9.9	-11.5	9	0	10	0	3	0	2002	…
59	Ethiopia	169	133 - 202	-1.2	-1.7	-1.4	0	2	0	4	0	1	…	2000
60	Fiji	20	17 - 24	-4.3	-2.5	-2.5	8	0	8	0	1	0	2000	…
61	Finland	4	3 - 5	-6.2	-2.6	-1.8	10	0	10	0	4	0	2003	…
62	France	5	4 - 6	-7.1	-2.3	-4.6	10	0	10	0	3	0	2002	…
63	Gabon	91	82 - 100	-0.2	0.0	0.0	0	0	0	0	0	1	…	2000
64	Gambia	123	105 - 141	-2.3	-1.3	-1.3	0	1	0	3	0	1	…	2000
65	Georgia	45	40 - 49	-0.9	0.0	0.0	9	0	9	1	2	0	2001	1999
66	Germany	5	4 - 5	-6.1	-3.9	-4.4	10	0	10	0	2	0	2001	…
67	Ghana	95	85 - 104	-2.5	-1.9	-1.6	0	1	1	3	0	0	1999	1998
68	Greece	6	5 - 6	-3.4	-5.3	-6.0	10	0	10	0	2	0	2001	…
69	Grenada	23	17 - 28	-2.3	-4.7	-4.7	3	0	7	0	0	0	1996	…
70	Guatemala	47	40 - 54	-4.8	-3.7	-3.9	9	4	10	2	0	0	1999	1999
71	Guinea	160	145 - 175	-2.8	-3.4	-2.9	0	0	0	2	0	0	…	1999
72	Guinea-Bissau	204	183 - 224	-1.5	-1.8	-1.8	0	0	0	1	0	1	…	2000
73	Guyana	69	42 - 96	-1.4	-2.5	-2.5	3	0	5	0	0	0	1996	…
74	Haiti	119	102 - 135	-1.8	-1.8	-1.8	3	3	2	1	0	1	1999	2000
75	Honduras	41	36 - 46	-3.6	-2.6	-1.4	4	4	0	2	0	2	1983	2001
76	Hungary	9	7 - 10	-6.3	-2.2	-8.0	10	0	10	0	4	0	2003	…
77	Iceland	3	3 - 4	-3.1	-10.2	-1.7	10	0	10	0	4	0	2003	…
78	India	87	76 - 99	-3.3	-2.0	-2.4	0	2	10	2	1	0	2000	1998
79	Indonesia	41	32 - 54	-6.2	-6.2	-5.3	0	2	0	7	0	3	…	2002
80	Iran, Islamic Republic of	39	31 - 47	-5.3	-4.4	-3.8	2	1	1	9	2	1	2001	2000
81	Iraq	125	96 - 157	19.5	0.5	0.0	0	2	0	4	0	0	…	1999
82	Ireland	6	5 - 7	-5.3	-1.4	-5.9	10	0	10	0	4	0	2003	…
83	Israel	6	6 - 7	-6.7	-4.3	-2.6	10	0	10	0	4	0	2003	…
84	Italy	5	4 - 6	-4.7	-6.4	-3.3	10	0	10	0	2	0	2001	…
85	Jamaica	20	17 - 23	0.0	0.0	0.0	10	2	6	0	0	1	1999	2000
86	Japan	4	4 - 4	-1.6	-5.3	-4.0	10	0	10	0	4	0	2003	…
87	Jordan	28	22 - 34	-2.6	-3.0	-2.7	1	2	1	6	1	1	2001	2002
88	Kazakhstan	73	56 - 90	1.3	1.7	0.0	9	0	10	2	4	0	2003	1999
89	Kenya	123	108 - 138	2.7	1.6	0.8	0	3	0	3	0	1	…	2003
90	Kiribati	66	58 - 74	-2.7	-1.9	-1.9	0	0	9	0	2	0	2001	…
91	Kuwait	12	11 - 13	…	-4.0	2.1	10	2	9	0	4	0	2003	1987
92	Kyrgyzstan	68	53 - 84	-1.6	-1.1	-0.9	9	0	10	1	4	0	2003	1997
93	Lao People's Democratic Republic	91	81 - 99	-3.8	-4.8	-4.8	0	0	0	3	0	0	…	1995
94	Latvia	13	10 - 15	3.7	-9.2	-1.1	10	0	10	0	4	0	2003	…
95	Lebanon	31	27 - 35	-1.7	-1.2	-1.2	0	0	3	1	0	1	1999	2000
96	Lesotho	84	74 - 95	-3.0	-2.4	-2.4	0	1	0	1	0	1	…	2001
97	Liberia	235	177 - 310	0.0	0.0	0.0	0	1	0	0	0	0	…	1986
98	Libyan Arab Jamahiriya	16	14 - 18	-7.1	-7.2	-7.2	1	0	0	1	0	0	1981	1995
99	Lithuania	9	7 - 10	2.8	-6.4	-8.0	9	0	10	0	4	0	2003	…
100	Luxembourg	4	4 - 6	-11.1	-0.3	-5.4	10	0	10	0	4	0	2003	…

Annex Table 2a Under-five mortality rates: estimates for 2003,[a] annual average percent change 1990–2003, and availability of data 1980–2003

Figures computed by WHO to ensure comparability; they are not necessarily the official statistics of Member States, which may use alternative rigorous methods.

	Member State	Under-5 mortality rate (both sexes)[a]					Data from available sources							
		per 1000 live births		Annual average percent change			1980–1989		1990–1999		2000–2003		Latest available ye	
		2003	Uncertainty	1990–1994	1995–1999	2000–2003	VR/SRS[b]	Survey/Census[c]	VR/SRS[b]	Survey/Census[c]	VR/SRS[b]	Survey/Census[c]	VR/SRS	Survey/Censu
101	Madagascar	126	109 - 143	-1.5	-2.6	-2.7	0	0	0	2	0	1	…	200
102	Malawi	178	157 - 201	-2.2	-2.7	-1.7	0	3	0	2	0	1	…	200
103	Malaysia	7	6 - 8	-9.7	-6.5	-6.5	8	0	10	0	1	0	2000	..
104	Maldives	72	63 - 81	-3.8	-3.4	-3.4	10	0	10	0	4	0	2003	.
105	Mali	220	180 - 260	-1.4	-0.8	-0.5	0	2	0	1	0	2	…	200
106	Malta	6	5 - 7	-0.4	-8.2	-4.7	10	0	10	0	3	0	2002	..
107	Marshall Islands	61	50 - 72	-2.5	-3.4	-3.4	4	0	8	0	0	0	1997	
108	Mauritania	184	161 - 207	0.0	0.0	0.0	0	2	0	2	0	2	…	200
109	Mauritius	17	11 - 23	-1.7	-3.4	-2.9	10	0	10	0	3	0	2002	..
110	Mexico	28	24 - 32	-4.6	-3.7	-2.0	10	2	10	2	3	0	2002	199
111	Micronesia, Federated States of	23	18 - 28	-3.6	-1.5	-1.6	4	0	5	0	0	0	1994	..
112	Monaco	4	4 - 5	…	-2.3	-5.3	5	0	0	0	0	0	1987	..
113	Mongolia	68	54 - 81	-3.0	-3.4	-3.4	3	0	10	2	4	0	2003	199
114	Morocco	39	32 - 45	-6.4	-5.5	-5.5	0	4	8	3	0	0	1998	199
115	Mozambique	158	142 - 175	-2.0	-3.4	-3.9	0	1	0	4	0	0	…	199
116	Myanmar	106	80 - 133	-2.1	-1.2	-0.9	3	1	10	2	2	0	2001	199
117	Namibia	65	54 - 75	-2.2	-2.2	-2.1	0	0	0	1	0	2	…	200
118	Nauru	30	26 - 35	…	0.0	0.0	0	0	3	1	0	0	1995	199
119	Nepal	82	69 - 96	-3.7	-4.6	-4.6	0	3	0	3	0	1	…	200
120	Netherlands	6	5 - 6	-5.5	-1.2	-3.1	10	0	10	0	4	0	2003	..
121	New Zealand	6	5 - 7	-4.8	-1.8	-6.6	10	0	10	0	4	0	2003	..
122	Nicaragua	38	32 - 45	-5.2	-3.7	-3.7	3	1	9	2	3	1	2002	200
123	Niger	262	219 - 303	-1.6	-1.8	-1.0	0	1	0	3	0	1	…	200
124	Nigeria	198	173 - 227	0.3	-2.9	-1.1	0	1	0	4	0	1	…	200
125	Niue	33	14 - 73	…	…	…	10	0	10	0	1	0	2000	..
126	Norway	4	4 - 5	-10.0	-1.1	-4.5	10	0	10	0	3	0	2002	..
127	Oman	12	11 - 15	-9.7	-4.9	-4.9	0	0	0	2	0	0	…	199
128	Pakistan	103	90 - 115	-1.9	-1.8	-1.7	0	11	0	9	0	2	…	200
129	Palau	28	22 - 35	-1.8	-1.3	-1.3	5	0	10	0	0	0	1999	..
130	Panama	24	21 - 26	-2.5	-2.8	-2.8	10	1	10	1	3	0	2002	199
131	Papua New Guinea	93	76 - 110	-0.6	-0.6	-0.6	1	1	0	2	0	0	1980	199
132	Paraguay	29	23 - 35	-1.7	-1.8	-1.8	10	1	9	2	2	0	2001	199
133	Peru	34	31 - 37	-5.6	-6.9	-6.9	10	3	9	3	1	1	2000	200
134	Philippines	36	29 - 44	-4.5	-4.4	-3.6	10	2	9	2	1	0	2000	199
135	Poland	8	7 - 9	-4.0	-8.8	-5.1	10	0	10	0	3	0	2002	..
136	Portugal	6	5 - 7	-7.9	-5.1	-6.5	10	0	10	0	3	0	2002	..
137	Qatar	13	10 - 16	-8.9	0.0	-6.0	8	0	9	1	3	0	2002	199
138	Republic of Korea	5	4 - 5	-6.6	-3.4	-3.3	9	2	10	0	4	0	2003	198
139	Republic of Moldova	32	24 - 40	-0.6	-1.7	-1.0	9	0	10	0	4	1	2003	200
140	Romania	20	19 - 21	-3.3	-2.9	-4.0	10	0	10	0	3	0	2002	..
141	Russian Federation	16	16 - 16	1.2	-2.4	-6.4	10	0	10	0	4	0	2003	..
142	Rwanda	203	183 - 222	3.9	-0.6	0.0	0	1	0	3	0	1	…	200
143	Saint Kitts and Nevis	22	19 - 26	-3.6	-3.6	-3.6	10	0	10	0	1	0	2000	..
144	Saint Lucia	14	12 - 17	-7.6	0.0	-6.3	10	0	10	0	2	0	2001	..
145	Saint Vincent and the Grenadines	22	19 - 26	-2.7	0.7	-0.5	10	0	10	0	0	0	1999	..
146	Samoa	24	21 - 28	-7.1	-2.1	-2.2	1	0	2	1	2	1	2002	200
147	San Marino	4	3 - 5	-10.2	-11.6	-4.3	10	0	10	0	4	0	2003	..
148	Sao Tome and Principe	118	95 - 141	0.0	0.0	0.0	3	0	0	0	0	1	1987	200
149	Saudi Arabia	27	23 - 33	-5.0	-3.1	-3.1	0	1	0	2	0	0	…	199
150	Senegal	137	118 - 156	-0.7	-0.6	-0.6	0	1	0	6	0	1	…	200

Member State	Under-5 mortality rate (both sexes)[a]					Data from available sources							
	per 1000 live births		Annual average percent change			1980–1989		1990–1999		2000–2003		Latest available year	
	2003	Uncertainty	1990–1994	1995–1999	2000–2003	VR/SRS[b]	Survey/Census[c]	VR/SRS[b]	Survey/Census[c]	VR/SRS[b]	Survey/Census[c]	VR/SRS	Survey/Census
Serbia and Montenegro	14	13 - 15	-5.8	-4.0	-4.0	8	0	10	0	1	0	2000	...
Seychelles	15	12 - 19	-1.0	-3.2	-3.2	10	0	10	0	1	0	2000	...
Sierra Leone	283	240 - 331	-0.6	-0.5	-0.3	0	1	0	0	0	1	...	2000
Singapore	3	3 - 3	-10.7	-3.9	-8.3	10	0	10	0	2	0	2001	...
Slovakia	8	7 - 9	-2.5	-4.1	-6.5	8	0	10	0	3	0	2002	...
Slovenia	5	3 - 6	-7.6	-3.5	-5.3	8	0	10	0	4	0	2003	...
Solomon Islands	22	18 - 26	-3.6	-3.6	-3.6	0	0	3	1	0	0	1999	1999
Somalia	225	181 - 283	0.0	0.0	0.0	0	0	0	0	0	1	...	2000
South Africa	66	58 - 74	-0.3	1.3	1.6	9	0	10	2	0	0	1999	1998
Spain	5	4 - 5	-6.4	-3.5	-6.0	10	0	10	0	2	0	2001	...
Sri Lanka	15	13 - 17	-4.9	-4.7	-8.5	10	1	6	1	0	0	1996	1993
Sudan	93	81 - 104	-2.5	-1.8	-1.5	0	1	0	3	0	0	...	1999
Suriname	39	35 - 44	-1.7	-1.4	-1.4	9	0	8	0	0	1	1997	2000
Swaziland	153	140 - 166	0.0	5.2	2.5	0	1	0	0	0	1	...	2000
Sweden	4	3 - 4	-8.8	-2.8	-0.8	10	0	10	0	4	0	2003	...
Switzerland	5	4 - 6	-6.4	-1.2	-4.3	10	0	10	0	4	0	2003	...
Syrian Arab Republic	18	16 - 19	-6.8	-6.6	-6.8	5	1	1	3	2	1	2001	2002
Tajikistan	118	100 - 136	-0.8	-0.5	-0.5	7	0	9	0	2	1	2001	2000
Thailand	26	23 - 29	-3.2	-3.1	-3.1	10	6	10	2	3	1	2002	2000
The former Yugoslav Republic of Macedonia	12	11 - 13	-6.0	-11.1	-3.6	8	0	10	0	3	0	2002	...
Timor-Leste	125	104 - 146	-2.0	-2.1	-1.6	0	0	0	0	0	1	...	2000
Togo	140	124 - 155	-0.8	-0.6	-0.6	0	1	0	1	0	0	...	1998
Tonga	19	16 - 23	-2.7	-2.4	-2.7	0	0	6	0	1	0	2002	...
Trinidad and Tobago	20	17 - 23	-5.6	2.1	0.0	10	1	9	0	0	0	1998	1987
Tunisia	24	21 - 26	-6.6	-5.4	-5.4	4	3	9	1	1	0	2000	1994
Turkey	39	37 - 41	-5.1	-5.6	-4.7	0	5	10	3	1	0	2000	1998
Turkmenistan	102	93 - 112	-1.7	2.2	1.0	7	0	9	0	0	1	1998	2000
Tuvalu	51	39 - 62	0.0	-1.1	-1.1	0	0	9	0	1	0	2000	...
Uganda	140	113 - 167	-0.5	-1.5	-1.3	0	1	0	3	0	1	...	2000
Ukraine	20	18 - 22	1.8	-2.6	-1.0	9	0	10	0	3	0	2002	...
United Arab Emirates	8	6 - 10	-4.7	-3.9	-3.9	0	2	8	1	3	0	2002	1995
United Kingdom	6	5 - 7	-5.6	-2.2	-2.5	10	0	10	0	3	0	2002	...
United Republic of Tanzania	165	149 - 180	0.1	0.1	0.0	0	1	0	7	0	1	...	2000
United States of America	8	7 - 9	-4.3	-1.4	-2.9	10	0	10	0	3	0	2002	...
Uruguay	15	13 - 17	-2.9	-5.8	-3.0	10	1	10	0	2	0	2001	1985
Uzbekistan	69	63 - 76	-1.1	-1.1	-1.0	9	0	10	1	2	1	2001	2000
Vanuatu	38	29 - 46	-4.4	-4.7	-4.7	0	1	0	0	0	0	...	1989
Venezuela, Bolivarian Republic of	21	19 - 23	-0.8	-2.4	-2.4	10	1	10	1	1	0	2000	1990
Viet Nam	23	20 - 26	-3.7	-7.4	-8.0	0	2	0	3	0	1	...	2002
Yemen	113	88 - 137	-2.4	-1.5	-1.2	0	0	0	3	0	0	...	1997
Zambia	182	154 - 210	0.2	0.0	0.0	0	1	1	3	1	1	2000	2002
Zimbabwe	126	111 - 141	2.4	5.4	2.5	0	4	5	4	0	0	1995	1999

der-five mortality rate is the probability (expressed as per 1000 live births) of a child born in a specific year dying before reaching five years of age, if subjected to current age-specific
ortality rates. The estimates presented here are the same as those published in Annex Table 1. See explanatory notes for sources and methods.
e column "VR/SRS" – vital registration/sample registration system – shows the number of years of data from either system available at WHO.
e column "Survey/Census" shows the number of surveys and censuses available at WHO.
Not available.

Annex Table 2b Under-five mortality rates (per 1000) directly obtained from surveys and vital registration, by age and latest availab
period or year[a]

Figures are not necessarily the official statistics of Member States, which may use alternative rigorous methods. Totals are not equivalent to the sum of the rates of the component age grou
since the figures provided are probabilities of dying rather than rates in the strict sense.

Member State	Period or year[d]	Source[e]	Under-5 0–4 years	Infant Neonatal 0–27 days	Infant Postneonatal[b] 28 days–5 months	Infant Postneonatal[b] 6–11 months	Infant Postneonatal[b] Total[c]	Infant Total[c] 0–11 months	Child 12–23 months	Child 24–59 months	Child Total[c]
Albania	2003	VR	14	3	…	…	6	8	1.9	4	6
Argentina	2002	VR	19	11	…	…	6	17	1.1	1.5	3
Armenia	1996-2000	DHS	39	19	14	3	17	36	0	3	3
Australia	2001	VR	6	4	…	…	1.6	5	0.4	0.6	1.0
Austria	2003	VR	6	3	…	…	1.4	4	0.5	0.7	1.1
Bahamas	2000	VR	12	5	…	…	4	8	1.5	1.6	3
Bahrain	2000	VR	10	4	…	…	3	7	0.7	1.9	3
Bangladesh	1996-2000	DHS	94	42	18	8	24	66	11	19	30
Barbados	2000	VR	17	11	…	…	5	16	0.9	0.6	1.5
Belgium	1992	VR	10	4	…	…	4	8	0.5	0.9	1.4
Belize	2000	VR	30	14	…	…	9	23	3	2	6
Benin	1997-2001	DHS	160	38	23	30	51	89	30	50	78
Bolivia	1994-1998	DHS	92	34	20	15	33	67	15	11	26
Brazil	2000	VR	23	13	…	…	8	20	1.7	1.8	3
Bulgaria	2003	VR	15	7	…	…	5	12	1.0	1.4	2
Burkina Faso	1995-1999	DHS	219	41	36	32	65	105	48	83	127
Burundi	1983-1987	DHS	153	35	25	16	38	74	28	59	85
Cambodia	1996-2000	DHS	124	37	44	17	58	95	11	22	32
Cameroon	1994-1998	DHS	151	37	20	22	40	77	32	50	80
Canada	2000	VR	6	4	…	…	1.7	5	0.3	0.5	0.8
Central African Republic	1990-1994	DHS	158	42	34	23	55	97	26	42	67
Chad	1993-1997	DHS	194	44	30	33	59	103	42	63	102
Chile	2002	VR	8	4	…	…	3	7	0.6	1.0	1.6
Colombia	1996-2000	DHS	25	15	4	3	7	21	1	2	4
Comoros	1992-1996	DHS	104	38	21	20	39	77	13	16	29
Costa Rica	2002	VR	12	8	…	…	4	11	0.9	1.0	1.9
Côte d'Ivoire	1994-1998	DHS	181	62	28	25	50	112	33	46	77
Croatia	2003	VR	7	5	…	…	1.4	6	0.3	0.7	1.0
Cuba	2002	VR	8	4	…	…	2	7	0.6	1.0	1.6
Czech Republic	2003	VR	5	2	…	…	1.5	4	0.4	0.6	1.0
Denmark	1996	VR	7	4	…	…	1.6	6	0.6	0.6	1.2
Dominican Republic	1998-2002	DHS	38	22	6	3	9	31	3	3	7
Ecuador	2000	VR	26	8	…	…	8	16	4	3	7
Egypt	1996-2000	DHS	54	24	11	9	20	44	5	6	11
El Salvador	1999	VR	15	4	…	…	7	11	2	1.7	4
Eritrea	1998-2002	DHS	93	24	14	11	24	48	19	29	48
Estonia	2002	VR	8	4	…	…	2	6	0.6	1.3	1.9
Ethiopia	1996-2000	DHS	166	49	28	24	48	97	29	50	77
Fiji	1978	VR	39	18	…	…	10	28	3	4	7
Finland	2003	VR	4	2	…	…	1.1	3	0.2	0.6	0.8
France	2000	VR	5	3	…	…	1.6	4	0.4	0.6	1.0
Gabon	1996-2000	DHS	89	30	13	15	27	57	15	19	33
Germany	2001	VR	5	3	…	…	1.6	4	0.4	0.6	1.0
Ghana	1994-1998	DHS	108	30	13	15	27	57	20	34	54
Greece	2001	VR	5	4	…	…	1.6	5	0.3	0.4	0.7
Guatemala	1995-1999	DHS	59	23	12	11	22	45	8	6	14
Guinea	1995-1999	DHS	177	48	32	21	50	98	35	55	87
Guyana	1996	VR	31	14	…	…	10	25	4	3	7
Haiti	1996-2000	DHS	119	32	27	23	48	80	20	22	42
Honduras	1981	VR	40	7	…	…	16	23	9	9	17

Member State	Period or year[d]	Source[e]	Under-5 0–4 years	Infant Neonatal 0–27 days	Infant Postneonatal[b] 28 days–5 months	Infant Postneonatal[b] 6–11 months	Infant Postneonatal[b] Total[c]	Infant Total[c] 0–11 months	Child 12–23 months	Child 24–59 months	Child Total[c]
Hungary	2003	VR	9	5	…	…	3	7	0.5	0.8	1.3
Iceland	2001	VR	3	2	…	…	0.7	3	0.5	0.2	0.7
India	1995-1999	DHS	95	43	15	11	24	68	12	18	29
Indonesia	1993-1997	DHS	58	22	15	10	24	46	5	8	13
Ireland	2001	VR	7	4	…	…	1.9	6	0.6	0.9	1.4
Israel	2003	VR	6	3	…	…	1.8	5	0.5	0.7	1.3
Italy	2001	VR	6	3	…	…	1.3	5	0.3	0.5	0.8
Jamaica	1991	VR	9	3	…	…	4	6	1.6	1.2	3
Japan	2000	VR	5	1.8	…	…	1.5	3	0.5	0.7	1.2
Jordan	1998-2002	DHS	27	16	4	3	7	22	2	3	5
Kazakhstan	1995-1999	DHS	71	34	17	12	28	62	6	4	10
Kenya	1994-1998	DHS	111	28	25	22	45	74	20	21	41
Kuwait	2002	VR	13	7	…	…	3	10	0.7	1.1	1.8
Kyrgyzstan	2003	VR	28	11	…	…	10	21	4	3	7
Latvia	2003	VR	13	6	…	…	4	9	1.1	2	3
Liberia	1982-1986	DHS	222	68	48	36	76	144	49	44	91
Lithuania	2003	VR	9	4	…	…	3	7	0.6	1.2	1.8
Luxembourg	2003	VR	5	3	…	…	2	5	0.4	0.0	0.4
Madagascar	1993-1997	DHS	159	40	30	29	56	96	32	38	70
Malawi	1996-2000	DHS	189	42	32	34	62	104	42	55	95
Mali	1997-2001	DHS	229	57	29	32	56	113	50	85	130
Malta	2003	VR	6	5	…	…	0.5	6	0.2	0.2	0.5
Mauritania	1999-2003	DHS	168	37	30	31	58	95	38	45	81
Mauritius	2000	VR	18	12	…	…	3	16	1.0	1.3	2
Mexico	2001	VR	20	8	…	…	5	13	1.5	1.6	3
Mongolia	1994	VR	57	10	…	…	25	35	8	10	18
Morocco	1988-1992	DHS	76	31	17	10	26	57	12	8	20
Mozambique	1993-1997	DHS	201	54	41	46	81	135	21	57	77
Namibia	1996-2000	DHS	62	20	13	6	18	38	8	17	25
Nepal	1996-2000	DHS	91	39	16	10	26	64	12	17	29
Netherlands	2003	VR	6	4	…	…	1.2	5	0.4	0.6	1.0
New Zealand	2000	VR	8	4	…	…	3	7	0.5	1.0	1.6
Nicaragua	1997-2001	DHS	39	16	9	6	15	31	5	4	9
Niger	1994-1998	DHS	274	44	35	49	79	123	71	109	172
Nigeria	1999-2003	DHS	201	48	25	30	52	100	50	65	112
Norway	2002	VR	4	2	…	…	1.0	3	0.5	0.7	1.2
Pakistan	1987-1991	DHS	112	49	24	15	37	86	16	13	29
Panama	2002	VR	17	8	…	…	6	14	2	2	4
Papua New Guinea	1977	VR	12	2	…	…	4	6	2	3	5
Paraguay	2000	VR	14	6	…	…	5	10	1.6	1.5	3
Peru	1996-2000	DHS	47	18	9	6	15	33	7	7	14
Philippines	1994-1998	DHS	48	18	9	8	17	35	6	8	14
Poland	2002	VR	9	5	…	…	2	8	0.5	0.7	1.2
Portugal	2002	VR	7	3	…	…	1.6	5	0.6	1.0	1.6
Republic of Moldova	2003	VR	18	7	…	…	7	14	1.4	2	3
Romania	2002	VR	21	8	…	…	9	17	1.5	1.8	3
Rwanda	1996-2000	DHS	196	44	33	35	64	107	43	59	100
Saint Lucia	1999	VR	25	15	…	…	2	17	1.4	3	4
Saint Vincent and the Grenadines	1999	VR	26	14	…	…	8	21	3	4	7
Sao Tome and Principe	1985	VR	122	23	…	…	43	65	32	36	67

Annex Table 2b Under-five mortality rates (per 1000) directly obtained from surveys and vital registration, by age and latest available period or year[a]

Figures are not necessarily the official statistics of Member States, which may use alternative rigorous methods. Totals are not equivalent to the sum of the rates of the component age groups since the figures provided are probabilities of dying rather than rates in the strict sense.

Member State	Period or year[d]	Source[e]	Under-5 0–4 years	Infant Neonatal 0–27 days	Postneonatal[b] 28 days–5 months	Postneonatal[b] 6–11 months	Postneonatal[b] Total[c]	Total[c] 0–11 months	Child 12–23 months	Child 24–59 months	Child Total[c]
Senegal	1993-1997	DHS	139	37	17	14	30	68	27	51	77
Serbia and Montenegro	2000	VR	16	9	…	…	4	13	1.4	1.1	2
Singapore	2001	VR	3	1.1	…	…	1.0	2	0.6	0.6	1.2
Slovakia	2002	VR	9	4	…	…	3	8	0.7	0.7	1.4
Slovenia	2003	VR	5	3	…	…	1.0	4	0.2	0.6	0.8
South Africa	1994-1998	DHS	59	20	16	11	26	45	8	6	15
Spain	2001	VR	5	3	…	…	1.3	4	0.4	0.6	1
Sri Lanka	1983-1987	DHS	34	16	5	4	8	25	2	7	10
Sudan	1986-1990	DHS	124	44	13	14	26	70	25	33	58
Suriname	1992	VR	19	7	…	…	6	13	2	2	5
Sweden	2001	VR	4	3	…	…	1.2	4	0.3	0.5	0.8
Switzerland	2000	VR	6	4	…	…	1.3	5	0.4	0.5	0.9
Thailand	1983-1987	DHS	44	20	12	3	15	35	5	5	9
The former Yugoslav Republic of Macedonia	2000	VR	15	9	…	…	3	12	0.9	1.0	1.9
Togo	1994-1998	DHS	146	41	19	22	38	80	23	51	72
Trinidad and Tobago	1983-1987	DHS	32	23	3	3	5	28	3	1	4
Tunisia	1984-1988	DHS	62	26	13	10	22	48	5	9	15
Turkey	1994-1998	DHS	52	26	9	8	17	43	5	5	10
Uganda	1996-2000	DHS	151	33	25	33	55	88	32	39	69
United Kingdom	2002	VR	6	4	…	…	1.7	5	0.4	0.5	0.9
United Republic of Tanzania	1995-1999	DHS	147	40	32	30	59	99	25	28	53
United States of America	2001	VR	8	5	…	…	2	7	0.5	0.8	1.3
Uruguay	2000	VR	16	8	…	…	6	14	1.0	1.2	2
Uzbekistan	1992-1996	DHS	59	23	15	12	26	49	6	5	11
Venezuela, Bolivarian Republic of	2000	VR	21	12	…	…	6	18	2	1.9	4
Viet Nam	1998-2002	DHS	24	12	4	2	6	18	3	3	6
Zambia	1998-2002	DHS	168	37	30	31	58	95	38	45	81
Zimbabwe	1995-1999	DHS	102	29	23	15	36	65	19	21	40

[a] Results are computed from nationally representative surveys based on a standard method or vital registration without any adjustment. Care should be exercised when making inter-country comparisons as the results are not directly comparable since the method of calculation varies depending on sources and there are different degrees of completeness of vital registration data submitted by Member States. See explanatory notes for definition of age groups.

[b] Data from vital registration reported to WHO are not sufficiently detailed to permit the calculation of postneonatal mortality rates for 28 days–5 months and 6–11 months.

[c] Totals are not equivalent to the sum of the rates of the component age groups since the figures provided are probabilities of dying rather than rates in the strict sense.

[d] Data from national vital registration systems refer to specific years whereas for surveys the results refer to a five-year period.

[e] VR: vital registration; DHS: Demographic and Health Survey.

… Not available.

Annex Table 3 Annual number of deaths by cause for children under five years of age in WHO regions, estimates for 2000–2003[a]

Figures computed by WHO to ensure comparability; they are not necessarily the official statistics of Member States, which may use alternative rigorous methods.

| Cause | ALL MEMBER STATES | | AFRICA | | THE AMERICAS | | | | | | SOUTH-EAST AS | |
					All		Member States with low mortality (Canada and USA)		Others			
Population (000)	616 764		110 944		77 885		22 978		54 908		178 987	
	(000)	% total	(000)	% total	(000)	% total	(000)	% total	(000)	% total	(000)	% tota
TOTAL Deaths	10 596	100	4 396	100	439	100	50	100	389	100	3 070	100
HIV/AIDS	321	3	285	6	6	1	0	0	6	2	22	1
Diarrhoeal diseases[c]	1762	17	701	16	51	12	0	0	51	13	552	18
Measles	395	4	227	5	1	0	0	0	1	0	103	3
Malaria	853	8	802	18	1	0	0	0	1	0	12	0
Acute respiratory infections	2 027	19	924	21	54	12	1	2	53	14	590	19
Neonatal causes[d]	3 910	37	1 148	26	195	44	29	58	166	43	1 362	44
Injuries	305	3	76	2	23	5	5	10	18	5	71	2
Unintentional	291	…	…	…	…	…	…	…	…	…	…	…
Road traffic accidents	50	…	…	…	…	…	…	…	…	…	…	…
Drowning	60	…	…	…	…	…	…	…	…	…	…	…
Intentional	14	…	…	…	…	…	…	…	…	…	…	…
Others	1 022	10	233	5	109	25	15	30	94	24	359	12

[a] See explanatory notes for sources and methods.

[b] Andorra, Austria, Belgium, Croatia, Cyprus, Czech Republic, Denmark, Finland, France, Germany, Greece, Iceland, Ireland, Israel, Italy, Luxembourg, Malta, Monaco, Netherlands, Norway, Portug San Marino, Slovenia, Spain, Sweden, Switzerland and United Kingdom.

[c] Includes only deaths from diarrhoea during the postneonatal period.

[d] Neonatal causes include diarrhoea during the neonatal period (see Annex Table 4). Globally the proportion of all deaths due to diarrhoea among all children under five years of age is 18%.

… Not available.

Annex Table 4 Annual number of deaths by cause for neonates in WHO regions, estimates for 2000–2003[a]

Figures computed by WHO to ensure comparability; they are not necessarily the official statistics of Member States, which may use alternative rigorous methods.

| Cause | ALL MEMBER STATES | | AFRICA | | THE AMERICAS | | | | | | SOUTH-EAST AS | |
					All		Member States with low mortality (Canada and USA)		Others			
	(000)	% total	(000)	% total	(000)	% total	(000)	% total	(000)	% total	(000)	% tota
TOTAL Neonatal deaths	3 910	100	1 148	100	195	100	29	100	166	100	1 362	100
Neonatal tetanus	257	7	108	9	2	1	0	0	2	1	58	4
Severe infection[c]	1 016	26	313	27	34	17	2	6	32	19	374	27
Birth asphyxia	894	23	274	24	36	19	4	14	33	20	314	23
Diarrhoeal diseases	108	3	40	3	1	1	0	0	1	1	37	3
Congenital anomalies	294	8	70	6	31	16	8	29	22	13	77	6
Preterm birth[d]	1 083	28	265	23	78	40	13	45	65	39	413	30
Others	258	7	78	7	13	7	2	7	11	7	89	7

[a] See explanatory notes for sources and methods.

[b] Andorra, Austria, Belgium, Croatia, Cyprus, Czech Republic, Denmark, Finland, France, Germany, Greece, Iceland, Ireland, Israel, Italy, Luxembourg, Malta, Monaco, Netherlands, Norway, Portug San Marino, Slovenia, Spain, Sweden, Switzerland and United Kingdom.

[c] Includes deaths from pneumonia, meningitis, sepsis/septicaemia and other infections during the neonatal period.

[d] Includes only deaths directly attributed to prematurity and to specific complications of preterm birth such as surfactant deficiency, but not all deaths in preterm infants.

EUROPE						EASTERN MEDITERRANEAN		WESTERN PACIFIC					
All		Member States with low mortality[b]		Others				All		Member States with low mortality (Australia, Japan and New Zealand)		Others	
50 738		22 050		28 688		67 918		130 292		7 833		122 459	
(000)	% total	(000)	% total	(000)	% total	(000)	% total	(000)	% total	(000)	% total	(000)	% total
263	100	25	100	238	100	1 409	100	1 020	100	7	100	1 013	100
1	0	0	0	1	0	4	0	3	0	0	0	3	0
35	13	0	0	35	15	245	17	178	17	0	0	178	18
2	1	0	0	1	1	52	4	11	1	0	0	11	1
0	0	0	0	0	0	37	3	1	0	0	0	1	0
32	12	0	2	31	13	292	21	137	13	0	4	137	13
116	44	14	55	102	43	610	43	480	47	3	43	477	47
17	7	2	7	16	7	45	3	73	7	1	12	72	7
...	...	...	...	...	...	...	...	...	...	...	...	...	...
...	...	...	...	...	...	...	...	...	...	...	...	...	...
...	...	...	...	...	...	...	...	...	...	...	...	...	...
...	...	...	...	...	...	...	...	...	...	...	...	...	...
61	23	9	36	52	22	124	9	137	13	3	40	134	13

EUROPE						EASTERN MEDITERRANEAN		WESTERN PACIFIC					
All		Member States with low mortality[b]		Others				All		Member States with low mortality (Australia, Japan and New Zealand)		Others	
(000)	% total	(000)	% total	(000)	% total	(000)	% total	(000)	% total	(000)	% total	(000)	% total
116	100	14	100	102	100	610	100	480	100	3	100	477	100
1	1	0	0	1	1	72	12	16	3	0	0	16	3
21	18	1	6	20	20	174	28	101	21	0	6	101	21
21	18	2	15	19	18	122	20	127	26	0	14	126	26
1	1	0	0	1	1	22	4	7	1	0	0	7	1
21	19	4	32	17	17	54	9	40	8	1	31	39	8
44	38	6	41	38	37	132	22	152	32	1	44	151	32
7	6	1	6	6	6	35	6	36	8	0	7	36	8

Annex Table 5 Selected national health accounts indicators: measured levels of expenditure on health, 1998–2002

Figures computed by WHO to assure comparability;[a] they are not necessarily the official statistics of Member States, which may use alternative rigorous methods.

	Member State	Total expenditure on health as % of gross domestic product					General government expenditure on health as % of total expenditure on health[b]					Private expenditure on health as % of total expenditure on health[b]					General government expenditure on health as % of total government expenditure				
		1998	1999	2000	2001	2002	1998	1999	2000	2001	2002	1998	1999	2000	2001	2002	1998	1999	2000	2001	2002
1	Afghanistan	6	5.9	6	6.5	8	8.9	7.7	6.3	9	39.2	91.1	92.3	93.7	91	60.8	8.8	9	10.5	14.3	23.1
2	Albania	6.4	6.5	6.1	6.4	6.1	35.9	37.7	39.2	36	38.7	64.1	62.3	60.8	64	61.3	7	7.3	7.8	7.5	8.1
3	Algeria	3.8	3.7	3.6	3.9	4.3	65.6	66.4	69.6	74.2	74	34.4	33.6	30.4	25.8	26	8.1	8.4	8.8	9.4	9.1
4	Andorra	9.2	6.8	7	6.8	6.5	78.6	71.6	70.1	71	70.5	21.4	28.4	29.9	29	29.5	39.1	29.5	25.7	26.3	26.6
5	Angola	3.1	3.1	3.3	5.3	5	33	41.4	54	51.8	41.9	67	58.6	46	48.2	58.1	1.8	2.1	3.1	5.4	4.1
6	Antigua and Barbuda	4.6	4.5	4.6	4.8	4.8	71.7	72.2	72	70.8	68.6	28.3	27.8	28	29.2	31.4	14.5	13.9	14.1	15	14.1
7	Argentina	8.2	9	8.9	9.5	8.9	55.2	56.2	55.1	53.5	50.2	44.8	43.8	44.9	46.5	49.8	14.6	14.8	14.5	14.2	15.3
8	Armenia	5.8	7.1	5.2	7	5.8	24.7	30.8	29.8	21.5	22.9	75.3	69.2	70.2	78.5	77.1	5.7	7.6	6.1	6.2	6
9	Australia	8.7	8.9	9.2	9.3	9.5	68.3	69.8	69.1	68.3	67.9	31.7	30.2	30.9	31.7	32.1	15.7	16.3	16.4	16.7	17.1
10	Austria	7.7	7.8	7.7	7.6	7.7	69.7	69.6	69.6	68.5	69.9	30.3	30.4	30.4	31.5	30.1	9.9	10.1	10.3	10.2	10.5
11	Azerbaijan	4.7	4.6	3.9	3.8	3.7	19.3	21.6	22	23	22.1	80.7	78.4	78	77	77.9	3.8	4.2	4.2	4.3	2.9
12	Bahamas	7.5	7	7	6.8	6.9	44.9	46.8	47.2	47.5	48.6	55.1	53.2	52.8	52.5	51.4	13.8	14.4	14.3	13.6	14.6
13	Bahrain	4.9	4.7	4.1	4.3	4.4	70.6	70	69.3	70.4	72	29.4	30	30.8	29.6	28	11.5	11.4	10.8	10.8	9.5
14	Bangladesh	3.1	3.2	3.2	3.2	3.1	30.7	27.2	25.6	25.8	25.2	69.3	72.8	74.4	74.2	74.8	5.4	4.7	4.3	4.7	4.4
15	Barbados	6	6.1	6.2	6.7	6.9	65.4	65.4	65.8	67.6	68.4	34.6	34.6	34.2	32.4	31.6	11.8	12	12	12.2	12.3
16	Belarus	6	6.1	6.1	6.6	6.4	82.1	81.1	80.1	75.5	73.9	17.9	18.9	19.9	24.5	26.1	10.9	10.4	10.7	10.7	10.5
17	Belgium	8.6	8.7	8.8	9	9.1	70.2	70.6	70.5	71.4	71.2	29.8	29.4	29.5	28.6	28.8	11.9	12.3	12.6	13	12.8
18	Belize	4.9	5.1	5	5.2	5.2	51.7	48.6	48	45.1	47.3	48.3	51.4	52	54.9	52.7	5.6	5.5	5.3	5	5.3
19	Benin	4.5	4.3	4.6	4.9	4.7	40.9	37	43.4	46.2	44.4	59.1	63	56.6	53.8	55.6	11.2	9	9.8	11.9	11.1
20	Bhutan	3.8	3.5	3.9	3.6	4.5	90.3	89.6	90.6	91.2	92.2	9.7	10.4	9.4	8.8	7.8	9.2	8.3	9.3	7.8	12
21	Bolivia	5	6.2	6.1	6.4	7	62.9	58.1	60.1	59.3	59.8	37.1	41.9	39.9	40.7	40.2	10.2	10.5	9.9	10.4	11.6
22	Bosnia and Herzegovina	6.5	10.7	9.7	9.2	9.2	27.3	56.7	52	48.8	49.8	72.7	43.3	48	51.2	50.2	2.9	8.9	7.8	7.9	8.8
23	Botswana	4.8	5.1	5.1	5.4	6	53.3	54.1	54.3	56.7	61.9	46.7	45.9	45.7	43.3	38.1	5.6	5.6	5.9	6.3	7.5
24	Brazil	7.4	7.8	7.6	7.8	7.9	44	42.8	41	42.9	45.9	56	57.2	59	57.1	54.1	9	9.3	8.5	9.2	10.1
25	Brunei Darussalam	3.8	3.5	3.6	3.5	3.5	81.3	79.4	80	78.3	78.2	18.7	20.6	20	21.7	21.8	5.1	4.8	5.1	4.6	4.7
26	Bulgaria	5.1	6.2	6.5	7.1	7.4	67.9	66.5	61.2	55.8	53.4	32.1	33.5	38.8	44.2	46.6	9.1	10.3	9.3	9.5	10.1
27	Burkina Faso	4.3	4.6	4.5	4.1	4.3	38.7	42	40	39.7	45.9	61.3	58	60	60.3	54.1	8.7	8.2	7.8	8.7	10.6
28	Burundi	3.1	3	3.1	3.2	3	20.5	19.9	17.9	20.8	21.5	79.5	80.1	82.1	79.2	78.5	2.4	2.1	2	2.2	2
29	Cambodia	10.5	10.8	11.8	11.8	12	10.1	10.1	14.2	14.9	17.1	89.9	89.9	85.8	85.1	82.9	11.8	11.3	15.7	16	18.6
30	Cameroon	4.4	4.9	4.7	4.5	4.6	17	24.4	27.8	26.2	26.2	83	75.6	72.2	73.8	73.8	4.6	7.2	9.5	7.4	7.9
31	Canada	9.2	9	8.9	9.4	9.6	70.6	70.3	70.4	70.1	69.9	29.4	29.7	29.6	29.9	30.1	14.3	14.7	15.2	15.8	15.9
32	Cape Verde	5.1	4.5	4.6	5	5	75.3	73.9	73.5	75.8	75.1	24.7	26.1	26.5	24.2	24.9	10.2	9	9.6	12.4	11.1
33	Central African Republic	3.4	3.5	3.8	3.7	3.9	34	38	41.1	39.4	41.6	66	62	58.9	60.6	58.4	6.7	7.7	7.5	9.6	7.4
34	Chad	5.4	6.2	6.9	6.6	6.5	31.4	33.2	41.2	41.5	41.9	68.6	66.8	58.8	58.5	58.1	11.2	10.5	12.9	13.6	12.2
35	Chile	6.1	6	5.7	5.7	5.8	36.4	38.4	42.2	43.7	45.1	63.6	61.6	57.8	56.3	54.9	8.3	8.3	9	9.7	10.2
36	China	4.8	5.1	5.6	5.7	5.8	39	38	34.6	35.5	33.7	61	62	65.4	64.5	66.3	13.3	11.8	10.3	10	10
37	Colombia	9.9	9.7	8	8.3	8.1	67.5	73.2	77.9	80.7	82.9	32.5	26.8	22.1	19.3	17.1	24.9	23.2	21.4	20.1	20.4
38	Comoros	3.4	3.2	2.7	2.3	2.9	63.4	60.8	54.9	46.9	58	36.6	39.2	45.1	53.1	42	8.8	11.2	9.6	6	8.2
39	Congo	3.3	2.7	2.1	2.1	2.2	72.4	68.4	70.2	69	70.3	27.6	31.6	29.8	31	29.7	5.6	5.7	5.6	5.7	6
40	Cook Islands	4.2	3.5	3.8	5.2	4.6	91.7	89.6	90.9	93.8	93	8.3	10.4	9.1	6.2	7	10	7.7	8.2	12.4	11.6
41	Costa Rica	8.1	7.9	8.3	8.8	9.3	69.3	68.1	66.7	65.2	65.4	30.7	31.9	33.3	34.8	34.6	24.1	24.6	24.2	23.3	24.4
42	Côte d'Ivoire	6.4	6.1	6.3	6.2	6.2	24.6	23.2	21.3	20.1	22.4	75.4	76.8	78.7	79.9	77.6	7.6	7.2	7.5	7.5	7.2
43	Croatia	7.9	8.6	9	8.2	7.3	85.1	86.1	86.4	85.5	81.4	14.9	13.9	13.6	14.5	18.6	12.9	13.5	14.5	13.8	12
44	Cuba	6.6	7.1	7.1	7.3	7.5	84.7	85.5	85.8	86	86.5	15.3	14.5	14.2	14	13.5	10.3	11.1	10.8	11.4	11.3
45	Cyprus	6.1	6.2	6.3	6.6	7	39.5	38.7	37.6	38.4	41.3	60.5	61.3	62.4	61.6	58.7	6.2	6.2	6.1	6.3	6.8
46	Czech Republic	6.6	6.6	6.6	6.9	7	91.8	91.5	91.4	91.4	91.4	8.2	8.5	8.6	8.6	8.6	15.8	15.6	15	15.1	14.7
47	Democratic People's Republic of Korea	3.5	4.2	4.5	4.6	4.6	76.9	75.3	73.5	73.4	76.6	23.1	24.7	26.5	26.6	23.4	3.3	5	5	5	5
48	Democratic Republic of the Congo	3.8	3.2	3.8	3.5	4.1	9.9	7.2	7.4	18.2	30.2	90.1	92.8	92.6	81.8	69.8	3.7	2.6	3.7	13.5	16.4
49	Denmark	8.4	8.5	8.4	8.6	8.8	82	82.2	82.4	82.7	82.9	18	17.8	17.6	17.4	17.1	11.9	12.4	12.6	12.9	13.1
50	Djibouti	6.3	6.2	6.3	6.1	6.3	52.5	52.9	52.8	51.5	52.9	47.5	47.1	47.2	48.5	47.1	10	10	10.1	10.6	10.1
51	Dominica	5.8	6.2	5.8	6	6.4	73.3	74.3	71.5	71.3	71.3	26.7	25.7	28.5	28.7	28.7	11.8	12.8	12.8	10.5	12.2
52	Dominican Republic	5.8	5.7	6.2	6.1	6.1	31.4	32.1	35.2	35.6	36.4	68.6	67.9	64.8	64.4	63.6	11.8	11.3	14.6	13.5	11.7
53	Ecuador	4.4	4.7	4.1	4.8	4.8	38.3	39.4	31.2	33.5	36	61.7	60.6	68.8	66.5	64	9.3	9.8	6.4	8.5	8.8
54	Egypt	5	4.9	5	5.1	4.9	34.7	35.9	35.3	37.8	36.6	65.3	64.1	64.7	62.2	63.4	6.8	5.9	5.8	6.4	6
55	El Salvador	8.2	8	8	7.7	8	42.5	43.5	45.1	42.4	44.7	57.5	56.5	54.9	57.6	55.3	24.2	25.1	25	21.2	22.8

	Member State	External resources for health as % of total expenditure on health					Social security expenditure on health as % of general government expenditure on health					Out-of-pocket expenditure as % of private expenditure on health					Private prepaid plans as % of private expenditure on health				
		1998	1999	2000	2001	2002	1998	1999	2000	2001	2002	1998	1999	2000	2001	2002	1998	1999	2000	2001	2002
1	Afghanistan	1.7	1.9	2.4	5.3	42.6	0	0	0	0	0	99	99	99	99	80	0	0	0	0	0
2	Albania	5.8	6.9	8.7	4.9	3.8	24.8	23.4	20.1	20	22.5	99.7	99.8	99.7	99.8	99.7	0	0	0	0	0
3	Algeria	0	0.1	0.1	0.1	0.1	46.1	44.1	36.2	33.8	51.1	84	83.4	80.2	80	76.6	2.6	2.7	2.6	3.2	4.6
4	Andorra	0	0	0	0	0	60	87.5	88.1	86.2	84.9	95.2	95.6	96.1	92.6	96.6	n/a	n/a	n/a	n/a	n/a
5	Angola	6.2	9.2	14.9	11.8	7.9	0	0	0	0	0	100	100	100	100	100	0	0	0	0	0
6	Antigua and Barbuda	3.9	3.8	3.8	3.4	1.1	0	0	0	0	0	100	100	100	100	100	n/a	n/a	n/a	n/a	n/a
7	Argentina	0.3	0.3	0.3	0.3	0.3	60.3	59.2	59.9	58.4	56.7	63.8	64	63.3	62.4	62.4	32	31.9	32.6	31.1	31.1
8	Armenia	11.7	19.6	20.9	24.8	18.6	0	0	0	0	0	89.5	78	79.5	75.1	83.5	n/a	n/a	n/a	n/a	n/a
9	Australia	0	0	0	0	0	56.2	58	61.1	60.9	61.4	25.2	24.2	23.9	23.6	24.6	23.7	21.6	21.8	23.8	22.7
10	Austria	0	0	0	0	0	56.6	57.3	58	59.2	58.9	59	60	61.3	58	58	25.2	24.2	23.9	23.6	24.6
11	Azerbaijan	0.8	1.1	2.2	4.2	4	0	0	0	0	0	100	100	100	100	100	0	n/a	n/a	n/a	n/a
12	Bahamas	n/a	n/a	n/a	0.2	n/a	2.2	1.8	1.8	2.3	2.1	40.3	40.3	40.3	40.3	40.3	58.6	58.6	58.6	58.6	58.6
13	Bahrain	0	0	0	0	0	0.3	0.3	0.4	0.4	0.4	74.1	73.5	70.2	70.4	69.2	22.6	23.2	26	25.9	26.9
14	Bangladesh	12.3	12.2	12.9	13.3	13.5	0	0	0	0	0	93	88.8	86.5	86	85.9	0	0	0	0	0.1
15	Barbados	4.5	4.2	4	4.4	4.2	0	0	0	0	0	76.5	77.2	77.3	76.9	77.2	23.5	22.8	22.7	23.1	22.8
16	Belarus	0	0.1	0.1	0.2	0.1	6.6	7.6	8.1	7.4	7.7	74	70.6	70.4	74.7	79.7	n/a	n/a	0.3	0.1	0.2
17	Belgium	0	0	0	0	0	89.3	86.6	82.2	77.7	77.7	84.4	83.9	84.2	86.8	86.3	6.8	6.8	6.5	6.7	6.7
18	Belize	3.6	3.1	2.9	8.5	8	0	0	0	12.5	21.6	100	100	100	100	100	0	0	0	0	0
19	Benin	25.9	14.4	23.4	61.8	65.9	n/a	n/a	n/a	n/a	n/a	91.1	91	91	90.6	90.3	8.3	8.4	8.4	8.7	9
20	Bhutan	17.9	36.8	17.1	18.5	18.7	0	0	0	0	0	100	100	100	100	100	0	0	0	0	0
21	Bolivia	6.2	5.7	6	7.1	7	63.3	60.9	62	65.2	65	74.2	83.8	81.6	77.9	81.3	10.9	5.5	8.1	12	9.5
22	Bosnia and Herzegovina	9.5	3.9	5.2	3	1.8	78	79	78	79	80	100	100	100	100	100	0	0	0	0	0
23	Botswana	2.4	2.2	1.9	2.5	3.8	n/a	n/a	n/a	n/a	n/a	28.8	30.3	31.3	31.9	30.8	23.8	22.7	20.6	20.2	19.9
24	Brazil	0.3	0.5	0.5	0.5	0.5	0	0	0	0	0	66.9	67.1	64.9	64.1	64.2	33.1	32.9	35.1	35.9	35.8
25	Brunei Darussalam	n/a	n/a	n/a	n/a	n/a	0	0	0	0	0	100	100	100	100	100	0	0	0	0	0
26	Bulgaria	0.1	0.5	1.9	1.5	1.4	0	9.4	11.8	36.2	34.1	98.6	99.0	99.0	99.2	98.4	0	0	0	0.1	0.9
27	Burkina Faso	13.2	13.2	11.8	6.6	5.8	0.8	0.4	0.9	1.4	0.9	99	99	99	98.9	98.9	n/a	n/a	n/a	n/a	n/a
28	Burundi	18.6	18	14.5	15.8	16.2	n/a	n/a	n/a	n/a	n/a	100	100	100	100	100	n/a	n/a	n/a	n/a	n/a
29	Cambodia	12.4	13.4	18.8	19.7	4.9	0	0	0	0	0	89.6	90.1	85.4	84.6	85.2	0	0	0	0	0
30	Cameroon	5.9	5.2	6.1	7	6.4	0.1	0.1	0.1	0.1	0.1	94.1	94.2	93.7	93.6	93.7	n/a	n/a	n/a	n/a	n/a
31	Canada	0	0	0	0	0	1.8	1.9	2	2	2.1	55.2	55.1	53.7	51	50.3	38.1	37.9	38.9	41.4	42.1
32	Cape Verde	7.6	8.4	13.5	15.1	19.3	30.2	36.9	36.1	35.1	33.6	99.9	99.7	99.6	99.5	99.8	0.1	0.3	0.4	0.5	0.2
33	Central African Republic	23.2	20	20	15.7	17	n/a	n/a	n/a	n/a	n/a	95.3	95.1	95.5	95.4	95.4	n/a	n/a	n/a	n/a	n/a
34	Chad	23.3	22.3	28.4	22.8	27.9	n/a	n/a	n/a	n/a	n/a	96.4	96.7	96.6	96.5	96.5	0.4	0.3	0.4	0.4	0.4
35	Chile	0.1	0.1	0.1	0.1	0	93.6	92.8	36.8	37.7	37.1	71.4	71	47.1	48	48.7	28.6	28.9	52.9	52	51.3
36	China	0.2	0.3	0.2	0.1	0.1	53	51.4	50.7	50.7	50.8	94	94.9	95.6	95.7	96.3	0.6	0.4	0.4	0.4	0.4
37	Colombia	0.3	0.3	0.3	0.1	0	62.3	63.2	60.2	61	59.3	84	76.5	66.1	61.1	57	10.7	15.3	22.8	26.2	31.4
38	Comoros	50.8	47.6	35.9	25.7	43	0	0	0	0	0	100	100	100	100	100	0	0	0	0	0
39	Congo	3.4	2.5	2.1	2.3	2.2	0	0	0	0	0	100	100	100	100	100	n/a	n/a	n/a	n/a	n/a
40	Cook Islands	42.6	37	29.3	19.1	5.4	0	0	0	0	0	100	100	100	100	100	0	0	0	0	0
41	Costa Rica	0.8	0.7	0.8	1.5	1.3	78.7	79.8	80.7	82.2	82.9	98.4	98.7	98.8	98.9	99	1.6	1.3	1.2	1.1	1
42	Côte d'Ivoire	3.1	3.3	3.4	2.7	2.2	22.3	23.7	22.6	22.6	23.5	94.5	94.5	94.7	94.7	94.6	5.5	5.5	5.3	5.3	5.4
43	Croatia	0.5	1	1	1.1	1.1	97.6	97.4	97.6	97.7	97.7	100	100	100	100	100	0	0	0	0	0
44	Cuba	0.1	0.2	0.2	0.3	0.2	0	0	0	0	0	78.5	76	75.6	75.2	75.2	0	0	0	0	0
45	Cyprus	0	0	0	2.6	2.3	0	0	0	0.1	0	98.7	98.4	97.8	97.9	97.9	1.3	1.6	2.2	2.1	2.1
46	Czech Republic	0	0	0	0	0	90.1	89.4	89.4	90.4	89.2	100	100	100	100	100	0	0	0	0	0
47	Democratic People's Republic of Korea	0.2	0.2	0.3	0.4	59	0	0	0	0	0	100	100	100	100	100	0	0	0	0	0
48	Democratic Republic of the Congo	6.4	3.6	4.8	16.4	27.8	0	0	0	0	0	100	100	100	100	100	n/a	n/a	n/a	n/a	n/a
49	Denmark	0	0	0	0	0	0	0	0	0	0	92	90.4	90.3	90.8	89.8	8	9.6	9	9.2	9.4
50	Djibouti	10.2	10.5	11.8	15.5	20.3	0	0	0	0	0	54.5	53.6	53.4	53.3	52.9	n/a	n/a	n/a	n/a	n/a
51	Dominica	2.3	2.1	1.3	0.9	0.5	0	0	0	0	0	100	100	100	100	100	n/a	n/a	n/a	n/a	n/a
52	Dominican Republic	3.2	3.2	2.4	1.8	1.4	21.4	20.3	22.4	22.6	20.3	88.4	88.4	88.4	88.4	88.2	0.3	0.4	0.4	0.4	0.4
53	Ecuador	2.4	3.2	4.1	1.8	0.9	15.4	31.7	28	32.2	35.4	79.1	84.2	85.3	87.6	88.4	6.4	5.4	4.8	3	2.3
54	Egypt	1.4	1.6	1.9	1.9	1.6	20.9	20.3	20	19.9	22	92.5	92.3	92.3	92.3	92	0.6	0.6	0.6	0.6	0.6
55	El Salvador	2.9	1.5	0.9	0.8	0.7	41.7	44	44.2	36.3	44.5	94	90.2	95.6	93.6	93.9	5.8	9.6	4.2	6.4	6.1

Annex Table 5 Selected national health accounts indicators: measured levels of expenditure on health, 1998–2002

Figures computed by WHO to assure comparability;[a] they are not necessarily the official statistics of Member States, which may use alternative rigorous methods.

	Member State	Total expenditure on health as % of gross domestic product					General government expenditure on health as % of total expenditure on health[b]					Private expenditure on health as % of total expenditure on health[b]					General government expenditure on health as % of total government expenditure				
		1998	1999	2000	2001	2002	1998	1999	2000	2001	2002	1998	1999	2000	2001	2002	1998	1999	2000	2001	2002
56	Equatorial Guinea	4.1	2.7	2	1.7	1.8	62	62.4	66.5	70.1	72.2	38	37.6	33.5	29.9	27.8	8.3	9.9	9.9	9.8	9.8
57	Eritrea	4.7	4.2	4.8	5.1	5.1	66.1	59.7	62.7	61.5	63.7	33.9	40.3	37.3	38.5	36.3	4.1	2.7	4.5	5.3	5.6
58	Estonia	5.6	6.1	5.5	5.1	5.1	86.3	80.4	76.7	77.8	76.3	13.7	19.6	23.3	22.2	23.7	13.4	12.1	11.7	11.5	11
59	Ethiopia	4.8	4.9	5.6	5.4	5.7	47.6	48.1	45.9	41.4	44.9	52.4	51.9	54.1	58.6	55.1	9.4	7.9	7.7	7.6	7.6
60	Fiji	4.1	3.7	3.9	3.9	4.2	65.4	65.2	65.2	67.1	64.6	34.6	34.8	34.8	32.9	35.4	6.9	7.5	7.2	6.7	7.5
61	Finland	6.9	6.9	6.7	7	7.3	76.3	75.3	75.1	75.4	75.7	23.7	24.7	24.9	24.6	24.3	10	10	10.2	10.7	11
62	France	9.3	9.3	9.3	9.4	9.7	76	76	75.8	75.9	76	24	24	24.2	24.1	24	13.1	13.2	13.4	13.7	13.8
63	Gabon	4.3	3.5	3.5	4.2	4.3	60.7	49.2	39.5	43.5	41.3	39.3	50.8	60.5	56.5	58.7	5.4	6.1	6.2	5.9	6.3
64	Gambia	6.8	6.6	7.2	7.2	7.3	24.5	34.2	44.2	43.7	44.6	75.5	65.8	55.8	56.3	55.4	7.2	10	14.4	9.4	12
65	Georgia	2.4	2.5	3.4	3.7	3.8	45.4	37.6	33.3	37.4	27.1	54.6	62.4	66.7	62.6	72.9	5.1	4.3	5.9	6.8	5.8
66	Germany	10.6	10.6	10.6	10.8	10.9	78.6	78.6	78.8	78.6	78.5	21.4	21.4	21.2	21.4	21.5	17.1	17.1	18.2	17.5	17.6
67	Ghana	5.5	5.7	5.7	5.6	5.6	42	40.2	40.6	40.9	41	58	59.8	59.4	59.1	59	8.9	9.3	7.8	8.5	8.4
68	Greece	9.4	9.6	9.7	9.4	9.5	52.1	53.4	53.9	53.1	52.9	47.9	46.6	46.1	46.9	47.1	10.2	10.8	10.5	10.5	10.8
69	Grenada	4.8	4.8	4.8	5.3	5.7	65.8	69.7	70.1	71.9	71	34.2	30.3	29.9	28.1	29	11.3	12.3	12.3	13.9	14.7
70	Guatemala	4.4	4.7	4.8	4.8	4.8	47.4	48.3	48.6	48.3	47.5	52.6	51.7	51.4	51.7	52.5	15.4	17	17	17.2	16.6
71	Guinea	5.3	5.5	5.3	5.3	5.8	14.8	16.3	16.9	16.8	15.5	85.2	83.7	83.1	83.2	84.5	5.1	5.4	4.9	4.8	4.8
72	Guinea-Bissau	5.1	5	5.6	6.1	6.3	35	41.8	47.7	46.6	48.2	65	58.2	52.3	53.4	51.8	7.1	6.6	6.1	6.6	8.5
73	Guyana	5	4.8	5.1	5.3	5.6	83.4	84	82.7	79.9	76.3	16.6	16	17.3	20.1	23.7	9.3	9.1	9.9	11.6	11.1
74	Haiti	7.2	6.8	6.8	7.1	7.6	35.4	36.3	36	37.7	39.4	64.6	63.7	64	62.3	60.6	19.7	18.5	20.7	23.8	23.8
75	Honduras	5.6	5.7	5.9	6.2	6.2	51.9	50.8	52.5	52.1	51.2	48.1	49.2	47.5	47.9	48.8	14.1	13.7	13.6	14	14
76	Hungary	7.3	7.4	7.1	7.4	7.8	74.8	72.4	70.7	69	70.2	25.2	27.6	29.3	31	29.8	10.1	11.4	11.7	10.4	10.4
77	Iceland	8.6	9.4	9.2	9.2	9.9	83	83.9	83.6	83.2	84	17	16.1	16.4	16.8	16	16.8	18.1	17.8	17.4	18.1
78	India	5.2	5.7	6.3	6.1	6.1	26.5	23.6	20.9	20.7	21.3	73.5	76.4	79.1	79.3	78.7	5.2	4.8	4.6	4.4	4.4
79	Indonesia[c]	2.5	2.6	2.8	3	3.2	27.8	29.6	25.4	35.8	36	72.2	70.4	74.6	64.2	64	3.3	3.8	3.5	4.7	5.4
80	Iran, Islamic Republic of	5.8	5.9	5.7	6.1	6	45.3	43.4	41.6	44.3	47.8	54.7	56.6	58.4	55.7	52.2	10.9	10.9	11	11.1	9
81	Iraq[d]	2	1.9	1.7	1.6	1.5	51	39.6	29.1	27.1	16.9	49	60.4	70.9	72.9	83.1	1.9	1.2	1.3	1.2	0.7
82	Ireland	6.2	6.3	6.4	6.9	7.3	76.5	72.8	73.3	75.6	75.2	23.5	27.2	26.7	24.4	24.8	13.6	13.2	14.5	15.5	16.4
83	Israel	8.4	8.5	8.5	9.6	9.1	72.1	69.4	67.2	66.5	65.7	27.9	30.6	32.8	33.5	34.3	11.5	11.2	11.1	11.8	10.9
84	Italy	7.7	7.8	8.1	8.3	8.5	71.8	72.3	73.7	76	75.6	28.2	27.7	26.3	24	24.4	11.1	11.5	12.8	13	13.3
85	Jamaica	5.9	5.5	6.4	6	6	58.6	50.3	52.6	43.4	57.4	41.4	49.7	47.4	56.6	42.6	7.4	5.6	6.6	4.3	5.9
86	Japan[e]	7.2	7.4	7.6	7.8	7.9	80.8	81.1	81.3	81.7	81.7	19.2	18.9	18.7	18.3	18.3	14	15.9	16.1	16.9	17
87	Jordan	8.6	8.9	9.2	9.4	9.3	53.6	48.2	45.2	45.7	46.1	46.4	51.8	54.8	54.3	53.9	12.5	12.1	12.1	12.5	12.5
88	Kazakhstan	3.8	4.3	4.1	3.4	3.5	55.1	51.9	50.9	56.4	53.2	44.9	48.1	49.1	43.6	46.8	9.7	9.6	9	8.2	8.9
89	Kenya	4.9	4.6	5.3	4.9	4.9	45.2	41.1	46.5	42.8	44	54.8	58.9	53.5	57.2	56	8	6.5	10.2	7.7	8.4
90	Kiribati	8.3	7.5	7.8	7.3	8	99	98.9	98.8	98.7	98.8	1	1.1	1.2	1.3	1.2	10.9	9.7	10	9.3	10.2
91	Kuwait	4.4	3.8	3.1	3.7	3.8	78.4	77.7	76.4	77.1	75.2	21.6	22.3	23.6	22.9	24.8	6.6	6.6	6.3	6.2	5.6
92	Kyrgyzstan	5.8	5.1	4.4	4.1	4.3	50.5	49.4	50	50.2	51.2	49.5	50.6	50	49.8	48.8	10.5	10.6	10.1	9.5	10.2
93	Lao People's Democratic Republic	2.5	3	2.9	3.1	2.9	48.6	49.4	53.3	55.5	50.9	51.4	50.6	46.7	44.5	49.1	5.7	8.8	7.6	8.7	8.7
94	Latvia	5.8	5.9	5.6	5.4	5.1	65.5	64	58.8	58.3	64.1	34.5	36	41.2	41.7	35.9	9.4	9.2	8.9	9.1	9.3
95	Lebanon	12.2	11.7	12	11.9	11.5	27.5	27.5	30.1	29.9	30.1	72.5	72.5	69.9	70.1	69.9	10.4	9.5	8.6	10.5	9.1
96	Lesotho	5.5	5.3	5.7	5.6	6.2	83.8	83	84.4	83.7	84.9	16.2	17	15.6	16.3	15.1	9.4	7.2	10	10.3	10.9
97	Liberia	5.3	5.2	3.7	2.9	2.1	80.4	81.4	74.7	71	68	19.6	18.6	25.3	29	32	9.9	11.4	7.8	5.9	5.5
98	Libyan Arab Jamahiriya	3.7	3.5	2.8	3.2	3.3	49.6	49.1	51.5	50.9	47.2	50.4	50.9	48.5	49.1	52.8	5.3	5.6	4.9	5	5
99	Lithuania	6.2	6.3	6.5	6.3	5.9	76˙	74.9	69.7	72.6	72.6	24	25.1	30.3	27.4	27.4	14.8	12.2	14.6	15.2	14
100	Luxembourg	5.9	6.2	5.5	5.9	6.2	90.9	89.7	89.7	89.8	85.4	9.1	10.1	10.3	10.2	14.6	12.8	13.5	12.9	13.5	12
101	Madagascar	2.2	2.2	2.1	1.9	2.1	56.5	53.7	52.7	64.1	55	43.5	46.3	47.3	35.9	45	7.4	6.9	6.5	7.1	8
102	Malawi	8.5	8.5	8.2	9.4	9.8	35.5	33.7	34.4	43.6	41.1	64.5	66.3	65.6	56.4	58.9	10.6	9.7	7.6	9.9	9.7
103	Malaysia	3	3.1	3.3	3.8	3.8	51.6	52.9	53.1	53.7	53.8	48.4	47.1	46.9	46.3	46.2	5.1	6	6.1	6.5	6.9
104	Maldives	5.5	5.6	5.9	6	5.8	85	85.2	86.9	87.5	87.7	15	14.8	13.1	12.5	12.3	13.3	13.2	13.7	13.8	12.5
105	Mali	4.2	4.1	4.7	4.4	4.5	45.7	42.9	49.7	50.1	50.8	54.3	57.1	50.3	49.9	49.2	7.6	6.6	8.5	8.2	9
106	Malta	8.4	8.3	8.8	9	9.7	69	67.5	68.4	71.3	71.8	31	32.5	31.6	28.7	28.2	11.9	11.8	13.1	13.6	14.3
107	Marshall Islands	9.7	9.5	9.8	9.8	10.6	66.4	65.2	65	64.7	67.3	33.6	34.8	35	35.3	32.7	10.9	10.8	9.6	9.6	10.9
108	Mauritania	2.7	2.7	2.5	2.9	3.9	63.9	64.2	63.3	67.9	74.2	36.1	35.8	36.7	32.1	25.8	6.9	7	6.5	8	10.1
109	Mauritius	2.8	3	2.8	2.8	2.9	68	71.5	72.8	75	76.9	32	28.5	27.2	25	23.1	7	7.2	6.6	7.6	8.3
110	Mexico	5.4	5.6	5.6	6	6.1	46	47.8	46.6	44.8	44.9	54	52.2	53.4	55.2	55.1	15.8	17.3	16.6	16.7	16.6

	Member State	External resources for health as % of total expenditure on health					Social security expenditure on health as % of general government expenditure on health					Out-of-pocket expenditure as % of private expenditure on health					Private prepaid plans as % of private expenditure on health				
		1998	1999	2000	2001	2002	1998	1999	2000	2001	2002	1998	1999	2000	2001	2002	1998	1999	2000	2001	2002
56	Equatorial Guinea	16.4	9.4	7.8	5.9	4.8	0	0	0	0	0	95.1	91.3	84.1	81.4	80.5	0	0	0	0	0
57	Eritrea	41.5	47.9	47.9	39.1	49.2	0	0	0	0	0	100	100	100	100	100	0	0	0	0	0
58	Estonia	1.5	3.5	0.9	0	0	77.1	82.1	86	86.1	86	96.6	71.3	84.9	84.7	83.9	n/a	4.1	4.1	4.8	4.4
59	Ethiopia	22.9	24.4	25.9	29.3	29.5	0.4	0.4	0.5	0.4	0.5	77.6	78.2	66.4	66.8	65.9	0.4	0.4	0.4	0.4	0.4
60	Fiji	7.7	11.1	10.9	10.1	5.6	0	0	0	0	0	100	100	100	100	100	0	0	0	0	0
61	Finland	0	0	0	0	0	19.4	19.8	20.4	20.7	21	81.9	82.2	81.9	82.2	82.2	11.1	10.8	10.5	10.1	9.8
62	France	0	0	0	0	0	96.8	96.7	96.6	96.5	96.8	43.1	43	43.4	42.1	40.9	52.6	52.6	52.2	53.6	54.9
63	Gabon	3.6	3.1	1.2	1.6	2.8	2.2	3.1	3.1	2.8	2.8	100	100	100	100	100	n/a	n/a	n/a	n/a	n/a
64	Gambia	26.2	31.6	39	33.5	40.6	0	0	0	0	0	68.5	65.1	64.4	64.6	64.3	n/a	n/a	n/a	n/a	n/a
65	Georgia	5	8.1	11	13.8	12.6	39.3	54.4	47.9	42.3	27.6	99.6	99.4	98.9	96.9	98.7	0.4	0.6	1.1	3.1	1.3
66	Germany	0	0	0	0	0	87	87.2	87.3	87.1	87.4	52.4	50.8	49.7	49.6	48.2	37.3	38.2	39.2	39.2	39.9
67	Ghana	6.2	6.1	12.1	17.6	18.5	n/a	n/a	n/a	n/a	n/a	100	100	100	100	100	0	0	0	0	0
68	Greece	n/a	n/a	n/a	n/a	n/a	37.5	35.4	32.3	36.5	35.6	71	69.5	69.1	68.8	66.9	4.2	4.1	4.1	4.1	3.9
69	Grenada	0.9	n/a	n/a	n/a	13.2	0	0	0	0	0	100	100	100	100	100	0	0	0	0	0
70	Guatemala	5.4	5.3	4.5	1.4	4.4	55.3	54.8	54.8	54.1	56.4	93.2	85.6	86.2	85.7	86.2	4.5	5.4	5.2	5.3	5.2
71	Guinea	12.7	13.5	13.8	12.5	9.5	1.6	1.5	1.4	1.5	1.4	99.4	99.4	99.4	99.4	99.5	0	0	0	0	0
72	Guinea-Bissau	25.2	29.4	30.7	31.8	35.9	0.2	0.2	0.1	0.1	0.1	100	100	100	100	100	0	0	0	0	0
73	Guyana	3.6	4	3.1	2.2	2.6	0	0	0	0	0	100	100	100	100	100	0	0	0	0	0
74	Haiti	26	27.3	27.9	23.6	15.6	0	0	0	0	0	67.1	68.9	68.9	71	69.5	n/a	n/a	n/a	n/a	n/a
75	Honduras	10.1	13.1	9.5	6.3	8	15.9	16.6	16.5	17.3	17.3	85.5	85.6	85.4	85.4	85.4	7.2	7.2	7.3	7.2	7.3
76	Hungary	0	0	0	0	0	83.4	83.8	83.9	83.3	81.3	88.4	90	89.8	89.3	88.2	0.2	0.3	0.6	1	1.3
77	Iceland	0	0	0	0	0	29.8	26.8	29.2	28	27	100	100	100	100	100	0	0	0	0	0
78	India	2.8	1.1	1.7	0.4	1	3.8	4.2	4.1	4.1	4.6	98.4	98.6	98.8	98.5	98.5	0.4	0.5	0.5	0.6	0.7
79	Indonesia[c]	8.3	8.3	6.6	2.9	1.8	8.7	6.8	6.8	8	9.3	74.3	70.6	72.8	76	76.1	6.7	10.4	8.2	4.1	5.2
80	Iran, Islamic Republic of	0	0	0.1	0.4	0.3	41.6	41.1	42.8	41	37	97.4	96.2	96.6	97.3	96.4	1.7	2.7	2.5	1.9	2.9
81	Iraq[d]	0.3	1	0.9	1.5	0.6	n/a	n/a	n/a	n/a	n/a	100	100	100	100	100	n/a	n/a	n/a	n/a	n/a
82	Ireland	0	0	0	0	0	1.1	1.1	1.2	0.9	0.8	45.6	51.4	50.5	48.8	53	38.1	29.3	28.4	26	21.6
83	Israel	0	1.6	2.6	3.6	3.9	65.1	63.4	62.5	61.7	62.4	100	94.8	92.1	89.3	87.8	0	0	0	0	0
84	Italy	0	0	0	0	0	0.1	0.1	0.1	0.3	0.1	86.9	86.7	86.2	83.9	83.3	3.3	3.4	3.4	3.7	3.7
85	Jamaica	2.6	2.6	1.8	3.3	4.1	0	0	0	0	0	66.6	69.5	65	69.3	61.8	27.3	25.1	30	26.2	32.5
86	Japan[e]	0	0	0	0	0	80.9	81.2	80.9	80.5	80.5	91.1	90.6	90.1	89.9	89.8	1.5	1.5	1.7	1.5	1.5
87	Jordan	7.1	6.6	5.9	5.7	5.2	0.8	0.8	0.9	0.7	0.7	86.7	73.5	74.7	74.5	74.3	5.1	5.3	5.5	7.3	7.1
88	Kazakhstan	0.7	0.8	0.7	0.7	0.6	28.6	0	0	0	0	100	100	100	100	100	0	0	0	0	0
89	Kenya	12.8	13.3	13.2	17.2	16.4	6.2	16.7	11.7	14.8	9.2	79.6	79.3	80.1	80.5	80	7.4	7.4	7.1	6.8	6.9
90	Kiribati	n/a	n/a	2.2	4.7	3	0	0	0	0	0	100	100	100	100	100	0	0	0	0	0
91	Kuwait	0	0	0	0	0	0	0	0	0	0	96.8	96.5	95.3	95.3	94.3	3.2	3.5	4.7	4.7	5.7
92	Kyrgyzstan	10.3	15.4	16.4	15.6	14	3.4	8	9.2	9.7	9	100	100	100	100	100	n/a	n/a	n/a	n/a	n/a
93	Lao People's Democratic Republic	20.4	19.5	19.7	21.1	9.6	n/a	n/a	n/a	n/a	n/a	80	80	80	80	80	n/a	n/a	n/a	n/a	n/a
94	Latvia	0.8	0.7	0.6	0.6	0.5	49.3	50	57	52	49.6	100	100	100	99.1	99	0	0	0	0.9	1
95	Lebanon	2	1	0.5	0.5	0.5	45.5	45.5	43.9	43	43.7	82.3	82.3	80.3	80.3	80	15.4	15.4	17.2	17.2	17.5
96	Lesotho	4.2	3.7	11.1	16.5	20.8	0	0	0	0	0	9.1	8	7.5	8.5	7	n/a	n/a	n/a	n/a	n/a
97	Liberia	67.1	67	56.4	44	40.8	0	0	0	0	0	97.1	97.2	96.2	96.2	95.7	0	0	0	0	0
98	Libyan Arab Jamahiriya	0	0	0	0	0	0	0	0	0	0	100	100	100	100	100	0	0	0	0	0
99	Lithuania	0	0.6	0.7	0.7	0.6	89.9	89.8	88.3	84.3	86.2	95.8	99.6	86.2	97	98.2	0.1	0.1	0.3	0.2	0.5
100	Luxembourg	0	0	0	0	0	82.7	93.1	94	94.4	94	82.4	72.6	72.7	74.2	81.8	17.6	13.7	14	13.6	9.4
101	Madagascar	34.8	40.5	43.1	38.8	32.2	n/a	n/a	n/a	n/a	n/a	89.2	89.7	89.7	85	88.8	10.8	10.3	10.3	15	11.2
102	Malawi	29.8	37	39.2	32.9	37.6	0	0	0	0	0	40.4	43.1	42.3	42.8	42.6	1.8	1.8	1.8	1.9	1.7
103	Malaysia	1.1	1	0.8	0	0	0.9	1	0.9	1.1	1	94.2	93.9	93.4	92.8	92.8	5.8	6.1	6.6	7.2	7.2
104	Maldives	12.6	7.7	3.3	1.8	3.4	24.1	21.3	20.5	24.9	23.8	100	100	100	100	100	0	0	0	0	0
105	Mali	24.2	18.8	24.2	20.8	18.2	18	24	21.8	22.9	27.7	89.3	89.3	89.4	89.1	88.8	0	0	0	0	0
106	Malta	0	0	0	0	0	78.5	78.3	75.5	72.1	66.7	82.5	82.7	73.7	88.5	81.2	7.2	7	6.9	7.4	7.2
107	Marshall Islands	13.5	38.2	36.5	25.4	22.7	0	0	0	0	0	100	100	100	100	100	0	0	0	0	0
108	Mauritania	5.8	5.5	5.7	4.9	3.3	0	0	0	0	0	100	100	100	100	100	0	0	0	0	0
109	Mauritius	1.4	1.2	1.1	1.6	1.8	6.3	5.8	7.3	7.7	7.2	100	100	100	100	100	4.1	4.1	4.7	5	5.4
110	Mexico	0.9	1.2	1	0.9	0.8	72.4	69.1	67.6	66.3	66	95.9	95.9	95.3	95	94.6	4.1	4.1	4.7	5	5.4

Annex Table 5 Selected national health accounts indicators: measured levels of expenditure on health, 1998–2002

Figures computed by WHO to assure comparability;[a] they are not necessarily the official statistics of Member States, which may use alternative rigorous methods.

	Member State	Total expenditure on health as % of gross domestic product					General government expenditure on health as % of total expenditure on health[b]					Private expenditure on health as % of total expenditure on health[b]					General government expenditure on health as % of total government expenditure				
		1998	1999	2000	2001	2002	1998	1999	2000	2001	2002	1998	1999	2000	2001	2002	1998	1999	2000	2001	2002
111	Micronesia, Federated States of	6.6	6.4	6.5	6.5	6.5	88.2	88	86.8	86.9	88.2	11.8	12	13.2	13.1	11.8	7.9	7.9	8	8.8	8.8
112	Monaco	10.5	8.5	10.2	9.8	11	75.7	73.5	75.7	76.6	79.6	24.3	26.5	24.3	23.4	20.4	13.2	10.3	12.9	12.5	14.6
113	Mongolia	6.2	6.1	6.3	6.4	6.6	65.4	66.5	70.3	72.3	70.4	34.6	33.5	29.7	27.7	29.6	9	9.8	10.5	10.5	10.6
114	Morocco	4.4	4.4	4.7	4.6	4.6	28.3	29.1	33.9	32.5	32.8	71.7	70.9	66.1	67.5	67.2	4.1	4	4.6	4.2	4.9
115	Mozambique	4.1	4.5	5.1	5.5	5.8	57.7	61.9	66.5	69.8	71	42.3	38.1	33.5	30.2	29	12.2	14.2	16.3	18.2	19.9
116	Myanmar	1.8	1.8	2.2	2.1	2.2	10.6	11	13.7	12.5	18.5	89.4	89	86.3	87.5	81.5	0.7	0.8	1.2	1.3	2.3
117	Namibia	6.8	7	6.9	6.9	6.7	72.4	73.3	68.9	71.1	70.1	27.6	26.7	31.1	28.9	29.9	13.2	13.1	12.4	13	12.9
118	Nauru	7.9	7.7	7.7	7.5	7.6	89	89.1	88.9	88.7	88.8	11	10.9	11.1	11.3	11.2	9.1	9.2	9.2	9.1	9.2
119	Nepal	5.1	4.8	4.7	4.9	5.2	25.6	21.4	21	24.7	27.2	74.4	78.6	79	75.3	72.8	7	5.9	5.6	6.2	7.5
120	Netherlands	7.9	8	7.9	8.3	8.8	67.2	65.9	66.5	65.9	65.6	32.8	34.1	33.5	34.1	34.4	11.2	11.2	11.5	11.7	12.2
121	New Zealand	7.9	7.8	7.9	8	8.5	77	77.5	78	76.4	77.9	23	22.5	22	23.6	22.1	13.5	13.9	14.5	14.5	15.5
122	Nicaragua	7.3	6.9	7.6	7.6	7.9	49.3	45.8	49.3	49.2	49.1	50.7	54.2	50.7	50.8	50.9	15.3	11.2	13.1	12.9	15.2
123	Niger	3.9	4.5	4.5	4.3	4	40.2	50.2	50.8	49	50.8	59.8	49.8	49.2	51	49.2	9.2	12.5	12.3	10.8	10
124	Nigeria	5.5	5.4	4.4	4.5	4.7	26.1	29.1	33.5	31.4	25.6	73.9	70.9	66.5	68.6	74.4	7.1	5.4	5.9	3.4	3.3
125	Niue	7.8	7.9	7.6	9.3	9.7	98.4	98.4	98.4	98.4	98.4	1.6	1.6	1.6	1.6	1.6	12.8	12.9	12.4	15.2	16
126	Norway	8.5	8.5	7.7	8.9	9.6	84.7	85.2	85	83.4	83.5	15.3	14.8	15	16.6	16.5	15.6	16.3	16.5	18.1	18.1
127	Oman	3.7	3.6	3.2	3.1	3.4	81.6	83.2	78.8	82.1	81.6	18.4	16.8	21.2	17.9	18.4	7.3	7.9	7.3	6.9	7.3
128	Pakistan	3.5	3.6	3.3	3.2	3.2	35.6	30.3	32.4	32.7	34.9	64.4	69.7	67.6	67.3	65.1	4.2	3.7	3.3	3.5	3.2
129	Palau	8.9	9	9	9.2	9.1	92.9	91.4	91.7	92	91	7.1	8.6	8.3	8	9	11.3	11.3	11.3	11.6	11.4
130	Panama	9	7.7	9	8.6	8.9	73.5	69.4	71.9	71.4	71.7	26.5	30.6	28.1	28.6	28.3	27.4	22.3	26	23.4	23.1
131	Papua New Guinea	3.8	4.2	4.3	4.4	4.3	90.9	89.9	89.7	89	88.6	9.1	10.1	10.3	11	11.4	12.3	13.3	12.9	13	13
132	Paraguay	6.5	7.2	8.4	8.4	8.4	45.5	44.9	40.2	35.2	38.1	54.5	55.1	59.8	64.8	61.9	16.2	16.7	17.5	15.9	17.5
133	Peru	4.5	4.9	4.7	4.6	4.4	52.6	53.1	53	52	49.9	47.4	46.9	47	48	50.1	12	12.3	12.1	12.4	12.4
134	Philippines	3.5	3.5	3.4	3.2	2.9	42.5	43.7	47.1	43.6	39.1	57.5	56.3	52.9	56.4	60.9	6.5	6.5	7	5.8	4.7
135	Poland	6	5.9	5.7	6	6.1	65.4	71.1	70	71.9	72.4	34.6	28.9	30	28.1	27.6	9.4	10.6	10.2	10.9	9.8
136	Portugal	8.4	8.7	9.2	9.3	9.3	67.1	67.6	69.5	70.6	70.5	32.8	32.3	30.4	29.3	29.3	12.8	13	14.1	14.3	14.2
137	Qatar	4	3.5	2.8	2.9	3.1	76.9	76.2	75.6	75.5	78.2	23.1	23.8	24.4	24.5	21.8	6.8	6.9	6.7	6.8	6.8
138	Republic of Korea	4.3	4.6	4.4	5.1	5	46.9	46.9	49	54.5	52.9	53.1	53.1	51	45.5	47.1	8.4	9.4	9.7	11.5	10.7
139	Republic of Moldova	6.9	6.8	6.4	6.3	7	63.3	45.9	51.8	51.9	58.2	36.7	54.1	48.2	48.1	41.8	9.7	8.5	9.8	11.2	12.9
140	Romania	5.2	5.8	5.8	6.1	6.3	59.6	64.9	67.9	67.8	65.9	40.4	35.1	32.1	32.2	34.1	8.8	10.6	11.2	12.4	12.7
141	Russian Federation	6.1	5.2	5.7	6	6.2	55.9	56	56.5	54.4	55.8	44.1	44	43.5	45.6	44.2	8	7.9	9.4	9.5	9.5
142	Rwanda	5	5.5	5.6	5.5	5.5	51.3	54	52.9	55.4	57.2	48.7	46	47.1	44.6	42.8	13.8	13.5	14.8	14	13.4
143	Saint Kitts and Nevis	5.2	5.5	5.6	5.4	5.5	62.5	60.1	63.7	64.2	62.1	37.5	39.9	36.3	35.8	37.9	10.8	10.4	10.4	10.9	9.7
144	Saint Lucia	4.5	4.6	4.8	5.1	5	67.5	68.8	69.8	68.9	68.4	32.5	31.2	30.2	31.1	31.6	10.1	10.2	10.7	11.8	11.5
145	Saint Vincent and the Grenadines	5.6	5.7	5.7	5.7	5.9	60.4	60.8	64	64.1	65.5	39.6	39.2	36	35.9	34.5	8.5	9	9.4	11.8	11.9
146	Samoa	5.8	6.2	5.8	5.6	6.2	73.5	74.1	77	82.2	75.9	26.5	25.9	23.1	17.8	24.1	13.1	12.9	14.7	13.9	13.9
147	San Marino	7	7.3	7.4	7.7	7.7	77.5	77.8	77.4	79.4	79.2	22.5	22.2	22.6	20.6	20.8	16.7	18.2	18	15.2	20.4
148	Sao Tome and Principe	8.8	10	9.4	10.5	11.1	82	87.3	86.2	87.6	87.7	18	12.7	13.8	12.4	12.3	12.1	12.5	12.3	11.4	14.5
149	Saudi Arabia	5	4.2	3.9	4.5	4.3	79.3	75.5	74.9	77.6	77.1	20.7	24.5	25.1	22.4	22.9	11.2	11.5	11.3	11.1	11.6
150	Senegal	4.2	4.5	4.7	5.2	5.1	36.8	38	42.1	45.1	45.2	63.2	62	57.9	54.9	54.8	8.3	8.3	10.3	10.8	11.2
151	Serbia and Montenegro	10.4	9.6	9.3	8.3	8.1	62.1	59.5	55.1	60	62.8	37.9	40.5	44.9	40	37.2	13.8	12.4	13.5	12.4	10.7
152	Seychelles	5.7	5.5	5.2	5.3	5.2	77.3	76.6	75.3	75.7	74.3	22.7	23.4	24.7	24.3	25.7	7.5	7.4	6.8	8.1	6.6
153	Sierra Leone	3	3.7	4.3	3.7	2.9	44.2	53.8	60.4	61	60.3	55.8	46.2	39.6	39	39.7	9.4	9.4	9.3	8.8	6.8
154	Singapore	4.2	4.1	3.6	3.9	4.3	41.6	38.3	35.2	33.5	30.9	58.4	61.7	64.8	66.5	69.1	8.7	8.2	6.7	5.9	5.9
155	Slovakia	5.7	5.9	5.7	5.7	5.9	91.6	89.9	89.7	89.6	89.4	8.4	10.1	10.3	10.4	10.6	8.6	9.4	8.5	10	10.3
156	Slovenia	7.8	7.7	8	8.3	8.3	75.7	75.5	76	74.9	74.9	24.3	24.5	24	25.1	25.1	14.3	14	13.5	14.6	14.7
157	Solomon Islands	4.5	4.9	4.9	5	4.8	93	93.4	93.4	93.5	93.2	7	6.6	6.6	6.5	6.8	11.4	11.1	11.4	11.5	11.8
158	Somalia	2.7	2.7	2.6	2.6	n/a	46.1	45	44.8	44.6	n/a	53.9	55	55.2	55.4	n/a	4.4	4.2	4.2	4.2	n/a
159	South Africa	8.4	8.8	8.4	8.7	8.7	44.8	41.1	42.4	41.2	40.6	55.2	58.9	57.6	58.8	59.4	11.5	10.8	11	11	10.7
160	Spain	7.5	7.5	7.5	7.5	7.6	72.2	72	71.6	71.4	71.3	27.8	28	28.4	28.6	28.7	13.1	13.4	13.3	13.6	13.6
161	Sri Lanka	3.4	3.5	3.6	3.6	3.7	51.3	49	49.2	48.9	48.7	48.7	51	50.8	51.1	51.3	5.8	5.7	6.1	6.1	6
162	Sudan	5.2	5.3	4.6	4.5	4.9	17.6	15.8	17.3	19.7	20.7	82.4	84.2	82.7	80.3	79.3	8.5	7.2	5.2	5.4	6.3
163	Suriname	7.3	5	9.4	8	8.6	61.7	59.6	43.3	39.6	41.8	38.3	40.4	56.7	60.4	58.2	10.2	8.9	9.9	9	10.3
164	Swaziland	7.1	6.4	6.1	6	6	56.6	59	58.6	57.9	59.5	43.4	41	41.4	42.1	40.5	13.5	11.8	11.6	11.3	10.9
165	Sweden	8.3	8.4	8.4	8.8	9.2	85.8	85.7	84.9	84.9	85.3	14.2	14.3	15.1	15.1	14.7	11.8	12	12.5	13.1	13.5

	Member State	External resources for health as % of total expenditure on health					Social security expenditure on health as % of general government expenditure on health					Out-of-pocket expenditure as % of private expenditure on health					Private prepaid plans as % of private expenditure on health				
		1998	1999	2000	2001	2002	1998	1999	2000	2001	2002	1998	1999	2000	2001	2002	1998	1999	2000	2001	2002
111	Micronesia, Federated States of	n/a	27.5	26.7	19.6	n/a	0	0	0	0	0	35.7	35.7	35.7	35.7	40	0	0	0	0	0
112	Monaco	0	0	0	0	0	98	98	98.2	98.3	98.5	79.2	81.5	77.8	77.8	81.5	20.8	18.5	22.2	22.2	18.5
113	Mongolia	9	18.9	17.2	15.4	0.7	39.9	39.7	40.2	40.3	40	74.5	74.1	73.9	73.4	74	0	0	0	0	0
114	Morocco	2.2	1.8	1.8	1.8	1.9	9	8.8	7.1	7.6	7.6	74.4	74.3	74.3	74.1	74	22.5	22.7	22.6	22.7	23
115	Mozambique	32.1	41.9	47.2	44.7	39.3	0	0	0	0	0	39	37.8	37.8	36	36.5	0.6	0.6	0.6	0.6	0.6
116	Myanmar	1.2	3.1	1.9	1.9	1	1.6	2.1	2	3.4	1.2	99.7	99.8	99.7	99.7	99.7	0	0	0	0	0
117	Namibia	2.5	2.4	3.8	4.3	5.2	1.4	1.2	1.8	1.9	1.5	21.9	21.3	18.2	20	20.5	74.5	74.7	77.3	75.2	74.8
118	Nauru	n/a	n/a	n/a	n/a	n/a	0	0	0	0	0	100	100	100	100	100	0	0	0	0	0
119	Nepal	10.9	9.3	13.8	13.3	9	0	0	0	0	0	92.4	92.5	92.2	92.2	92.2	0	0	0	0	0
120	Netherlands	0	0	0	0	0	93.9	93.8	93.9	93.8	93.8	26.9	27.7	28.2	26.7	24.5	52.1	51.1	49.8	49.8	52.3
121	New Zealand	0	0	0	0	0	0	0	0	0	0	70.8	70.7	69.9	72	72.6	27.7	27.6	28.5	26.5	25.9
122	Nicaragua	9.1	8.5	7.9	7.9	9.3	23	31.5	27	31.3	28.1	98.1	95.6	92.9	92.9	96	1.9	4.4	7.1	7.1	4
123	Niger	17.4	28.9	45.2	33.5	37.7	3.5	2.6	2.8	3.1	2.9	84.2	90.5	82.8	83	94.6	4.9	5.1	4.8	4.9	5.4
124	Nigeria	13.1	13.8	16.2	5.6	6.1	0	0	0	0	0	95	94.8	92.7	91.4	90.4	2.4	3.4	5.1	6.5	6.7
125	Niue	n/a	n/a	n/a	n/a	n/a	0	0	0	0	0	100	100	100	100	100	0	0	0	0	0
126	Norway	0	0	0	0	0	0	0	0	0	0	96.6	96.6	96.7	97.1	97.2	0	0	0	0	0
127	Oman	0	0	0.1	0	0	0.1	0.1	0.1	0.1	0.1	51	49.8	55.9	46.5	51.4	49	50.2	44.1	53.5	48.6
128	Pakistan	2.7	2.2	3.5	3.5	1.8	41.6	44.9	39.6	43.3	42.9	98.4	98.6	98.5	98.4	98.3	n/a	n/a	n/a	n/a	n/a
129	Palau	13.5	11.9	11.4	11.8	n/a	0	0	0	0	0	100	100	100	100	100	0	0	0	0	0
130	Panama	0.9	1	0.9	0.5	0.9	39.5	43.5	41	45.3	45.7	83.5	82.4	81.5	84.5	81.8	16.5	17.6	18.5	15.5	18.2
131	Papua New Guinea	29	18.5	22.1	22.8	34.3	0	0	0	0	0	86.4	83.4	83.9	83.3	83.3	4.8	9.4	9.3	9.4	9.4
132	Paraguay	2.1	2.1	1.8	2.3	2.1	50.5	48.1	53	47.7	30.1	88.6	85.6	88.6	87	88.6	11.4	14.4	11.4	13	11.4
133	Peru	1.4	1.4	1.2	4.6	4.6	38.9	43.5	42.9	42.9	42.9	87.1	82.6	79.4	79.4	79.4	9.3	13.6	17.2	17.2	17.2
134	Philippines	2.8	3.7	3.5	3.7	2.8	8.9	11.5	14.9	18.2	23.4	80.6	77	76.6	77.8	77.9	15.5	18	18	17	17.9
135	Poland	0	0	0	0	0	0	83.5	82.6	83.8	87.4	100	100	100	100	100	n/a	n/a	n/a	n/a	n/a
136	Portugal	0	0	0	0	0	7.7	7.1	6.5	6.5	6.5	94.9	95.3	95.7	95.5	95.7	4.7	4.3	4.3	4.5	4.3
137	Qatar	0	0	0	0	0	0	0	0	0	0	87	86.7	86.2	85.7	85.4	0	0	0	0	0
138	Republic of Korea	0	0	0	0	0	80.8	78.7	79.6	81.4	81	85.8	84.4	81.5	81.3	82.3	5	4.1	5.9	4.9	4.2
139	Republic of Moldova	1.1	16.1	33	8.4	2.8	0	0	0	0	0	100	100	100	100	100	n/a	n/a	n/a	n/a	n/a
140	Romania	2.7	2.6	2	1.7	0.8	64.4	77.8	80.3	77.5	77.3	82.6	90.1	92	94.6	88.7	17.4	9.9	8	5.4	5.5
141	Russian Federation	0.7	0.9	0.2	0.2	0.2	34.4	32.9	40.6	40	41	57.1	69.7	72.5	68.8	63.6	3.9	3.7	3.8	10.3	14.7
142	Rwanda	50.5	27.8	36.8	29.6	32.8	0.6	0.6	0.6	0.6	0.6	67	64.6	61.3	66.1	65.2	0.3	0.3	0.3	0.3	0.3
143	Saint Kitts and Nevis	6.4	5.7	5.2	5	4.7	0	0	0	0	0	100	100	100	100	100	n/a	n/a	n/a	n/a	n/a
144	Saint Lucia	0.5	0.5	0.5	0.6	0.1	16.2	12.5	19.4	21	22.3	100	100	100	100	100	n/a	n/a	n/a	n/a	n/a
145	Saint Vincent and the Grenadines	0.2	0.2	0.2	0.2	0.2	0	0	0	0	0	100	100	100	100	100	n/a	n/a	n/a	n/a	n/a
146	Samoa	15.8	13.8	19.1	15.6	8.7	0.6	0.3	0.3	0.2	0.3	79.4	80.1	81.7	87.5	79.8	0	0	0	0	0
147	San Marino	0	0	0	0	0	96.5	97.6	94.5	96	95.5	96.4	96.5	96.7	96.7	96.8	3.6	3.5	3.3	3.3	3.2
148	Sao Tome and Principe	48.5	59.9	57.5	61.8	60.2	0	0	0	0	0	100	100	100	100	100	0	0	0	0	0
149	Saudi Arabia	0	0	0	0	0	0	0	0	0	0	34	32.5	30.1	30.4	30.1	38	39	40.5	39.9	40.1
150	Senegal	13.1	12.7	12.9	17.1	16.9	18.9	18.3	15.3	14.3	14	97.8	97.8	97.8	96.5	96.5	2.2	2.2	2.2	2.2	3.5
151	Serbia and Montenegro	0.1	1.1	1.7	1.1	0.3	98.4	96.3	93.8	94.5	94	100	100	100	100	100	0	0	0	0	0
152	Seychelles	8	7.5	6.8	6.8	7.5	5	11.3	5.2	5.1	5	62.8	62.8	61.4	63.6	60.4	0	0	0	0	0
153	Sierra Leone	18.8	22.2	25.4	25.1	16.5	0	0	0	0	0	100	100	100	100	100	0	0	0	0	0
154	Singapore	0	0	0	0	0	17.6	19	23.3	24.5	26.1	97.3	97.4	97.2	97	97.3	0	0	0	0	0
155	Slovakia	0.1	0.1	0	0	0	96.6	91.2	91.3	91.9	92.7	100	100	100	100	100	0	0	0	0	0
156	Slovenia	0	0	0.1	0.1	0.1	87.9	87.5	87.5	87.2	87.1	44.4	39.3	38.6	41.7	40.9	55.6	60.7	61.4	58.3	58.3
157	Solomon Islands	7.7	7.1	16.5	16.5	41	0	0	0	0	0	45.8	47.1	48.3	49.2	49.2	0	0	0	0	0
158	Somalia	5.3	6.1	9	9.3	0	0	0	0	0	n/a	100	100	100	100	n/a	0	0	0	0	n/a
159	South Africa	0.2	0.1	0.4	0.4	0.3	4	3.5	3.3	3.1	3.8	23.6	21	22.8	21.8	20.9	74.7	77.4	75.6	76.7	77.7
160	Spain	0	0	0	0	0	11.8	9.4	9.6	9.2	7.2	83.6	83.3	83.1	82.9	82.5	13.1	13.4	13.6	14	14.5
161	Sri Lanka	2.8	2.7	2.7	3.1	1.9	0	0	0	0	0	94.9	95.1	95	95	95.1	1	1	1.1	1.1	1
162	Sudan	1.7	2.9	2	2.5	2.6	0	0	0	0	0	99.6	99.6	99.5	99.5	99.5	0	0	0	0	0
163	Suriname	9.5	17.6	9.7	13.2	6.6	34.9	33.3	40.7	36.7	22.2	33.7	32.7	61.5	69.8	61.6	1.4	1.3	0.6	0.5	0.4
164	Swaziland	18.8	10.3	5.5	4.1	3.5	0	0	0	0	0	34.9	40.9	42.4	41.8	41.7	16.6	18.6	18.9	20	20
165	Sweden	0	0	0	0	0	0	0	0	0	0	100	100	100	100	100	0	0	0	0	0

Annex Table 5 Selected national health accounts indicators: measured levels of expenditure on health, 1998–2002

Figures computed by WHO to assure comparability;[a] they are not necessarily the official statistics of Member States, which may use alternative rigorous methods.

	Member State	Total expenditure on health as % of gross domestic product					General government expenditure on health as % of total expenditure on health[b]					Private expenditure on health as % of total expenditure on health[b]					General government expenditure on health as % of total government expenditure				
		1998	1999	2000	2001	2002	1998	1999	2000	2001	2002	1998	1999	2000	2001	2002	1998	1999	2000	2001	2002
166	Switzerland	10.3	10.5	10.4	10.9	11.2	54.9	55.3	55.6	57.1	57.9	45.1	44.7	44.4	42.9	42.1	15.7	16.7	17.1	17.9	18.7
167	Syrian Arab Republic	5.3	5.5	5.1	5	5.1	40.4	41	43	45	45.8	59.6	59	57	55	54.2	7.1	7.2	7.3	6.7	6.5
168	Tajikistan	3.3	3.8	3.3	3.3	3.3	34.6	27.6	28.1	28.9	27.7	65.4	72.4	71.9	71.1	72.3	7.2	6.3	6.4	6.5	5.7
169	Thailand	3.9	3.7	3.6	3.5	4.4	56.8	57.1	58.3	58.9	69.7	43.2	42.9	41.7	41.1	30.3	12.4	11.5	11.8	11.5	17.1
170	The former Yugoslav Republic of Macedonia	7.8	6.3	6	6.1	6.8	87.4	85.2	84.6	83.1	84.7	12.6	14.8	15.4	16.9	15.3	19.4	15.1	15	12.3	14
171	Timor-Leste	7.7	8.5	6.9	9.6	9.7	67.9	70.7	65.7	64.4	63.9	32.1	29.3	34.3	35.6	36.1	6.7	7.7	5.8	9	9
172	Togo	10.5	10.7	9.9	10.1	10.5	20.2	22.2	14.8	14.3	10.8	79.8	77.8	85.2	85.7	89.2	9.4	12.4	7.5	8.6	7.8
173	Tonga	6.4	6.2	6.5	6.9	6.9	70.9	71.6	73.7	73.6	73.5	29.1	28.4	26.3	26.4	26.5	12.2	15.6	15.9	15.9	15.8
174	Trinidad and Tobago	4.1	3.9	3.7	3.5	3.7	45.2	44.3	40.3	39.9	37.3	54.8	55.7	59.7	60.1	62.7	5.5	5.6	5.6	5.6	5.7
175	Tunisia	5.9	5.6	5.6	5.8	5.8	50.3	52.3	48.5	51	49.9	49.7	47.7	51.5	49	50.1	7.8	7.8	6.9	8	7.5
176	Turkey	4.8	6.4	6.6	6.5	6.5	71.9	61.1	62.9	62.5	65.8	28.1	38.9	37.1	37.5	34.2	11.5	10.3	9.8	8.1	10.3
177	Turkmenistan	4	3.5	4.4	4.1	4.3	73.7	69.2	71.6	69.4	70.7	26.3	30.8	28.4	30.6	29.3	12.1	12.3	12.1	12.1	12.1
178	Tuvalu	5.2	5.4	5.5	5	4.4	59.3	57.3	53.5	53.4	46.7	40.7	42.7	46.5	46.6	53.3	3.7	3.6	1.8	2.9	1.5
179	Uganda	5.4	6.2	6.5	7.3	7.4	28.8	30.6	26.8	27.3	27.9	71.2	69.4	73.2	72.7	72.1	8.3	9.4	9	9.6	9.1
180	Ukraine	4.9	4.3	4.2	4.4	4.7	71.7	68.8	69	69.3	71.1	28.3	31.2	31	30.7	28.9	9.3	8.6	8.4	8.9	9.4
181	United Arab Emirates	4	3.5	3.4	3.4	3.1	77	75	75.5	75.1	73.4	23	25	24.5	24.9	26.6	7.7	7.2	7.3	6.9	7.3
182	United Kingdom	6.9	7.2	7.3	7.5	7.7	80.4	80.6	80.9	83	83.4	19.6	19.4	19.1	17	16.6	13.9	14.8	15	15.5	15.8
183	United Republic of Tanzania	4.6	4.6	4.8	5.2	4.9	49.3	47.8	51.6	55.3	54.8	50.7	52.2	48.4	44.7	45.2	14.3	14.8	14.6	16.9	14.9
184	United States of America	13	13	13.1	13.9	14.6	44.5	44.3	44.4	44.9	44.9	55.5	55.7	55.6	55.1	55.1	18.5	18.4	18.2	20	23.1
185	Uruguay	10.6	10.6	10.5	10.8	10	37.8	34.8	33.4	33.8	29	62.2	65.2	66.6	66.2	71	12	10.6	10.3	10.8	7.9
186	Uzbekistan	6.6	5.9	5.6	5.6	5.5	48.6	49.2	46.4	46.4	45.5	51.4	50.8	53.6	53.6	54.5	7.1	7	6.6	7.1	6.8
187	Vanuatu	3.7	3.7	3.7	3.6	3.8	70.4	71.8	71.8	73.1	73.6	29.6	28.2	28.2	26.9	26.4	11.9	12	12.6	12.6	12.8
188	Venezuela, Bolivarian Republic of	5.3	5.9	6	5.1	4.9	54.7	51.8	54.4	43.8	46.9	45.3	48.2	45.6	56.2	53.1	13	13.1	11.5	7.3	8
189	Viet Nam	4.9	4.9	5.2	5.1	5.2	32.7	32.7	28.1	28.2	29.2	67.3	67.3	71.9	71.8	70.8	7.1	6.7	6	6	6.1
190	Yemen	4.9	4.3	4.3	4.5	3.7	34.7	33.7	35.9	33.5	27.2	65.3	66.3	64.1	66.5	72.8	5.1	5	4.9	4.6	3.5
191	Zambia	6.6	5.5	5.4	5.7	5.8	53.7	51.2	52.2	52.8	52.9	46.3	48.8	47.8	47.2	47.1	11.5	9.9	8.5	9.4	11.3
192	Zimbabwe	11.4	8.1	7.9	7.7	8.5	55.9	48.9	52.2	47.4	51.6	44.1	51.1	47.8	52.6	48.4	12.2	10.4	8.3	9.6	12.2

[a] See explanatory notes for sources and methods.

[b] In some cases, sum of the ratios of general government and private expenditures on health may not add to 100 because of rounding.

[c] Information on expenditures by parastatals and other ministries (except the national family planning coordinating board (BKKBN)) was available for only 2001 and 2002.

[d] These are preliminary estimates while awaiting final confirmation of Oil for Food programme expenditures. Data do not include expenditures in the three northern governorates.

[e] Health data for 2002 have been largely developed by WHO, as they are not yet available through the OECD Health Data 2004.

n/a Used when the information accessed indicates that a cell should have an entry but no estimates could be made.

0 Used when no evidence of the schemes to which the cell relates exists. Some estimates yielding a ratio inferior to 0.04% are shown as 0.

	Member State	External resources for health as % of total expenditure on health					Social security expenditure on health as % of general government expenditure on health					Out-of-pocket expenditure as % of private expenditure on health					Private prepaid plans as % of private expenditure on health				
		1998	1999	2000	2001	2002	1998	1999	2000	2001	2002	1998	1999	2000	2001	2002	1998	1999	2000	2001	2002
166	Switzerland	0	0	0	0	0	72.3	72.1	72.6	70.4	69.1	72.6	74.5	74.1	73.9	74.8	25.2	23.3	23.6	23.8	22.9
167	Syrian Arab Republic	0.2	0.1	0.1	0.1	0.2	0	0	0	0	0	100	100	100	100	100	0	0	0	0	0
168	Tajikistan	13.7	14.5	18.3	16.9	14.9	0	0	0	0	0	100	100	100	100	100	0	0	0	0	0
169	Thailand	0.1	0.4	0.1	0.2	0.2	26.8	26.9	27.6	31	21.8	78.2	76.4	76.8	75.7	75.8	11.6	12.6	12.8	13.6	14.2
170	The former Yugoslav Republic of Macedonia	3.2	4.2	1.3	4	0.9	98	97.4	97.4	97.1	97.4	100	100	100	100	100	0	0	0	0	0
171	Timor-Leste	76.2	63.4	56.5	60.6	35.7	n/a	n/a	n/a	n/a	n/a	39.5	39.5	39.5	51.9	51.9	0	0	0	0	0
172	Togo	3.7	2.7	3.6	2.7	4.7	10.6	8.1	13.4	11.6	14.4	92.8	92.8	92.8	92.4	93.4	2.5	2.4	2.5	3	2.3
173	Tonga	21.3	23.9	24.6	23.7	24	0	0	0	0	0	100	100	100	100	100	0	0	0	0	0
174	Trinidad and Tobago	9	8.3	7.3	7.3	6.6	0	0	0	0	0	86.4	85.8	86.3	86.4	85.8	7.2	7.5	7.2	7.2	7.5
175	Tunisia	0.7	0.7	0.8	0.8	0.7	23.7	26.1	26.7	22.9	22.7	86.3	83	81.7	82.5	83	12	15.1	16.6	15.9	15.5
176	Turkey	0	0	0	0	0	50.6	53	55.5	56.9	49.6	99.6	74.8	74.6	88	88	0.2	10.9	11.8	12	12
177	Turkmenistan	0.9	2.1	1	0.8	0.7	6.4	6.3	6.4	6.4	6.4	100	100	100	100	100	0	0	0	0	0
178	Tuvalu	7.1	6.4	6.4	29.5	n/a	0	0	0	0	0	100	100	100	100	100	0	0	0	0	0
179	Uganda	30.9	27.6	28.3	27.4	28.8	0	0	0	0	0	71.2	61.5	56.7	51.8	52.3	0.3	0.2	0.1	0.2	0.2
180	Ukraine	0.4	0.3	0.7	0.7	3.6	0	0	0	0	0	97.8	96.9	95.4	95.4	95.5	1.7	2	2.3	2.5	2.4
181	United Arab Emirates	0	0	0	0	0	0	0	0	0	0	69.5	67.2	65.2	65.6	65.2	16.9	18.5	19.5	19.1	19.1
182	United Kingdom	0	0	0	0	0	0	0	0	0	0	55.7	55.2	54.7	58.1	55.9	17.4	16.8	16.6	18	18.6
183	United Republic of Tanzania	25.1	27	29.7	29.6	26.9	0	0	0	3.8	2.7	87.5	83.5	83	83.1	82.5	n/a	4.5	4.4	4.4	4.4
184	United States of America	0	0	0	0	0	33.4	33.1	33.7	32.8	30.8	28	27.6	27.1	26.2	25.4	61.1	61.8	63.2	64.7	65.7
185	Uruguay	0.6	0.1	0.5	0.8	0.6	49	52.6	50	47.7	53.7	30.1	26.6	25.9	24.9	25	69.9	73.4	74.1	75.1	75
186	Uzbekistan	0.1	0.9	1.8	2.9	5	0	0	0	0	0	100	100	100	100	100	0	0	0	0	0
187	Vanuatu	26	26.4	26.7	19.5	19.5	0	0	0	0	0	51	47.8	49.9	46.3	45.8	0	0	0	0	0
188	Venezuela, Bolivarian Republic of	1.2	1	0.4	0.1	0.1	18.6	25	28.5	33.6	30.8	89.7	88.5	87	87.4	87.2	4.8	4	3.7	3.7	4.1
189	Viet Nam	2.8	3.4	2.7	2.6	1.8	11.5	9.5	10.5	10.4	10.3	89.7	86.5	87.7	87.6	87.6	3.4	3.7	4.2	4.2	4.2
190	Yemen	7.7	5.3	4.7	3.6	3	n/a	n/a	n/a	n/a	n/a	87.7	86.6	85.9	86.8	85.8	n/a	n/a	n/a	n/a	n/a
191	Zambia	23.9	20.3	18.5	14	18.6	0	0	0	0	0	62.7	81.3	79.2	76.4	75.3	0	0	0	0	0
192	Zimbabwe	17.5	15.7	11.4	6.6	2.5	0	0	0	0	0	75.2	44.9	42.8	47.4	47.3	16.4	39.6	42.2	38.5	38.8

Annex Table 6 Selected national health accounts indicators: measured levels of per capita expenditure on health, 1998–2002

Figures computed by WHO to assure comparability;[a] they are not necessarily the official statistics of Member States, which may use alternative rigorous methods.

	Member State	Per capita total expenditure on health at average exchange rate (US$)					Per capita total expenditure on health at international dollar rate					Per capita government expenditure on health at average exchange rate (US$)					Per capita government expenditure on health at international dollar rate				
		1998	1999	2000	2001	2002	1998	1999	2000	2001	2002	1998	1999	2000	2001	2002	1998	1999	2000	2001	2002
1	Afghanistan	8	8	8	8	14	41	35	20	22	34	1	1	1	1	6	4	3	1	2	13
2	Albania	58	75	75	87	94	229	258	264	299	302	21	28	30	31	36	82	97	104	108	117
3	Algeria	62	61	65	70	77	139	141	139	158	182	41	41	45	52	57	91	93	97	118	135
4	Andorra	1654	1277	1205	1261	1382	2038	1642	1743	1854	1908	1301	914	845	895	975	1602	1175	1222	1316	1345
5	Angola	17	16	25	37	38	48	49	54	87	92	6	7	13	19	16	16	20	29	45	39
6	Antigua and Barbuda	404	412	424	456	470	433	448	466	507	527	290	297	305	323	322	311	323	335	359	361
7	Argentina	679	699	680	680	238	1061	1128	1110	1149	956	375	392	375	364	120	586	634	611	614	480
8	Armenia	34	42	32	48	45	155	200	161	246	232	9	13	10	10	10	38	62	48	53	53
9	Australia	1739	1889	1872	1776	1995	2110	2253	2439	2558	2699	1188	1319	1293	1213	1354	1441	1573	1684	1747	1832
10	Austria	2040	2047	1831	1806	1969	1953	2069	2147	2174	2220	1422	1426	1275	1238	1375	1362	1441	1495	1490	1551
11	Azerbaijan	26	26	25	26	27	102	107	104	111	120	5	6	6	6	6	20	23	23	26	27
12	Bahamas	1000	1042	1069	1084	1127	1032	1031	1089	1043	1074	450	488	505	515	548	464	482	514	495	522
13	Bahrain	474	474	483	490	517	760	752	684	749	792	334	332	334	345	372	537	526	474	527	570
14	Bangladesh	11	11	11	11	11	45	47	50	54	54	3	3	3	3	3	14	13	13	14	14
15	Barbados	533	571	601	634	669	821	876	922	993	1018	348	374	396	429	458	537	573	607	671	696
16	Belarus	90	73	64	82	93	411	438	478	556	583	74	59	51	62	69	337	355	383	419	430
17	Belgium	2109	2139	1952	1983	2159	2041	2139	2288	2441	2515	1481	1510	1376	1416	1537	1433	1510	1613	1743	1790
18	Belize	133	149	156	167	176	228	251	263	291	300	69	72	75	75	83	118	122	126	131	142
19	Benin	18	17	17	18	20	35	34	39	44	44	7	6	7	8	9	14	13	17	20	19
20	Bhutan	8	8	9	9	12	52	52	60	59	76	7	7	8	8	11	47	46	54	54	70
21	Bolivia	53	63	61	61	63	120	149	150	161	179	33	37	37	36	38	75	87	90	96	107
22	Bosnia and Herzegovina	76	135	114	113	130	170	304	291	293	322	21	76	59	55	65	46	172	151	143	161
23	Botswana	137	141	144	151	171	238	265	285	331	387	73	76	78	85	106	127	143	155	188	240
24	Brazil	348	246	266	227	206	519	550	567	596	611	153	105	109	98	94	228	236	232	255	280
25	Brunei Darussalam	463	448	470	429	430	644	601	646	644	653	376	356	376	336	336	524	477	517	504	510
26	Bulgaria	79	99	101	121	145	264	336	381	450	499	54	66	62	67	77	179	224	233	251	267
27	Burkina Faso	12	12	10	9	11	33	37	37	35	38	5	5	4	4	5	13	16	15	14	17
28	Burundi	5	4	3	3	3	16	15	15	16	16	1	1	1	1	1	3	3	3	3	3
29	Cambodia	25	28	30	30	32	134	146	172	181	192	3	3	4	4	5	14	15	24	27	33
30	Cameroon	28	31	28	28	31	55	62	62	64	68	5	8	8	7	8	9	15	17	17	18
31	Canada	1842	1916	2064	2124	2222	2291	2400	2541	2743	2931	1300	1348	1452	1488	1552	1617	1688	1788	1922	2048
32	Cape Verde	64	63	57	64	69	157	150	166	188	193	48	46	42	48	52	118	111	122	142	145
33	Central African Republic	10	10	10	10	11	40	43	47	48	50	3	4	4	4	4	14	16	19	19	21
34	Chad	12	12	11	12	14	35	39	43	45	47	4	4	5	5	6	11	13	18	19	20
35	Chile	325	293	281	253	246	607	598	595	621	642	118	112	119	110	111	221	230	251	271	290
36	China	36	40	48	52	63	154	175	212	233	261	14	15	17	18	21	60	67	73	82	88
37	Colombia	240	203	158	159	151	639	598	509	536	536	162	148	123	128	125	431	438	396	433	444
38	Comoros	11	10	8	7	10	32	30	25	22	27	7	6	4	3	6	20	18	14	10	16
39	Congo	20	19	19	17	18	36	28	23	24	25	14	13	13	12	13	26	19	16	17	18
40	Cook Islands	169	155	170	241	256	389	406	515	751	697	155	139	155	226	238	357	364	468	705	648
41	Costa Rica	304	324	339	358	383	572	597	642	685	743	211	221	226	234	250	397	406	428	446	486
42	Côte d'Ivoire	54	49	42	41	44	114	110	111	110	107	13	11	9	8	10	28	25	24	22	24
43	Croatia	387	387	374	366	369	575	628	689	674	630	330	333	323	313	300	490	541	595	576	513
44	Cuba	143	163	175	186	197	170	196	209	225	236	121	139	150	160	171	144	167	180	194	204
45	Cyprus	718	739	710	764	882	715	743	712	768	883	284	286	267	293	364	283	288	268	295	364
46	Czech Republic	391	380	358	408	504	916	932	977	1083	1118	359	347	327	373	461	841	853	892	990	1022
47	Democratic People's Republic of Korea[b]	16	19	21	23	0.3	29	47	52	56	57	12	14	15	17	0.2	22	36	38	41	44
48	Democratic Republic of the Congo	5	9	11	5	4	15	12	12	12	15	1	1	1	1	1	2	1	1	2	4
49	Denmark	2725	2767	2478	2565	2835	2141	2297	2353	2520	2583	2235	2275	2043	2120	2352	1755	1888	1940	2083	2142
50	Djibouti	52	52	52	51	54	75	74	74	74	78	27	27	27	26	28	39	39	39	38	41
51	Dominica	197	214	200	203	205	287	310	296	302	310	144	159	143	145	146	210	230	212	215	221
52	Dominican Republic	114	121	146	155	154	219	232	273	281	295	36	39	51	55	56	69	75	96	100	107
53	Ecuador	84	65	53	80	91	170	172	156	192	197	32	25	17	27	33	65	68	49	64	71
54	Egypt	64	67	67	59	59	162	171	181	194	192	22	24	24	22	21	56	61	64	73	70
55	El Salvador	165	163	170	169	178	347	347	357	353	372	70	71	76	72	80	148	151	161	150	166

	Member State	Per capita total expenditure on health at average exchange rate (US$)					Per capita total expenditure on health at international dollar rate					Per capita government expenditure on health at average exchange rate (US$)					Per capita government expenditure on health at international dollar rate				
		1998	1999	2000	2001	2002	1998	1999	2000	2001	2002	1998	1999	2000	2001	2002	1998	1999	2000	2001	2002
56	Equatorial Guinea	42	44	52	65	83	132	113	92	117	139	26	28	35	46	60	82	70	61	82	100
57	Eritrea	10	8	8	9	8	35	30	29	34	36	7	5	5	6	5	23	18	18	21	23
58	Estonia	223	244	221	224	263	494	548	548	557	604	193	196	169	174	201	426	440	421	433	461
59	Ethiopia	5	5	5	5	5	15	16	19	20	21	2	2	2	2	2	7	8	9	8	9
60	Fiji	82	85	80	79	94	197	194	203	209	240	54	56	52	53	60	129	127	132	140	155
61	Finland	1732	1710	1543	1628	1852	1607	1640	1698	1841	1943	1321	1288	1159	1228	1401	1226	1235	1276	1389	1470
62	France	2306	2282	2061	2103	2348	2231	2306	2416	2588	2736	1753	1735	1563	1596	1786	1696	1754	1832	1964	2080
63	Gabon	162	130	138	151	159	272	197	193	240	248	98	64	55	66	66	165	97	76	105	102
64	Gambia	23	23	23	21	18	70	72	82	85	83	6	8	10	9	8	17	25	36	37	37
65	Georgia	16	13	20	22	25	61	66	96	111	123	7	5	7	8	7	28	25	32	41	33
66	Germany	2772	2727	2398	2418	2631	2470	2563	2640	2735	2817	2179	2143	1889	1901	2066	1942	2015	2080	2151	2212
67	Ghana	22	23	14	15	17	61	67	68	71	73	9	9	6	6	7	26	27	28	29	30
68	Greece	1083	1146	1043	1044	1198	1428	1517	1617	1670	1814	564	612	562	554	634	743	810	872	887	960
69	Grenada	205	225	245	262	285	330	366	394	426	465	135	157	171	188	202	217	255	276	307	330
70	Guatemala	78	78	81	86	93	170	185	192	197	199	37	38	39	41	44	80	89	93	95	94
71	Guinea	24	24	20	20	22	83	90	89	93	105	4	4	3	3	3	12	15	15	16	16
72	Guinea-Bissau	8	8	9	9	9	29	30	37	40	38	3	4	4	4	5	10	13	18	19	18
73	Guyana	48	44	48	50	53	182	184	196	211	227	40	37	40	40	40	152	154	162	169	173
74	Haiti	32	34	31	31	29	76	74	75	79	83	11	12	11	12	12	27	27	27	30	33
75	Honduras	48	49	56	60	60	134	131	143	153	156	25	25	29	31	31	69	67	75	79	80
76	Hungary	335	345	326	375	496	775	820	847	961	1078	251	250	231	258	348	579	593	599	663	757
77	Iceland	2509	2849	2746	2478	2916	2252	2543	2561	2680	2802	2084	2389	2296	2061	2449	1870	2133	2141	2230	2353
78	India	22	26	29	29	30	66	78	89	92	96	6	6	6	6	6	17	18	19	19	20
79	Indonesia	12	18	20	21	26	73	78	86	99	110	3	5	5	7	9	20	23	22	35	40
80	Iran, Islamic Republic of	55	51	63	79	104	340	352	364	415	432	25	22	26	35	50	154	153	151	184	206
81	Iraq[c]	11	14	17	12	11	34	29	29	35	44	6	6	5	3	2	18	12	8	9	7
82	Ireland	1454	1589	1579	1839	2255	1487	1623	1775	2059	2367	1112	1157	1157	1390	1695	1138	1182	1300	1557	1779
83	Israel	1511	1498	1617	1754	1496	1666	1703	1828	2048	1890	1089	1040	1086	1166	983	1201	1182	1229	1362	1242
84	Italy	1600	1597	1506	1562	1737	1800	1853	2001	2107	2166	1149	1154	1109	1187	1314	1293	1339	1474	1602	1639
85	Jamaica	175	162	191	178	180	217	202	239	231	234	102	81	100	77	103	127	101	126	100	134
86	Japan[d]	2222	2601	2827	2558	2476	1742	1829	1958	2077	2133	1795	2109	2298	2089	2022	1407	1483	1591	1696	1742
87	Jordan	144	148	154	163	165	345	360	385	410	418	77	71	70	74	76	185	174	174	187	193
88	Kazakhstan	53	46	48	48	56	179	212	231	223	261	29	24	24	27	30	99	110	117	126	139
89	Kenya	19	16	18	18	19	68	64	73	70	70	9	7	8	8	8	31	26	34	30	31
90	Kiribati	47	49	45	40	49	137	126	129	124	141	46	48	44	40	49	135	125	127	122	139
91	Kuwait	557	531	516	539	547	730	598	486	560	552	437	412	395	416	411	573	465	372	432	415
92	Kyrgyzstan	20	13	12	13	14	134	122	111	111	117	10	6	6	6	7	68	60	56	56	60
93	Lao People's Democratic Republic	6	8	9	10	10	33	43	43	50	49	3	4	5	6	5	16	21	23	28	25
94	Latvia	159	179	182	190	203	381	410	423	456	477	104	114	107	111	130	250	262	249	266	306
95	Lebanon	588	569	577	583	568	675	669	703	727	697	162	157	174	174	171	186	184	211	218	210
96	Lesotho	28	27	27	23	25	93	89	98	102	119	24	23	23	20	21	78	74	83	86	101
97	Liberia	7	8	7	5	4	20	23	19	15	11	6	7	5	4	2	16	19	14	11	7
98	Libyan Arab Jamahiriya	210	207	175	158	121	246	230	191	219	222	104	102	90	81	57	122	113	98	111	105
99	Lithuania	194	194	212	220	241	451	457	507	538	549	148	145	148	159	175	342	343	353	391	399
100	Luxembourg	2610	2848	2459	2614	2951	2326	2731	2680	2899	3066	2373	2555	2206	2347	2521	2115	2451	2404	2603	2620
101	Madagascar	6	5	5	5	5	20	20	20	19	18	3	3	3	3	3	11	11	11	12	10
102	Malawi	15	14	12	14	14	42	43	42	46	48	5	5	4	6	6	15	14	14	20	20
103	Malaysia	99	109	129	143	149	236	255	294	342	349	51	58	69	77	80	122	135	156	183	188
104	Maldives	108	116	126	125	120	248	268	293	306	307	92	99	110	109	105	211	229	255	268	269
105	Mali	11	10	10	11	12	25	26	31	29	33	5	4	5	5	6	12	11	15	15	17
106	Malta	765	784	806	830	957	762	782	802	830	965	528	529	551	591	687	526	528	549	591	693
107	Marshall Islands	187	182	188	190	210	353	346	355	368	415	124	118	122	123	141	235	225	231	238	279
108	Mauritania	11	10	9	10	14	32	33	33	39	54	7	7	6	7	10	21	22	21	26	40
109	Mauritius	102	109	109	107	113	251	272	285	305	317	69	78	79	80	87	171	195	208	229	244
110	Mexico	232	271	321	367	379	427	460	491	533	550	107	129	149	165	170	196	220	228	239	247

Annex Table 6 Selected national health accounts indicators: measured levels of per capita expenditure on health, 1998–2002

Figures computed by WHO to assure comparability;[a] they are not necessarily the official statistics of Member States, which may use alternative rigorous methods.

	Member State	Per capita total expenditure on health at average exchange rate (US$)					Per capita total expenditure on health at international dollar rate					Per capita government expenditure on health at average exchange rate (US$)					Per capita government expenditure on health at international dollar rate				
		1998	1999	2000	2001	2002	1998	1999	2000	2001	2002	1998	1999	2000	2001	2002	1998	1999	2000	2001	2002
111	Micronesia, Federated States of	137	138	140	143	143	281	283	297	308	311	121	121	121	124	126	248	249	257	268	275
112	Monaco	3342	3267	3053	3051	3656	3014	3156	3533	3722	4258	2528	2400	2312	2337	2909	2280	2318	2676	2851	3388
113	Mongolia	24	21	23	25	27	106	110	115	119	128	16	14	16	18	19	69	73	81	86	90
114	Morocco	56	54	54	53	55	161	160	175	183	186	16	16	18	17	18	46	47	59	59	61
115	Mozambique	9	10	10	10	11	27	31	36	44	50	5	6	7	7	8	16	19	24	31	36
116	Myanmar[e]	102	135	184	229	315	20	21	28	28	30	11	15	25	29	58	2	2	4	3	6
117	Namibia	129	128	126	114	99	317	333	342	347	331	93	94	87	81	70	230	244	236	247	232
118	Nauru	640	700	645	585	656	1222	1317	1334	1327	1334	569	624	574	519	582	1087	1174	1185	1176	1184
119	Nepal	10	10	11	11	12	55	53	55	61	64	3	2	2	3	3	14	11	12	15	17
120	Netherlands	1977	2003	1821	1974	2298	1955	2025	2112	2377	2564	1328	1321	1211	1300	1508	1314	1335	1404	1566	1683
121	New Zealand	1125	1155	1054	1056	1255	1441	1527	1611	1710	1857	866	895	823	807	978	1110	1183	1257	1307	1447
122	Nicaragua	54	52	59	59	60	168	168	191	199	206	27	24	29	29	29	83	77	94	98	101
123	Niger	8	9	7	7	7	26	29	29	28	27	3	4	4	3	3	11	15	15	14	14
124	Nigeria	17	17	18	20	19	47	47	39	42	43	4	5	6	6	5	12	14	13	13	11
125	Niue	298	350	288	327	373	94	117	114	145	149	293	344	283	321	367	92	116	113	143	147
126	Norway	2865	3024	2850	3352	4033	2313	2561	2747	3258	3409	2427	2576	2422	2795	3366	1959	2182	2335	2716	2845
127	Oman	209	221	245	232	246	377	360	340	354	379	171	184	193	191	201	308	299	268	291	309
128	Pakistan	16	15	14	12	13	61	63	60	60	62	6	5	4	4	5	22	19	19	19	21
129	Palau	502	447	456	424	439	720	687	684	735	730	466	408	418	390	400	669	628	627	677	664
130	Panama	345	307	353	336	355	545	484	574	554	576	254	213	254	240	254	400	336	413	395	413
131	Papua New Guinea	29	28	27	24	22	124	143	143	143	136	26	25	25	21	19	113	128	128	127	120
132	Paraguay	107	105	119	102	82	270	299	346	352	343	49	47	48	36	31	123	134	139	124	131
133	Peru	102	98	96	94	93	209	227	226	225	226	53	52	51	49	47	110	120	120	117	113
134	Philippines	32	36	34	30	28	163	164	169	163	153	13	16	16	13	11	69	72	80	71	60
135	Poland	264	249	247	292	303	563	571	584	635	657	172	177	173	210	219	368	406	409	457	476
136	Portugal	932	985	951	994	1092	1290	1424	1570	1662	1702	625	665	660	702	770	866	962	1091	1173	1201
137	Qatar	736	759	844	862	935	920	822	716	797	894	566	578	638	650	731	707	626	542	601	700
138	Republic of Korea	319	438	483	524	577	571	690	748	923	982	149	206	237	286	305	268	324	367	504	519
139	Republic of Moldova	27	18	19	22	27	121	117	115	124	151	17	8	10	11	16	77	54	60	64	88
140	Romania	96	91	96	109	128	319	359	378	429	469	57	59	65	74	85	190	233	256	291	309
141	Russian Federation	112	70	102	128	150	371	345	428	485	535	62	39	58	70	84	208	193	242	264	298
142	Rwanda	15	14	13	11	11	39	42	43	44	48	8	8	7	6	6	20	22	23	25	27
143	Saint Kitts and Nevis	345	393	435	443	467	512	576	624	637	667	216	236	277	284	290	320	346	397	409	414
144	Saint Lucia	199	213	225	227	229	263	283	298	303	306	134	147	157	156	157	177	194	208	209	209
145	Saint Vincent and the Grenadines	153	161	162	166	180	286	306	314	318	340	92	98	104	106	118	173	186	201	204	223
146	Samoa	76	84	80	74	88	181	200	215	211	238	56	62	61	61	67	133	148	165	173	181
147	San Marino	2159	2346	2118	2315	2475	2429	2723	2815	3124	3094	1673	1825	1639	1837	1959	1882	2118	2179	2479	2449
148	Sao Tome and Principe	25	32	29	33	36	77	89	86	100	108	21	28	25	29	32	64	78	74	88	95
149	Saudi Arabia	354	313	336	360	345	662	533	523	600	534	281	236	252	280	266	525	403	392	465	411
150	Senegal	22	23	22	25	27	44	49	54	62	62	8	9	9	11	12	16	19	23	28	28
151	Serbia and Montenegro	132	76	61	90	120	382	293	308	298	305	82	45	34	54	75	237	174	169	179	191
152	Seychelles	448	441	395	388	425	562	564	544	568	557	347	338	298	294	316	435	432	409	430	414
153	Sierra Leone	5	6	6	7	6	21	23	28	29	27	2	3	4	4	4	9	12	17	18	16
154	Singapore	900	849	824	816	898	943	967	933	995	1105	374	326	291	274	277	392	371	329	334	341
155	Slovakia	235	225	214	223	265	559	595	608	652	723	215	202	192	199	237	512	535	546	584	646
156	Slovenia	813	829	765	821	922	1223	1299	1356	1487	1547	616	626	582	615	690	927	981	1031	1114	1158
157	Solomon Islands	40	42	39	38	29	109	116	99	90	83	37	39	37	36	27	102	108	92	84	77
158	Somalia	6	7	6	6	n/a	15	14	13	13	n/a	3	3	3	3	n/a	7	6	6	6	n/a
159	South Africa	261	266	244	224	206	585	628	625	673	689	117	109	103	92	84	262	258	265	277	280
160	Spain	1112	1139	1028	1065	1192	1371	1467	1493	1569	1640	803	820	735	760	850	990	1057	1069	1120	1170
161	Sri Lanka	29	30	32	30	32	102	112	122	123	131	15	15	16	15	16	52	55	60	60	64
162	Sudan	20	18	17	18	19	49	53	49	51	58	3	3	3	3	4	9	8	9	10	12
163	Suriname	194	104	188	144	197	289	194	351	338	385	120	62	81	57	82	178	115	152	134	161
164	Swaziland	96	85	81	73	66	330	305	298	300	309	54	50	48	42	39	187	180	175	174	184
165	Sweden	2335	2395	2277	2169	2489	1960	2118	2241	2366	2512	2003	2053	1933	1841	2124	1682	1816	1902	2008	2144

	Member State	Per capita total expenditure on health at average exchange rate (US$)					Per capita total expenditure on health at international dollar rate					Per capita government expenditure on health at average exchange rate (US$)					Per capita government expenditure on health at international dollar rate				
		1998	1999	2000	2001	2002	1998	1999	2000	2001	2002	1998	1999	2000	2001	2002	1998	1999	2000	2001	2002
166	Switzerland	3908	3881	3572	3774	4219	2967	2985	3112	3287	3446	2144	2148	1986	2156	2443	1628	1652	1731	1878	1995
167	Syrian Arab Republic	57	60	60	61	58	111	112	105	106	109	23	25	26	27	27	45	46	45	48	50
168	Tajikistan	7	7	5	6	6	33	40	38	43	47	3	2	2	2	2	12	11	11	12	13
169	Thailand	73	75	72	66	90	234	231	237	241	321	42	43	42	39	63	133	132	138	142	223
170	The former Yugoslav Republic of Macedonia	139	115	107	102	124	349	297	303	296	341	122	98	91	85	105	305	253	257	246	289
171	Timor-Leste	40	32	32	51	47	113	132	117	194	195	27	23	21	33	30	77	94	77	125	125
172	Togo	35	35	26	26	36	134	138	125	128	163	7	8	4	4	4	27	31	18	18	18
173	Tonga	95	91	92	88	91	230	227	257	288	292	67	66	68	65	67	163	162	189	212	214
174	Trinidad and Tobago	192	207	234	244	264	337	361	388	381	428	87	92	95	97	98	152	160	156	152	160
175	Tunisia	126	124	115	120	126	347	350	369	405	415	64	65	56	61	63	175	183	179	207	207
176	Turkey	149	180	195	137	172	312	392	443	391	420	107	110	122	86	113	224	240	279	244	276
177	Turkmenistan	27	29	46	58	79	157	156	218	228	182	20	20	33	40	56	116	108	156	158	129
178	Tuvalu	68	75	74	66	78	68	83	94	87	77	41	43	39	35	36	40	48	50	46	36
179	Uganda	15	17	16	18	18	46	56	62	72	77	4	5	4	5	5	13	17	17	20	22
180	Ukraine	41	27	26	34	40	163	144	154	184	210	29	19	18	24	29	117	99	106	127	150
181	United Arab Emirates	724	704	787	824	802	724	759	759	798	750	557	527	594	619	589	557	569	573	600	551
182	United Kingdom	1688	1781	1784	1837	2031	1607	1725	1839	2012	2160	1356	1436	1442	1524	1693	1292	1391	1488	1669	1801
183	United Republic of Tanzania	12	12	13	14	13	24	25	27	31	31	6	6	6	8	7	12	12	14	17	17
184	United States of America	4096	4298	4539	4873	5274	4096	4298	4539	4873	5274	1823	1905	2017	2187	2368	1823	1905	2017	2187	2368
185	Uruguay	722	668	631	597	361	995	976	965	980	805	273	233	211	202	105	376	340	323	331	234
186	Uzbekistan	41	41	31	25	21	144	134	133	140	143	20	20	14	12	9	70	66	62	65	65
187	Vanuatu	50	48	46	42	44	123	117	122	116	121	35	35	33	31	32	86	84	88	85	89
188	Venezuela, Bolivarian Republic of	220	254	300	261	184	332	339	360	317	272	120	132	163	114	86	181	176	196	139	128
189	Viet Nam	18	18	21	21	23	108	112	129	136	148	6	6	6	6	7	35	37	36	38	43
190	Yemen	18	19	23	23	23	69	62	64	69	58	6	6	8	8	6	24	21	23	23	16
191	Zambia	21	17	17	20	20	51	40	38	50	51	11	9	9	10	11	28	21	20	26	27
192	Zimbabwe	59	35	46	55	118	278	189	174	157	152	33	17	24	26	61	155	92	91	74	78

[a] See explanatory notes for sources and methods.

[b] The exchange rate changed from 2.15 Won in 2001 to 152 Won in 2002, drastically affecting total health expenditure and general government health expenditure in US dollars between the two years.

[c] These are preliminary estimates while awaiting final confirmation of Oil for Food programme expenditures. Data do not include expenditures in the three northern governorates.

[d] Health data for 2002 have been largely developed by WHO, as they are not yet available through the OECD Health Data 2004.

[e] Official exchange rates have been used.

n/a Used when the information accessed indicates that a cell should have an entry but no figures were available.

Annex Table 7 Selected immunization indicators in all WHO Member States

Figures computed by WHO to assure comparability;[a] they are not necessarily the official statistics of Member States, which may use alternative rigorous methods.

	Member State	Newborns immunized with BCG 2003 (%)	1-year-olds immunized with 3 doses of DTP 2003 (%)	Children under 2 years immunized with 1 dose of measles 2003 (%)	1-year-olds immunized with 3 doses of hepatitis B 2003 (%)	1-year-olds immunized with 3 doses of Hib vaccine 2003 (%)	1-year-olds immunized with yellow fever vaccine 2003 (%)
1	Afghanistan	56	54	50	not in schedule	n/a	n/a
2	Albania	95	97	93	97	n/a	n/a
3	Algeria	98	87	84	in schedule no coverage estimates	at risk not in schedule	n/a
4	Andorra	n/a	99	96	84	91	n/a
5	Angola	62	46	62	not in schedule	at risk not in schedule	52
6	Antigua and Barbuda	n/a	99	99	99	99	n/a
7	Argentina	99	88	97	in schedule no coverage estimates	in schedule no coverage estimates	n/a
8	Armenia	92	94	94	93	n/a	n/a
9	Australia	n/a	92	93	95	94	n/a
10	Austria	n/a	84	79	44	84	n/a
11	Azerbaijan	99	97	98	98	n/a	n/a
12	Bahamas	n/a	92	90	88	in schedule no coverage estimates	n/a
13	Bahrain	n/a	97	100	98	97	n/a
14	Bangladesh	95	85	77	in schedule no coverage estimates	n/a	n/a
15	Barbados	n/a	86	90	91	86	n/a
16	Belarus	99	86	99	99	n/a	n/a
17	Belgium	n/a	90	75	50	in schedule no coverage estimates	n/a
18	Belize	99	96	96	96	96	n/a
19	Benin	99	88	83	81	at risk not in schedule	83
20	Bhutan	93	95	88	95	n/a	n/a
21	Bolivia	94	81	64	81	95	in schedule no coverage estimates
22	Bosnia and Herzegovina	94	87	84	in schedule no coverage estimates	in schedule no coverage estimates	n/a
23	Botswana	99	97	90	78	at risk not in schedule	n/a
24	Brazil	99	96	99	91	in schedule no coverage estimates	in schedule no coverage estimates
25	Brunei Darussalam	99	99	99	99	in schedule no coverage estimates	n/a
26	Bulgaria	98	96	96	96	n/a	n/a
27	Burkina Faso	83	84	76	not in schedule	at risk not in schedule	71
28	Burundi	84	74	75	not in schedule	at risk not in schedule	not in schedule
29	Cambodia	76	69	65	in schedule no coverage estimates	n/a	n/a
30	Cameroon	82	73	61	in schedule no coverage estimates	at risk not in schedule	not in schedule
31	Canada	n/a	91	95	in schedule no coverage estimates	83	n/a
32	Cape Verde	78	78	68	54	at risk not in schedule	not in schedule
33	Central African Republic	70	40	35	not in schedule	at risk not in schedule	33
34	Chad	72	47	61	not in schedule	at risk not in schedule	41
35	Chile	94	99	99	not in schedule	in schedule no coverage estimates	n/a
36	China	93	90	84	70	n/a	n/a
37	Colombia	96	91	92	93	93	in schedule no coverage estimates
38	Comoros	75	75	63	27	at risk not in schedule	n/a
39	Congo	60	50	50	not in schedule	at risk not in schedule	not in schedule
40	Cook Islands	99	96	99	93	at risk not in schedule	n/a
41	Costa Rica	87	88	89	86	87	n/a
42	Côte d'Ivoire	66	54	56	48	at risk not in schedule	51
43	Croatia	98	94	95	not in schedule	95	n/a
44	Cuba	99	71	99	99	99	n/a
45	Cyprus	n/a	98	86	88	58	n/a
46	Czech Republic	98	97	99	86	97	n/a
47	Democratic People's Republic of Korea	88	68	95	in schedule no coverage estimates	n/a	n/a
48	Democratic Republic of the Congo	68	49	54	not in schedule	at risk not in schedule	29
49	Denmark	n/a	96	96	not in schedule	96	n/a
50	Djibouti	63	68	66	not in schedule	at risk not in schedule	n/a

Districts achieving at least 80% DTP3 coverage 2003 (%)	Children born in 2003 protected against tetanus by vaccination of their mothers with tetanus toxoid (PAB) (%)	Pregnant women immunized with two or more doses of tetanus toxoid 2003 (%)	Number of diseases covered by routine immunization before 24 months 2003	Was a 2nd opportunity provided for measles immunization?	Vitamin A distribution linked with routine immunization 2003	Number of wild polio cases reported 2004 (as of 25/01/05)	Country polio eradication status 2004	Use of auto-disable (AD) syringes 2003	Use of vaccine of assured quality 2003	Total routine vaccine spending financed using government funds 2003 (%)
19	40	40	6	Yes	No	4	endemic	partial AD use	Yes	0
100	n/a	73	8	Yes	No	0	certified polio free	exclusive AD use	Yes	40
n.d.	n/a	55	7	Yes	No	0	non-endemic	partial AD use	Yes	100
n.d.	n/a	n/a	10	Yes	No	0	certified polio free	partial AD use	Yes	100
7	72	72	7	Yes	Yes	0	non-endemic	exclusive AD use	Yes	10
n.d.	n/a	n/a	9	Yes	No	0	certified polio free	no information provided	Yes	n.d.
n.d.	n/a	n.d.	10	Yes	No	0	certified polio free	no information provided	Yes	n.d.
100	n/a	n/a	9	Yes	No	0	certified polio free	partial AD use	Yes	65
n.d.	n/a	n/a	10	Yes	No	0	certified polio free	no AD use	Yes	100
n.d.	n/a	n/a	10	Yes	No	0	certified polio free	no AD use	Yes	100
91	n/a	n/a	9	Yes	Yes	0	certified polio free	partial AD use	Yes	51
n.d.	n/a	n/a	9	Yes	No	0	certified polio free	no information provided	Yes	n.d.
n.d.	n/a	56	9	Yes	No	0	non-endemic	no AD use	Yes	100
97	89	89	7	No	Yes	0	non-endemic	partial AD use	Yes	100
n.d.	n/a	n/a	9	Yes	No	0	certified polio free	no information provided	Yes	n.d.
100	n/a	n/a	9	Yes	No	0	certified polio free	no AD use	Yes	100
n.d.	n/a	n/a	10	Yes	No	0	certified polio free	no AD use	Yes	n.d.
100	n/a	n.d.	10	Yes	No	0	certified polio free	no AD use	Yes	100
77	56	72	8	Yes	Yes	6	importation	exclusive AD use	Yes	0
95	n/a	78	7	No	No	0	non-endemic	partial AD use	Yes	n.d.
83	n/a	n.d.	11	Yes	Yes	0	certified polio free	exclusive AD use	Yes	n.d.
78	n/a	n/a	10	Yes	No	0	certified polio free	partial AD use	Yes	70
100	n/a	55	7	Yes	No	1	importation	no AD use	Yes	100
84	n/a	n.d.	11	Yes	Yes	0	certified polio free	no AD use	Yes	100
100	n/a	n.d.	10	Yes	No	0	certified polio free	no AD use	Yes	100
100	n/a	n/a	9	Yes	No	0	certified polio free	partial AD use	Yes	100
43	50	50	7	Yes	No	8	re-established transmission	exclusive AD use	Yes	100
88	46	41	6	Yes	Yes	0	non-endemic	exclusive AD use	Yes	n.d.
16	43	43	7	Yes	Yes	0	certified polio free	exclusive AD use	Yes	7
31	65	53	7	Yes	Yes	10	importation	exclusive AD use	Yes	100
n.d.	n/a	n/a	10	Yes	No	0	certified polio free	no information provided	Yes	n.d.
53	n/a	72	7	No	No	0	certified polio free	no AD use	Yes	800
8	63	17	7	No	No	30	re-established transmission	partial AD use	Yes	n.d.
9	43	43	7	No	No	22	re-established transmission	partial AD use	Yes	n.d.
92	n/a	n/a	9	Yes	No	0	certified polio free	no AD use	Yes	n.d.
98	n.d.	n.d.	9	Yes	Yes	0	certified polio free	partial AD use	Yes	n.d.
57	n/a	n.d.	11	Yes	No	0	certified polio free	no AD use	Yes	100
24	46	n.d.	7	No	No	0	non-endemic	exclusive AD use	Yes	n.d.
15	59	60	6	No	Yes	0	non-endemic	exclusive AD use	Yes	n.d.
100	n/a	n/a	7	Yes	No	0	certified polio free	exclusive AD use	Yes	n.d.
86	n/a	n/a	10	Yes	No	0	certified polio free	no AD use	Yes	n.d.
20	80	41	8	No	No	16	re-established transmission	exclusive AD use	Yes	58
100	n/a	n/a	9	Yes	No	0	certified polio free	no AD use	Yes	100
43	n/a	n/a	10	Yes	No	0	certified polio free	no AD use	Yes	99
100	n/a	n/a	9	Yes	No	0	certified polio free	no AD use	Yes	n.d.
100	n/a	n/a	10	Yes	No	0	certified polio free	no AD use	Yes	100
0	n/a	97	7	Yes	Yes	0	non-endemic	exclusive AD use	Partial	n.d.
15	48	48	7	No	Yes	0	non-endemic	partial AD use	Yes	n.d.
100	n/a	n/a	8	Yes	No	0	certified polio free	no AD use	Yes	100
0	n/a	35	6	No	No	0	non-endemic	no AD use	Yes	n.d.

Annex Table 7 Selected immunization indicators in all WHO Member States
Figures computed by WHO to assure comparability;[a] they are not necessarily the official statistics of Member States, which may use alternative rigorous methods.

	Member State	Newborns immunized with BCG 2003 (%)	1-year-olds immunized with 3 doses of DTP 2003 (%)	Children under 2 years immunized with 1 dose of measles 2003 (%)	1-year-olds immunized with 3 doses of hepatitis B 2003 (%)	1-year-olds immunized with 3 doses of Hib vaccine 2003 (%)	1-year-olds immunized with yellow fever vaccine 2003 (%)
51	Dominica	99	99	99	not in schedule	at risk not in schedule	n/a
52	Dominican Republic	90	65	79	81	75	n/a
53	Ecuador	99	89	99	58	58	in schedule no coverage estimates
54	Egypt	98	98	98	98	at risk not in schedule	n/a
55	El Salvador	90	88	99	75	88	n/a
56	Equatorial Guinea	73	33	51	not in schedule	at risk not in schedule	not in schedule
57	Eritrea	91	83	84	83	at risk not in schedule	n/a
58	Estonia	99	94	95	in schedule no coverage estimates	in schedule no coverage estimates	n/a
59	Ethiopia	76	56	52	not in schedule	at risk not in schedule	not in schedule
60	Fiji	99	94	91	92	88	n/a
61	Finland	98	98	97	not in schedule	96	n/a
62	France	85	97	86	29	86	n/a
63	Gabon	89	38	55	not in schedule	at risk not in schedule	15
64	Gambia	99	90	90	90	90	90
65	Georgia	87	76	73	49	n/a	n/a
66	Germany	n/a	89	92	81	89	n/a
67	Ghana	92	80	80	80	80	77
68	Greece	n/a	88	88	88	in schedule no coverage estimates	n/a
69	Grenada	n/a	97	99	97	98	n/a
70	Guatemala	97	83	75	not in schedule	at risk not in schedule	n/a
71	Guinea	78	45	52	not in schedule	at risk not in schedule	47
72	Guinea-Bissau	84	77	61	not in schedule	at risk not in schedule	not in schedule
73	Guyana	95	90	89	90	90	in schedule no coverage estimates
74	Haiti	71	43	53	not in schedule	at risk not in schedule	n/a
75	Honduras	91	92	95	92	92	n/a
76	Hungary	99	99	99	not in schedule	100	n/a
77	Iceland	n/a	97	93	not in schedule	97	n/a
78	India	81	70	67	in schedule no coverage estimates	n/a	n/a
79	Indonesia	82	70	72	75	n/a	n/a
80	Iran, Islamic Republic of	99	99	99	98	at risk not in schedule	n/a
81	Iraq	93	81	90	70	at risk not in schedule	n/a
82	Ireland	90	85	78	not in schedule	86	n/a
83	Israel	n/a	97	95	98	96	n/a
84	Italy	n/a	96	83	97	95	n/a
85	Jamaica	88	81	78	19	16	n/a
86	Japan	n/a	97	99	not in schedule	n/a	n/a
87	Jordan	n/a	97	96	97	97	n/a
88	Kazakhstan	99	99	99	99	n/a	n/a
89	Kenya	87	73	72	73	73	56
90	Kiribati	99	99	88	99	at risk not in schedule	n/a
91	Kuwait	n/a	99	97	99	in schedule no coverage estimates	n/a
92	Kyrgyzstan	99	98	99	99	n/a	n/a
93	Lao People's Democratic Republic	65	50	42	50	n/a	n/a
94	Latvia	99	98	99	98	92	n/a
95	Lebanon	n/a	92	96	88	92	n/a
96	Lesotho	83	79	70	in schedule no coverage estimates	at risk not in schedule	n/a
97	Liberia	43	38	53	not in schedule	at risk not in schedule	7
98	Libyan Arab Jamahiriya	99	93	91	91	at risk not in schedule	n/a
99	Lithuania	99	94	98	95	n/a	n/a
100	Luxembourg	n/a	98	91	49	in schedule no coverage estimates	n/a

Districts achieving at least 80% DTP3 coverage in 2003 (%)	Children born in 2003 protected against tetanus by vaccination of their mothers with tetanus toxoid (PAB) (%)	Pregnant women immunized with two or more doses of tetanus toxoid in 2003 (%)	Number of diseases covered by routine immunization before 24 months 2003	Was a 2nd opportunity provided for measles immunization?	Vitamin A distribution linked with routine immunization 2003	Number of wild polio cases reported 2004 (as of 25/01/05)	Country polio eradication status 2004	Use of auto-disable (AD) syringes 2003	Use of vaccine of assured quality 2003	Total routine vaccine spending financed using government funds 2003 (%)
n.d.	n/a	n.d.	8	Yes	No	0	certified polio free	no information provided	Yes	n.d.
40	n/a	n.d.	10	Yes	Yes	0	certified polio free	partial AD use	Yes	65
13	n/a	n.d.	11	Yes	No	0	certified polio free	partial AD use	Yes	100
n.d.	71	66	9	Yes	Yes	1	endemic	no AD use	Partial	n.d.
71	n/a		10	Yes	No	0	certified polio free	no AD use	Yes	n.d.
0	53	33	6	No	No	0	non-endemic	partial AD use	Yes	n.d.
17	55	60	7	No	No	0	non-endemic	exclusive AD use	Yes	n.d.
100	n/a	n/a	10	Yes	No	0	certified polio free	no AD use	Yes	100
10	24	33	6	Yes	Yes	0	non-endemic	exclusive AD use	Yes	n.d.
100	n/a	98	9	Yes	No	0	certified polio free	partial AD use	Yes	100
n.d.	n/a	n/a	9	Yes	No	0	certified polio free	no AD use	Yes	n.d.
n.d.	n/a	n/a	10	Yes	No	0	certified polio free	no AD use	Yes	n.d.
32	54	30	7	No	No	0	non-endemic	no AD use	Yes	n.d.
14	n/a	95	9	Yes	Yes	0	non-endemic	exclusive AD use	Yes	63
48	n/a		8	Yes	No	0	certified polio free	partial AD use	Yes	19
n.d.	n/a	n/a	9	Yes	No	0	certified polio free	no AD use	Yes	10
48	70	66	9	Yes	Yes	0	non-endemic	partial AD use	Yes	n.d.
n.d.	n/a	n/a	9	Yes	No	0	certified polio free	no information provided	Yes	n.d.
100	n/a	n.d.	9	Yes	No	0	certified polio free	partial AD use	Yes	100
96	n/a	n.d.	8	Yes	Yes	0	certified polio free	exclusive AD use	Yes	100
18	74	58	7	Yes	Yes	4	importation	exclusive AD use	Yes	n.d.
55	66	38	6	No	Yes	0	non-endemic	partial AD use	Yes	n.d.
85	n/a	n.d.	11	Yes	No	0	certified polio free	partial AD use	Yes	n.d.
28	52	n.d.	6	Yes	Yes	0	certified polio free	exclusive AD use	Yes	n.d.
93	n/a	n.d.	10	Yes	Yes	0	certified polio free	partial AD use	Yes	100
100	n/a	n/a	9	Yes	No	0	certified polio free	no AD use	Yes	n.d.
n.d.	n/a	n/a	9	Yes	No	0	certified polio free	exclusive AD use	Yes	100
n.d.	78	69	7	No	Yes	130	endemic	partial AD use	Yes	100
72	51	84	7	No	Yes	0	non-endemic	exclusive AD use	Yes	90
100	n/a	n/a	7	Yes	No	0	non-endemic	no AD use	No	100
n.d.	70	n.d.	9	Yes	No	0	non-endemic	no information provided	Yes	n.d.
100	n/a	n/a	10	Yes	No	0	certified polio free	no information provided	Yes	n.d.
82	n/a	n/a	10	Yes	No	0	certified polio free	no AD use	Yes	100
n.d.	n/a	n/a	9	No	No	0	certified polio free	no AD use	Yes	n.d.
70	n/a	n.d.	10	Yes	No	0	certified polio free	no AD use	Yes	100
n.d.	n/a	n/a	8	No	No	0	certified polio free	no AD use	Yes	n.d.
100	n/a	24	9	Yes	No	0	non-endemic	no AD use	Yes	100
100	n/a	n/a	8	Yes	No	0	certified polio free	no AD use	Yes	100
37	66	66	9	Yes	Yes	0	non-endemic	exclusive AD use	Yes	36
n.d.	n/a	n.d.	7	Yes	No	0	certified polio free	no information provided	Yes	n.d.
n.d.	n/a	n.d.	9	Yes	No	0	non-endemic	no AD use	Yes	n.d.
100	n/a	n/a	9	Yes	No	0	certified polio free	partial AD use	Yes	40
20	36	36	7	Yes	Yes	0	certified polio free	partial AD use	Yes	0
100	n/a	n/a	10	Yes	No	0	certified polio free	no AD use	Yes	100
100	n/a	n/a	9	Yes	No	0	non-endemic	no AD use	Yes	100
21	n/a	27	7	Yes	No	0	non-endemic	exclusive AD use	Yes	10
0	56	24	7	No	Yes	0	non-endemic	partial AD use	Yes	n.d.
n.d.	n/a	n/a	7	Yes	No	0	non-endemic	no information provided	Yes	n.d.
98	n/a	n/a	9	Yes	No	0	certified polio free	partial AD use	Yes	100
n.d.	n/a	n/a	9	Yes	No	0	certified polio free	no information provided	Yes	n.d.

Annex Table 7 Selected immunization indicators in all WHO Member States
Figures computed by WHO to assure comparability;[a] they are not necessarily the official statistics of Member States, which may use alternative rigorous methods.

	Member State	Newborns immunized with BCG 2003 (%)	1-year-olds immunized with 3 doses of DTP 2003 (%)	Children under 2 years immunized with 1 dose of measles 2003 (%)	1-year-olds immunized with 3 doses of hepatitis B 2003 (%)	1-year-olds immunized with 3 doses of Hib vaccine 2003 (%)	1-year-olds immunized with yellow fever vaccine 2003 (%)
101	Madagascar	72	55	55	55	at risk not in schedule	n/a
102	Malawi	91	84	77	84	in schedule no coverage estimates	n/a
103	Malaysia	99	96	92	95	in schedule no coverage estimates	n/a
104	Maldives	98	98	96	98	n/a	n/a
105	Mali	63	69	68	79	at risk not in schedule	62
106	Malta	n/a	94	90	not in schedule	93	n/a
107	Marshall Islands	93	68	90	74	70	n/a
108	Mauritania	84	76	71	not in schedule	at risk not in schedule	not in schedule
109	Mauritius	92	92	94	92	at risk not in schedule	n/a
110	Mexico	99	91	96	91	98	n/a
111	Micronesia, Federated States of	64	92	91	89	in schedule no coverage estimates	n/a
112	Monaco	90	99	99	99	in schedule no coverage estimates	n/a
113	Mongolia	98	98	98	98	at risk not in schedule	n/a
114	Morocco	92	91	90	90	at risk not in schedule	n/a
115	Mozambique	87	72	77	72	at risk not in schedule	n/a
116	Myanmar	79	77	75	in schedule no coverage estimates	n/a	n/a
117	Namibia	92	82	70	not in schedule	at risk not in schedule	n/a
118	Nauru	95	80	40	75	at risk not in schedule	n/a
119	Nepal	91	78	75	15	n/a	n/a
120	Netherlands	n/a	98	96	not in schedule	in schedule no coverage estimates	n/a
121	New Zealand	n/a	90	85	90	in schedule no coverage estimates	n/a
122	Nicaragua	94	86	93	86	86	n/a
123	Niger	64	52	64	not in schedule	at risk not in schedule	31
124	Nigeria	48	25	35	not in schedule	at risk not in schedule	in schedule no coverage estimates
125	Niue	99	95	86	95	in schedule no coverage estimates	n/a
126	Norway	n/a	90	84	not in schedule	92	n/a
127	Oman	98	99	98	99	100	n/a
128	Pakistan	82	67	61	in schedule no coverage estimates	n/a	n/a
129	Palau	n/a	99	99	99	in schedule no coverage estimates	n/a
130	Panama	87	86	83	86	86	in schedule no coverage estimates
131	Papua New Guinea	60	54	49	53	at risk not in schedule	n/a
132	Paraguay	70	77	91	77	55	n/a
133	Peru	94	89	95	60	36	in schedule no coverage estimates
134	Philippines	91	79	80	40	at risk not in schedule	n/a
135	Poland	94	99	97	97	n/a	n/a
136	Portugal	81	99	96	94	99	n/a
137	Qatar	99	92	93	98	96	n/a
138	Republic of Korea	87	97	96	91	n/a	n/a
139	Republic of Moldova	98	98	96	99	n/a	n/a
140	Romania	99	97	97	98	n/a	n/a
141	Russian Federation	97	98	96	94	n/a	n/a
142	Rwanda	88	96	90	96	96	not in schedule
143	Saint Kitts and Nevis	99	99	98	99	99	n/a
144	Saint Lucia	95	90	90	14	81	n/a
145	Saint Vincent and the Grenadines	87	99	94	31	in schedule no coverage estimates	n/a
146	Samoa	73	94	99	97	at risk not in schedule	n/a
147	San Marino	n/a	96	91	96	96	n/a
148	Sao Tome and Principe	99	94	87	43	at risk not in schedule	34
149	Saudi Arabia	94	95	96	95	95	n/a
150	Senegal	77	73	60	not in schedule	at risk not in schedule	59

Districts achieving at least 80% DTP3 coverage 2003 (%)	Children born in 2003 protected against tetanus by vaccination of their mothers with tetanus toxoid (PAB) (%)	Pregnant women immunized with two or more doses of tetanus toxoid 2003 (%)	Number of diseases covered by routine immunization before 24 months 2003	Was a 2nd opportunity provided for measles immunization?	Vitamin A distribution linked with routine immunization 2003	Number of wild polio cases reported 2004 (as of 25/01/05)	Country polio eradication status 2004	Use of auto-disable (AD) syringes 2003	Use of vaccine of assured quality 2003	Total routine vaccine spending financed using government funds 2003 (%)
58	55	49	7	No	Yes	0	non-endemic	exclusive AD use	Yes	12
69	70	87	8	Yes	Yes	0	non-endemic	exclusive AD use	Yes	n.d.
100	n/a	84	10	Yes	No	0	certified polio free	no AD use	Yes	100
100	n/a	96	7	No	Yes	0	non-endemic	exclusive AD use	Yes	n.d.
43	32	46	8	Yes	Yes	18	importation	exclusive AD use	Yes	59
n.d.	n/a	n/a	9	Yes	No	0	certified polio free	no AD use	Yes	68
n.d.	n/a	72	10	Yes	Yes	0	certified polio free	partial AD use	Yes	n.d.
42	41	36	6	Yes	No	0	non-endemic	exclusive AD use	Yes	100
100	n/a	73	9	Yes	No	0	non-endemic	no AD use	Yes	100
98	n/a	n/a	10	Yes	No	0	certified polio free	exclusive AD use	Partial	100
100	n/a	n/a	10	Yes	No	0	certified polio free	no AD use	Yes	6
n.d.	n/a	n/a	12	Yes	No	0	certified polio free	no information provided	Yes	n.d.
100	n/a	n/a	7	Yes	Yes	0	certified polio free	no AD use	Yes	22
82	n/a	26	7	Yes	Yes	0	non-endemic	no AD use	Yes	100
n.d.	57	30	7	No	Yes	0	non-endemic	exclusive AD use	Yes	n.d.
50	77	73	7	Yes	No	0	non-endemic	partial AD use	Yes	0
56	85	63	6	Yes	Yes	0	non-endemic	no AD use	Yes	100
n.d.	n/a	n/a	9	Yes	No	0	certified polio free	no information provided	Yes	n.d.
49	69	30	7	No	Yes	0	non-endemic	partial AD use	Yes	65
n.d.	n/a	n/a	9	Yes	No	0	certified polio free	no AD use	Yes	n.d.
n.d.	n/a	n/a	9	Yes	No	0	certified polio free	no AD use	Yes	100
57	n/a	n/a	10	Yes	Yes	0	certified polio free	no AD use	Yes	74
10	36	40	7	No	Yes	25	endemic	exclusive AD use	Yes	n.d.
n.d.	51	n.d.	7	No	Yes	774	endemic	no information provided	Yes	n.d.
100	n/a	n/a	10	Yes	No	0	certified polio free	exclusive AD use	Yes	100
95	n/a	n/a	8	Yes	No	0	certified polio free	no AD use	Yes	100
100	n/a	53	10	Yes	Yes	0	non-endemic	no AD use	Yes	100
16	57	57	7	No	No	49	endemic	exclusive AD use	Yes	100
n.d.	n/a	n/a	10	Yes	No	0	certified polio free	no information provided	Yes	n.d.
62	n/a	n/a	11	Yes	No	0	certified polio free	partial AD use	Yes	n.d.
15	34	29	7	Yes	Yes	0	certified polio free	partial AD use	Yes	80
73	n/a	n.d.	11	Yes	No	0	certified polio free	no AD use	Yes	100
65	n/a	n.d.	10	Yes	No	0	certified polio free	no AD use	Yes	100
20	70	27	7	Yes	Yes	0	certified polio free	partial AD use	Yes	3
n.d.	n/a	n/a	9	Yes	No	0	certified polio free	no AD use	Partial	100
100	n/a	n/a	10	Yes	No	0	certified polio free	partial AD use	Yes	100
100	n/a	n/a	11	Yes	No	0	non-endemic	no AD use	Yes	100
100	n/a	n/a	10	Yes	No	0	certified polio free	no AD use	Yes	100
100	n/a	n/a	9	Yes	No	0	certified polio free	partial AD use	Yes	49
100	n/a	n/a	7	Yes	No	0	certified polio free	exclusive AD use	Yes	100
n.d.	n/a	n/a	9	Yes	No	0	certified polio free	no AD use	Yes	n.d.
67	76	51	8	Yes	No	0	non-endemic	partial AD use	Yes	50
n.d.	n/a	n.d.	10	Yes	No	0	certified polio free	no AD use	Yes	n.d.
50	n/a	n.d.	10	Yes	No	0	certified polio free	partial AD use	Yes	100
n.d.	n/a	n.d.	9	Yes	No	0	certified polio free	no information provided	Yes	n.d.
100	n/a	n/a	7	Yes	No	0	certified polio free	partial AD use	Yes	n.d.
100	n/a	n/a	9	Yes	No	0	certified polio free	exclusive AD use	Yes	100
71	n/a	97	8	Yes	Yes	0	non-endemic	exclusive AD use	Yes	n.d.
100	n/a	n/a	10	Yes	No	1	importation	no AD use	Yes	100
24	75	65	7	Yes	No	0	non-endemic	exclusive AD use	Yes	100

Annex Table 7 Selected immunization indicators in all WHO Member States

Figures computed by WHO to assure comparability;[a] they are not necessarily the official statistics of Member States, which may use alternative rigorous methods.

	Member State	Newborns immunized with BCG 2003 (%)	1-year-olds immunized with 3 doses of DTP 2003 (%)	Children under 2 years immunized with 1 dose of measles 2003 (%)	1-year-olds immunized with 3 doses of hepatitis B 2003 (%)	1-year-olds immunized with 3 doses of Hib vaccine 2003 (%)	1-year-olds immunized with yellow fever vaccine 2003 (%)
151	Serbia and Montenegro	94	89	87	in schedule no coverage estimates	n/a	n/a
152	Seychelles	99	99	99	99	at risk not in schedule	n/a
153	Sierra Leone	87	70	73	not in schedule	at risk not in schedule	76
154	Singapore	97	92	88	92	at risk not in schedule	n/a
155	Slovakia	98	99	99	99	99	n/a
156	Slovenia	98	92	94	not in schedule	in schedule no coverage estimates	n/a
157	Solomon Islands	76	71	78	78	at risk not in schedule	n/a
158	Somalia	65	40	40	not in schedule	at risk not in schedule	not in schedule
159	South Africa	97	94	83	94	94	n/a
160	Spain	n/a	98	97	83	98	n/a
161	Sri Lanka	99	99	99	in schedule no coverage estimates	n/a	n/a
162	Sudan	53	50	57	not in schedule	at risk not in schedule	not in schedule
163	Suriname	n/a	74	71	in schedule no coverage estimates	at risk not in schedule	in schedule no coverage estimates
164	Swaziland	97	95	94	95	at risk not in schedule	n/a
165	Sweden	n/a	98	94	not in schedule	98	n/a
166	Switzerland	n/a	95	82	not in schedule	91	n/a
167	Syrian Arab Republic	99	99	98	98	in schedule no coverage estimates	n/a
168	Tajikistan	99	82	89	57	n/a	n/a
169	Thailand	99	96	94	95	n/a	n/a
170	The former Yugoslav Republic of Macedonia	95	96	96	not in schedule	n/a	n/a
171	Timor-Leste	80	70	60	not in schedule	at risk not in schedule	n/a
172	Togo	84	64	58	not in schedule	at risk not in schedule	not in schedule
173	Tonga	99	98	99	93	at risk not in schedule	n/a
174	Trinidad and Tobago	n/a	91	88	76	93	88
175	Tunisia	93	95	90	92	96	n/a
176	Turkey	89	68	75	68	at risk not in schedule	n/a
177	Turkmenistan	99	98	97	97	n/a	n/a
178	Tuvalu	99	93	95	95	at risk not in schedule	n/a
179	Uganda	96	81	82	63	63	not in schedule
180	Ukraine	98	97	99	77	n/a	n/a
181	United Arab Emirates	98	94	94	92	94	n/a
182	United Kingdom	n/a	91	80	not in schedule	91	n/a
183	United Republic of Tanzania	91	95	97	95	at risk not in schedule	not in schedule
184	United States of America	n/a	96	93	92	94	n/a
185	Uruguay	99	91	95	91	91	n/a
186	Uzbekistan	98	98	99	99	n/a	n/a
187	Vanuatu	63	49	48	56	at risk not in schedule	n/a
188	Venezuela	91	68	82	75	54	in schedule no coverage estimates
189	Viet Nam	98	99	93	78	n/a	n/a
190	Yemen	67	66	66	42	at risk not in schedule	n/a
191	Zambia	94	80	84	not in schedule	at risk not in schedule	n/a
192	Zimbabwe	92	80	80	80	at risk not in schedule	n/a

[a] See explanatory notes for sources and methods.
n/a Not applicable.
n.d. No data reported.

Districts achieving at least 80% DTP3 coverage 2003 (%)	Children born in 2003 protected against tetanus by vaccination of their mothers with tetanus toxoid (PAB) (%)	Pregnant women immunized with two or more doses of tetanus toxoid 2003 (%)	Number of diseases covered by routine immunization before 24 months 2003	Was a 2nd opportunity provided for measles immunization?	Vitamin A distribution linked with routine immunization 2003	Number of wild polio cases reported 2004 (as of 25/01/05)	Country polio eradication status 2004	Use of auto-disable (AD) syringes 2003	Use of vaccine of assured quality 2003	Total routine vaccine spending financed using government funds 2003 (%)
99	n/a	n/a	9	Yes	No	0	certified polio free	no AD use	Partial	n.d.
100	n/a	100	10	Yes	No	0	non-endemic	no AD use	Yes	100
15	62	62	7	Yes	No	0	non-endemic	partial AD use	Yes	20
n.d.	n/a	n/a	9	Yes	No	0	certified polio free	no AD use	Yes	100
100	n/a	n/a	10	Yes	No	0	certified polio free	exclusive AD use	Yes	100
n.d.	n/a	n/a	9	Yes	No	0	certified polio free	no AD use	Yes	100
40	n/a	56	7	Yes	Yes	0	certified polio free	partial AD use	Yes	n.d.
3	65	49	6	No	Yes	0	non-endemic	exclusive AD use	Yes	n.d.
57	52	85	8	Yes	Yes	0	non-endemic	no AD use	Yes	n.d.
100	n/a	n/a	10	Yes	No	0	certified polio free	exclusive AD use	Yes	100
100	n/a	96	8	Yes	Yes	0	non-endemic	partial AD use	Yes	100
41	35	36	6	No	Yes	113	re-established transmission	exclusive AD use	Yes	0
n.d.	n/a	n.d.	9	Yes	No	0	certified polio free	no information provided	Yes	n.d.
50	n/a	75	7	Yes	No	0	non-endemic	no AD use	Yes	100
n.d.	n/a	n/a	8	Yes	No	0	certified polio free	no AD use	Yes	n.d.
n.d.	n/a	n/a	8	Yes	No	0	certified polio free	no information provided	Yes	n.d.
100	n/a	n.d.	10	Yes	Yes	0	non-endemic	no AD use	Yes	n.d.
100	n/a	n/a	7	Yes	No	0	certified polio free	partial AD use	Yes	0
n.d.	n/a	93	7	Yes	No	0	non-endemic	no AD use	Partial	100
100	n/a	n/a	8	Yes	No	0	certified polio free	no AD use	Yes	90
31	n/a	51	6	Yes	Yes	0	non-endemic	partial AD use	Yes	n.d.
29	47	56	6	Yes	Yes	0	non-endemic	exclusive AD use	Yes	0
100	n/a	86	8	Yes	No	0	certified polio free	exclusive AD use	Yes	100
100	n/a	n/a	10	Yes	No	0	certified polio free	no AD use	Yes	n.d.
97	n/a	n.d.	8	Yes	No	0	non-endemic	no AD use	Yes	100
4	37	37	7	Yes	No	0	certified polio free	no AD use	Yes	100
77	n/a	n/a	8	Yes	No	0	certified polio free	partial AD use	Yes	82
n.d.	n/a	n.d.	7	Yes	No	0	certified polio free	no AD use	Yes	100
54	48	48	8	Yes	Yes	0	non-endemic	partial AD use	Yes	7
100	n/a	n/a	9	Yes	No	0	certified polio free	partial AD use	Partial	96
100	n/a	n/a	10	Yes	No	0	non-endemic	no AD use	Yes	100
98	n/a	n/a	9	Yes	No	0	certified polio free	no AD use	Yes	100
84	83	80	7	Yes	Yes	0	non-endemic	exclusive AD use	Yes	30
n.d.	n/a	n/a	12	Yes	No	0	certified polio free	partial AD use	Yes	56
100	n/a	n/a	10	Yes	No	0	certified polio free	no AD use	Yes	100
100	n/a	n/a	9	Yes	Yes	0	certified polio free	partial AD use	Partial	77
17	n/a	63	7	Yes	No	0	certified polio free	partial AD use	Yes	100
45	n/a	n.d.	11	Yes	No	0	certified polio free	no AD use	Yes	100
94	79	91	8	Yes	Yes	0	certified polio free	partial AD use	Partial	55
24	31	31	7	Yes	Yes	0	non-endemic	exclusive AD use	Yes	100
76	60	81	6	Yes	Yes	0	non-endemic	exclusive AD use	Yes	0
10	60	60	7	Yes	Yes	0	non-endemic	no AD use	Yes	n.d.

Annex Table 8 Selected indicators related to reproductive, maternal and newborn health

These data are estimates from various international sources and may not be the same as Member States' own estimates. They have not been submitted to Member States for consideration

	Member State	Contraceptive prevalence rate (modern methods)		Pregnant women who received			Births attended by skilled health personnel		Births in health facili	
		(%)	Year	1+ ANC visit (%)	4+ ANC visits (%)	Year	(%)	Year	(%)	Yea
1	Afghanistan	4	2000	52	...	2003	14	2003	13	200
2	Albania	15	2000	81	42	2002	99	2000	94	200
3	Algeria	50	2000	79	...	2000	92	2000	92	200
4	Andorra	...	...	...	...	...	...	...	...	.
5	Angola	5	2001	...	...	...	45	2001	...	.
6	Antigua and Barbuda	51	1988	...	82	2001	100	2000	...	.
7	Argentina	...	...	...	95	2001	99	2001	...	.
8	Armenia	22	2000	82	65	2000	97	2000	91	200
9	Australia	72	1986	...	...	...	100	1999	...	.
10	Austria	47	1996	...	...	...	100	1993	...	.
11	Azerbaijan	12	2001	70	...	2001	84	2000	74	200
12	Bahamas	60	1988	...	...	...	99	2002	...	.
13	Bahrain	31	1995	63	61	1995	98	1995	...	.
14	Bangladesh	44	1999–00	39	11	1999–00	14	2003	6	1999–(
15	Barbados	53	1988	89	...	2001	91	1999	...	.
16	Belarus	42	1995	...	...	...	100	2002	...	.
17	Belgium	74	1992	...	...	...	100	1987	...	.
18	Belize	42	1991	...	96	2001	83	1999	...	.
19	Benin	7	2001	88	61	2001	66	2001	78	200
20	Bhutan	19	1994	...	...	...	24	2000	...	.
21	Bolivia	27	2000	84	69	2001	65	2002	56	199
22	Bosnia and Herzegovina	16	2000	99	...	2000	100	2000	...	.
23	Botswana	39	2000	99	97	2001	94	2000	...	.
24	Brazil	70	1996	84	76	1996	88	1996	92	199
25	Brunei Darussalam	...	...	...	100	2001	99	1999	...	.
26	Bulgaria	25	1997	...	...	...	...	...	...	.
27	Burkina Faso	5	1998–99	72	18	2003	38	2003	38	200
28	Burundi	10	2000	93	79	2001	25	2000	...	.
29	Cambodia	19	2000	44	9	2000	32	2000	10	200
30	Cameroon	7	1998	77	52	1998	60	2000	54	199
31	Canada	73	1995	...	...	...	98	2001	...	.
32	Cape Verde	46	1998	...	99	2001	89	1998	...	.
33	Central African Republic	7	2000	75	39	1994	44	2000	50	1994–9
34	Chad	2	2000	51	13	1997	16	2000	...	.
35	Chile	...	...	...	95	1995	100	2002	...	.
36	China	83	1997	...	...	...	97	1995	...	.
37	Colombia	64	2000	90	79	2000	86	2000	87	200
38	Comoros	19	2000	87	53	1996	62	2000	...	.
39	Congo	...	...	...	...	...	...	...	...	.
40	Cook Islands	60	1996	...	...	...	100	1998	...	.
41	Costa Rica	65	1993	...	70	2001	98	2001	...	.
42	Côte d'Ivoire	7	1998–99	84	35	1998–99	63	2000	48	1998–9
43	Croatia	...	...	...	...	...	100	2002	...	.
44	Cuba	72	2000	...	100	2001	100	1999	...	.
45	Cyprus	...	...	...	...	...	...	...	...	.
46	Czech Republic	63	1997	99	...	1993	100	2002	...	.
47	Democratic People's Republic of Korea	53	1992	98	...	2000	97	2000	...	.
48	Democratic Republic of the Congo	4	2001	72	...	...	61	2001	...	.
49	Denmark	72	1988	...	...	...	100	1987	...	.
50	Djibouti	...	...	...	...	...	61	2003	...	.
51	Dominica	48	1987	...	100	2001	100	1999	...	.
52	Dominican Republic	63	2000	100	93	1999	98	2002	97	199
53	Ecuador	50	1999	56	...	1999	69	1999	...	.
54	Egypt	54	2000	54	41	2000	69	2003	52	200
55	El Salvador	54	1998	...	76	2001	90	1998	...	.

Births by caesarean section		No. of midwives available		Annual number of live births, 2000	Maternal mortality ratio 2000	Stillbirth rate 2000	Early neonatal mortality rate 2000	Neonatal mortality rate 2000
(%)	Year	Total	Year	(000)	(per 100 000 live births)	(per 1000 total births)	(per 1000 live births)	(per 1000 live births)
...	...	...	...	1044	1900[b]	54[b]	45[b]	60[b]
15	2002	1891	1994	59	55[b]	11[b]	9[b]	12[b]
6	2000	...	...	701	140[b]	32	16[b]	20
24	1999	8	2002	...	...	6[b]	3[b]	4[b]
...	...	492	1997	655	1700[b]	48[b]	40[b]	54[b]
...	...	...	...	...	...	7[b]	6[b]	8[b]
...	...	...	...	721	70	6	8	10
7	2000	1483	2002	31	55[b]	16	13	17
21	1998	11649	2001	246	6	3	3	3
21	2002	1650	2002	75	5	4	2	3
4	2002	10033	2002	150	94[b]	32	27[b]	36
...	...	...	...	6	60[b]	3	8	10
16	1995	...	...	14	33	10[b]	9[b]	11
3	1999–00	15794	2001	4226	380	24	27	36
...	...	...	...	3	95	11	6	8
17	2002	6208	2002	87	36	6	3	5
16	1999	6603	1996	112	10	4	2	3
8	1991	...	...	7	140	18	16	18
4	2001	432	1995	265	850	37[b]	31	38
...	...	1016	1995	73	420[b]	22[b]	18	38
15	1998	...	...	257	420[b]	11	20	27
...	...	1220	2002	38	31	11[b]	9	11
...	...	...	...	54	100[b]	44[b]	37	40
36	1996	...	...	3474	260	8	12	15
...	...	404	2000	8	37	6	3	4
17	2002	3433	2002	62	32	8	5	8
1	2003	476	2001	580	1000	30[b]	25	36
...	...	...	...	276	1000[b]	33[b]	28	41
1	2000	3040	2000	461	450	37[b]	31	40
3	1998	69	1996	551	730	39[b]	32	40
19	1997–98	358	2000	332	5	3	3	4
6	1998	...	...	12	150[b]	22	8	10
2	1994–95	1018	1995	143	1100	45[b]	38	48
1	1996–97	161	2001	381	1100	35[b]	29	45
37	1994	...	...	288	30	4	4	6
...	...	44517	1999	19428	56	19[b]	16[b]	21
25	2000	...	...	980	130	11	12	14
5	1996	90	1997	27	480[b]	26[b]	22	29
...	...	164	1995	153	510[b]	29[b]	24[b]	32[b]
...	...	3	2001	...	...	11[b]	9[b]	12[b]
21	1992	...	...	79	25	8	6	7
3	1998–99	2203	1996	573	690[b]	53[b]	44	65
14	2002	1493	2002	49	10	5	4	5
...	...	...	...	137	33	11	3	4
...	...	...	...	10	47	4[b]	3[b]	4[b]
14	2002	4949	2002	88	9	3	2	2
...	...	12823	1995	388	67[b]	20[b]	17[b]	22[b]
...	...	...	...	2463	990[b]	42[b]	35[b]	47[b]
18	2001	1312	2002	65	7	5	3	4
...	...	...	...	27	730[b]	34[b]	29[b]	38[b]
...	...	...	...	...	...	7[b]	5[b]	7[b]
32	1999	...	...	199	150[b]	14	14	19
19	1999	1037	2000	300	130	7	12	16
11	2000	...	...	1808	84	10	16	21
16	1998	...	...	164	150[b]	12	9	16

Annex Table 8 Selected indicators related to reproductive, maternal and newborn health
These data are estimates from various international sources and may not be the same as Member States' own estimates. They have not been submitted to Member States for consideration

	Member State	Contraceptive prevalence rate (modern methods)		Pregnant women who received			Births attended by skilled health personnel		Births in health facili
		(%)	Year	1+ ANC visit (%)	4+ ANC visits (%)	Year	(%)	Year	(%)	Yea
56	Equatorial Guinea	...	...	...	37	2001	65	2001	...	..
57	Eritrea	5	2002	...	49	2001	28	2002	...	.
58	Estonia	56	1994	...	...	...	100	2002	...	..
59	Ethiopia	6	2000	27	10	2000	6	2000	5	200
60	Fiji	...	...	...	...	...	100	1998	...	.
61	Finland	75	1989	...	...	...	100	2002	...	.
62	France	69	1994	...	...	...	99	1993	...	.
63	Gabon	13	2000	94	63	2000	86	2000	84	200
64	Gambia	9	2000	92	...	2000	55	2000	...	.
65	Georgia	20	2000	91	...	1999	96	1999	92	199
66	Germany	72	1992	...	...	...	...	...	...	.
67	Ghana	13	1998	90	69	2003	47	2003	46	200
68	Greece	...	...	...	...	...	...	...	...	.
69	Grenada	...	1990	...	98	2001	100	2000	...	..
70	Guatemala	31	1998–99	86	68	1998–99	41	2003	42	1998–9
71	Guinea	4	1999	74	48	1999	35	1999	29	199
72	Guinea–Bissau	4	2000	89	62	2001	35	2000	...	..
73	Guyana	36	2000	88	...	2000	86	2000	...	..
74	Haiti	23	2000	79	42	2000	24	2000	18	200
75	Honduras	51	2001	...	84	2001	56	2001	...	..
76	Hungary	68	1993	...	...	...	...	...	...	..
77	Iceland	...	...	...	...	...	...	...	...	.
78	India	43	1998–99	65	30	1998–99	43	2000	34	1998–9
79	Indonesia	57	2003	97	81	2002–03	66	2002–03	40	2002–0
80	Iran, Islamic Republic of	56	1997	...	77	2001	90	2000	...	..
81	Iraq	10	1989	...	78	2001	72	2000	...	..
82	Ireland	...	...	...	...	...	100	2002	...	..
83	Israel	52	1987–88	...	...	...	99	1987	...	..
84	Italy	39	1995–96	...	...	...	...	...	...	..
85	Jamaica	63	1997	...	99	2001	95	1997	...	..
86	Japan	nd	2000	...	...	...	100	1996	...	..
87	Jordan	39	2002	99	91	2002	100	2002	97	200
88	Kazakhstan	57	1999	82	71	1999	99	1999	98	199
89	Kenya	32	1998	88	52	2003	42	2003	40	200
90	Kiribati	...	...	...	88	2001	85	1998	...	.
91	Kuwait	41	1996	83	81	1996	98	1995	...	..
92	Kyrgyzstan	49	1997	88	81	1997	98	1997	96	199
93	Lao People's Democratic Republic	29	2000	44	29	2001	19	2001	...	..
94	Latvia	39	1995	...	...	...	100	2002	...	..
95	Lebanon	37	1996	...	87	2001	88	1996	...	..
96	Lesotho	30	2000	91	88	2001	60	2000	...	.
97	Liberia	6	1986	...	84	2001	51	2000	...	..
98	Libyan Arab Jamahiriya	26	1995	...	81	2001	94	1995	...	..
99	Lithuania	31	1995	...	...	...	...	...	...	..
100	Luxembourg	...	...	...	...	...	100	2002	...	..
101	Madagascar	12	2000	91	38	1997	46	2000	...	..
102	Malawi	26	2000	94	55	2000	61	2002	54	200
103	Malaysia	30	1994	...	...	...	97	2001	...	.
104	Maldives	...	...	98	81	2001	70	2000	...	..
105	Mali	7	2001	53	30	2001	41	2001	24	200
106	Malta	...	...	...	...	...	98	1993	...	..
107	Marshall Islands	...	...	...	...	...	95	1998	...	..
108	Mauritania	5	1999–00	63	16	2000–01	57	2000–01	49	2000–0
109	Mauritius	49	1991	...	...	...	99	1999	...	..
110	Mexico	60	1997	...	86	2001	86	1997	...	..

Births by caesarean section		No. of midwives available		Annual number of live births, 2000	Maternal mortality ratio 2000	Stillbirth rate 2000	Early neonatal mortality rate 2000	Neonatal mortality rate 2000
(%)	Year	Total	Year	(000)	(per 100 000 live births)	(per 1000 total births)	(per 1000 live births)	(per 1000 live births)
...	...	9	1996	20	880[b]	36[b]	30[b]	40[b]
2	1995	72	1996	153	630	23[b]	19	25
15	2002	422	2002	12	38	5	4	6
1	2000	1142	2002	2865	850	20	38	51
...	...	...	...	20	75[b]	9	7	9
16	2002	3952	2002	57	5	4	2	2
16	1999	15122	2002	758	17	5	2	3
6	2000	...	...	41	420	33[b]	27	31
...	...	98	1997	49	540[b]	44[b]	37	46
12	2002	1500	2002	57	32[b]	23	19[b]	25
22	2001	9506	2001	749	9	4	2	3
4	2003	4094	2002	645	540[b]	19	26	27
...	...	1916	1993	101	10	5	3	4
...	...	...	...	...	...	12[b]	10[b]	13[b]
12	1998–99	...	...	406	240	9	14	19
2	1999	299	2000	361	740	45[b]	38	48
...	...	156	1996	69	1100[b]	43[b]	36[b]	48[b]
...	...	...	...	17	170	22[b]	19[b]	25[b]
2	2000	...	...	248	680	30[b]	25	34
12	1996	...	...	204	110	15	13	18
23	2002	2076	2002	92	11	6	5	6
17	2001	200	2002	4	0	5	2	2
7	1998–99	...	...	25780	540	39[b]	33	43
4	2002–03	11547	2000	4564	230[b]	17[b]	14	18
...	...	...	...	1258	76	17	17[b]	22
...	...	...	...	843	250[b]	32	46[b]	63
19	2000	...	...	54	4	6	3	4
17	2001	1147	2002	125	13	5	3	4
32	1999	...	...	518	5	3	2	3
...	...	...	...	54	87	9[b]	8[b]	10[b]
...	...	24511	2000	1196	10	5	1	2
16	2002	...	...	148	41	13	12	17
11	1998	8099	2002	257	210[b]	29	29	32
4	2003	...	...	1026	1000	29[b]	24	29
...	...	...	...	...	...	24[b]	20[b]	27[b]
11	1996	...	...	48	12	6	4	6
6	1997	2775	2002	110	110[b]	32	26	31
...	...	...	...	195	650[b]	32[b]	26[b]	35[b]
17	2002	493	2002	18	61	8	5	7
23	1998	...	...	68	150[b]	19[b]	16[b]	20
...	...	791	1995	56	550[b]	26[b]	21[b]	28[b]
...	...	103	1997	145	760[b]	58[b]	48	66
...	...	...	...	121	97[b]	11[b]	9[b]	11
15	2002	1239	2002	31	19	6	3	5
19	2000	95	2002	6	28	7	3	4
1	1997	1472	2001	687	550	29[b]	24	33
3	2000	...	...	526	1800	13	30	40
...	...	7711	2000	549	41	3	4	5
...	...	463	1995	11	110[b]	25	30	37
1	2001	284	2000	596	1200	12	40	55
25	2002	125	2002	5	...	4	4	5
...	...	...	...	...	...	24[b]	20[b]	26[b]
3	2000–01	232	1995	113	1000	63[b]	52[b]	70
...	...	...	...	20	24	9	9	12
12	1987	...	...	2324	83	11	11	15

Annex Table 8 Selected indicators related to reproductive, maternal and newborn health

These data are estimates from various international sources and may not be the same as Member States' own estimates. They have not been submitted to Member States for consideration

Member State	Contraceptive prevalence rate (modern methods)		Pregnant women who received			Births attended by skilled health personnel		Births in health facili†	
	(%)	Year	1+ ANC visit (%)	4+ ANC visits (%)	Year	(%)	Year	(%)	Yea
111 Micronesia, Federated States of	...	...	...	...	...	93	1999	...	.
112 Monaco	...	...	...	...	...	...	...	...	.
113 Mongolia	54	2000	...	97	2001	99	2000	...	.
114 Morocco	42	1995	32	8	1992	40	1995	30	199
115 Mozambique	5	1997	71	41	1997	48	1997	...	.
116 Myanmar	28	1997	...	76	2001	56	1997	...	.
117 Namibia	26	1992	85	69	2000	76	2000	75	200
118 Nauru	...	...	...	...	...	...	...	...	.
119 Nepal	35	2001	49	15	2001	11	2001	9	200
120 Netherlands	76	1993	...	...	...	100	1995	...	.
121 New Zealand	72	1995	...	...	...	100	1995	...	.
122 Nicaragua	66	2001	85	72	2001	67	2001	66	200
123 Niger	4	2000	39	11	1998	16	2000	18	199
124 Nigeria	9	1999	61	47	2003	35	2003	33	200
125 Niue	...	...	...	...	...	100	1996	...	.
126 Norway	69	1989	...	...	...	100	1988	...	.
127 Oman	18	1995	77	71	1995	95	2000	...	.
128 Pakistan	20	2001	36	16	1996–97	20	1998	17	1996–9
129 Palau	...	...	...	...	...	100	1998	...	.
130 Panama	54	1984	...	72	2001	90	1998	...	.
131 Papua New Guinea	20	1996	...	78	2001	53	1996	...	.
132 Paraguay	48	1998	...	89	2001	61	1998	...	.
133 Peru	50	2000	85	69	2000	59	2000	57	200
134 Philippines	28	1998	94	70	2003	60	2003	38	200
135 Poland	19	1991	...	...	...	100	2002	...	.
136 Portugal	33	1979–80	...	...	...	100	2000	...	.
137 Qatar	32	1998	62	58	1998	99	1998	...	.
138 Republic of Korea	67	1997	...	...	...	100	1997	...	.
139 Republic of Moldova	43	2000	99	...	1997	99	1997	99	199
140 Romania	30	1999	89	...	1999	98	1999	98	199
141 Russian Federation	...	...	96	...	1999	99	2002	98	199
142 Rwanda	6	2000	93	10	2001	31	2000	26	200
143 Saint Kitts and Nevis	37	1984	...	100	2001	100	1995	...	.
144 Saint Lucia	46	1988	...	100	2001	100	1995	...	.
145 Saint Vincent and Grenadines	55	1988	...	92	2001	100	1990	...	.
146 Samoa	...	...	...	...	...	100	1998	...	.
147 San Marino	...	...	...	...	...	...	...	...	.
148 Sao Tome and Principe	27	2000	91	...	2000	79	2000	...	.
149 Saudi Arabia	29	1996	77	73	1996	91	1996	...	.
150 Senegal	8	1997	82	64	1999	58	2000	99	199
151 Serbia and Montenegro	33	2000	...	...	...	93	2001	...	.
152 Seychelles	...	...	...	...	...	...	...	...	.
153 Sierra Leone	4	2000	82	68	2001	42	2000	...	.
154 Singapore	53	1997	...	...	...	100	1998	...	.
155 Slovakia	41	1991	...	...	...	99	2002	...	.
156 Slovenia	59	1994	...	...	...	100	2002	...	.
157 Solomon Islands	...	...	...	...	...	85	1999	...	.
158 Somalia	...	...	...	32	2001	34	1999	...	.
159 South Africa	55	1998	89	72	1998	84	1998	85	199
160 Spain	67	1995	...	...	...	...	...	...	.
161 Sri Lanka	44	1993	...	98	2001	97	2000	...	.
162 Sudan	7	1993	...	75	2001	87	2000	...	.
163 Suriname	41	2000	91	91	2001	85	2000	...	.
164 Swaziland	26	2000	...	...	...	70	2000	...	.
165 Sweden	72	1981	...	...	...	100	1987	...	.

Births by caesarean section		No. of midwives available		Annual number of live births, 2000	Maternal mortality ratio 2000	Stillbirth rate 2000	Early neonatal mortality rate 2000	Neonatal mortality rate 2000
(%)	Year	Total	Year	(000)	(per 100 000 live births)	(per 1000 total births)	(per 1000 live births)	(per 1000 live births)
...	...	7	2000	3	...	11[b]	9[b]	12[b]
...	...	232	1995	...	...	4[b]	2[b]	3[b]
5	2000	612	2002	58	110	25[b]	21	26
2	1992	...	...	691	220	17[b]	14	21
3	1997	1414	2000	753	1000[b]	42[b]	35[b]	48
...	...	10307	2000	1194	360[b]	36[b]	30[b]	40
7	1992	2038	1997	67	300[b]	26[b]	21	25
...	...	...	...	...	...	13[b]	11[b]	14[b]
1	2001	1549	1995	805	740	23	29	40
14	2002	1825	2002	195	16	5	3	4
19	1999	2288	1999	54	7	3	3	4
15	2001	...	...	170	230[b]	11	13	18
1	1998	461	2002	599	1600[b]	31[b]	26	43
2	2003	47847	1992	4645	800[b]	48[b]	40	53
...	...	2	1996	...	...	12[b]	10[b]	13[b]
16	2001	3089	2002	57	10	4	2	3
7	1995	...	...	82	87[b]	6[b]	5[b]	6
3	1990–91	...	...	5230	500[b]	22	38	57
...	...	1	1998	...	...	13[b]	10[b]	14[b]
...	...	...	...	69	160	8	8	11
...	...	...	...	180	300[b]	28[b]	24	32
18	1995–96	...	...	166	170	10	9	16
13	2000	...	...	639	410	8	12	16
7	2003	140675	2002	2029	200	11	12	15
...	...	21997	2000	380	10	4	4	6
30	2001	...	...	113	8	6	3	3
16	1998	...	...	12	7	6[b]	5[b]	5
...	...	8728	2000	597	20	2	2	3
6	1997	1138	2002	49	36	16	16	16
11	1999	6197	2002	231	58	6	6	9
12	1999	67527	2002	1246	65	18	7	9
2	2000	10	2002	323	1400	42[b]	35	45
...	...	...	...	...	...	11[b]	9[b]	12[b]
...	...	...	...	3	...	12	8	10
...	...	...	...	2	...	10[b]	9[b]	11[b]
...	...	3	1999	5	...	12[b]	10[b]	13[b]
...	...	6	1990	...	...	4[b]	2[b]	2[b]
...	...	40	1996	5	...	34[b]	28[b]	38[b]
8	1996	...	...	718	23	11[b]	10[b]	12
2	1997	550	1995	355	690[b]	27[b]	22	31
...	...	...	...	127	9	6	7	9
...	...	299	1996	...	...	8[b]	7[b]	9[b]
2	1997	193	1996	225	2000[b]	50[b]	42[b]	56[b]
...	...	447	1999	47	15	3	1	1
18	2002	1087	2002	55	10	4	4	5
14	2002	...	...	17	17	4	3	4
...	...	23	1999	15	130[b]	11[b]	9[b]	12[b]
...	...	...	...	461	1100[b]	44[b]	37[b]	49[b]
16	1998	...	...	1028	230[b]	18[b]	15	21
...	...	...	...	384	5	4	2	3
...	...	7725	1999	310	92	11[b]	9	11
4	1992–93	...	...	1092	590[b]	24[b]	20	29
...	...	...	...	10	110	16[b]	14[b]	18[b]
...	...	...	...	38	370[b]	34[b]	28[b]	38[b]
17	2001	5979	2000	88	8	3	2	2

Annex Table 8 Selected indicators related to reproductive, maternal and newborn health

These data are estimates from various international sources and may not be the same as Member States' own estimates. They have not been submitted to Member States for consideratio

	Member State	Contraceptive prevalence rate (modern methods)		Pregnant women who received			Births attended by skilled health personnel		Births in health facil	
		(%)	Year	1+ ANC visit (%)	4+ ANC visits (%)	Year	(%)	Year	(%)	Yea
166	Switzerland	78	1994–95	...	...	...	...	...	...	.
167	Syrian Arab Republic	28	1993	...	51	2001	76	1993	...	.
168	Tajikistan	27	2000	75	...	2000	71	2000	...	.
169	Thailand	70	1997	...	86	2001	99	2002	...	.
170	The former Yugoslav Republic of Macedonia	...	...	...	...	...	98	2002	...	.
171	Timor–Leste	...	...	...	...	...	24	2002	...	.
172	Togo	9	2000	78	46	1998	49	2000	49	199
173	Tonga	...	...	...	...	...	92	2000	...	.
174	Trinidad and Tobago	33	2000	96	98	2001	96	2000	...	.
175	Tunisia	51	1994	...	79	2001	90	2000	...	.
176	Turkey	38	1998	67	42	1998	83	2003	73	199
177	Turkmenistan	53	2000	87	83	2000	97	2000	96	200
178	Tuvalu	...	...	...	...	...	99	1997	...	.
179	Uganda	18	2000–01	92	40	2000–01	39	2000–01	37	200
180	Ukraine	38	1999	90	...	1999	99	1999	99	199
181	United Arab Emirates	24	1995	97	94	1995	99	1995	...	.
182	United Kingdom	81	2002	...	...	...	99	1998	...	.
183	United Republic of Tanzania	17	1999	96	69	1999	36	1999	42	199
184	United States of America	71	1995	...	...	...	99	1997	...	.
185	Uruguay	...	...	...	94	2001	100	1997	...	.
186	Uzbekistan	63	2000	95	...	1996	96	2000	94	199
187	Vanuatu	...	...	...	...	...	89	1995	...	.
188	Venezuela, Bolivarian Republic of	...	...	...	90	2001	94	2000	...	.
189	Viet Nam	56	2000	70	29	2002	85	2002	79	200
190	Yemen	10	1997	34	11	1997	22	1997	16	199
191	Zambia	23	2001–02	94	71	2001–02	43	2001–02	43	200
192	Zimbabwe	50	1999	82	64	1999	73	1999	72	199

[a] See explanatory notes for sources and methods.

[b] Estimates derived by regression and similar estimation methods.

Births by caesarean section		No. of midwives available		Annual number of live births, 2000	Maternal mortality ratio 2000	Stillbirth rate 2000	Early neonatal mortality rate 2000	Neonatal mortality rate 2000
(%)	Year	Total	Year	(000)	(per 100 000 live births)	(per 1000 total births)	(per 1000 live births)	(per 1000 live births)
10	2002	2033	2000	68	7	3	3	3
...	...	...	...	473	160[b]	9[b]	7[b]	9[b]
2	2002	3857	2002	160	100[b]	34[b]	29[b]	38[b]
...	...	...	...	1082	44	11[b]	9	13
10	2001	1456	2001	29	13	9	7	9
...	...	...	...	19	660[b]	36[b]	30[b]	40[b]
2	1998	402	1995	179	570	40[b]	33	40
...	...	27	2000	3	...	10[b]	8[b]	10[b]
...	...	...	...	17	110	16	10	13
8	2000	...	...	166	120	11	9	14
14	1998	41590	2001	1495	70[b]	17	19	22
4	2000	3642	1997	105	31[b]	13	26	35
...	...	10	2002	...	...	20[b]	16[b]	22[b]
3	2000–01	850	2002	1195	880	15	25	32
9	1999	24483	2002	418	38	28	9	9
10	1995	...	...	50	54[b]	5[b]	4[b]	5
17	1997	24801	1993	681	11	5	3	4
3	1999	13820	1995	1423	1500	38[b]	32	43
23	2000	...	...	4146	14	4	4	5
...	...	...	...	58	20	9	5	7
3	1996	20997	2002	567	24[b]	25	21	27
...	...	...	...	6	...	17[b]	14[b]	19[b]
...	...	...	...	578	78	9	9	12
10	2002	14662	2001	1593	130[b]	24	13	15
1	1997	...	...	820	570	17[b]	27	37
2	2001–02	...	...	450	750	31[b]	26	40
7	1999	...	...	419	1100	17	27	33

index